Testicular Autoimmunity

Histopathology of Testicular Autoimmunity

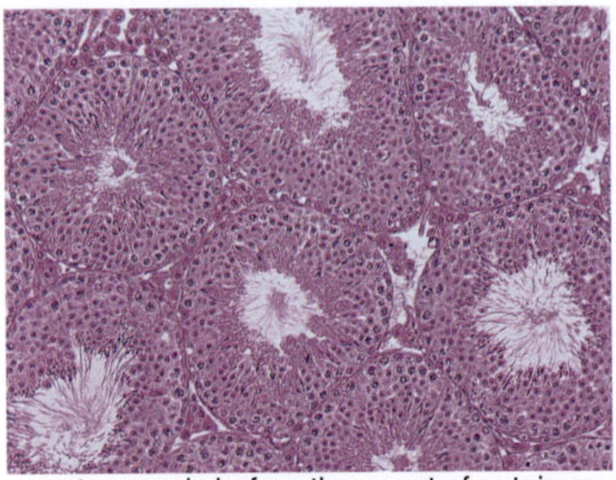

Normal spermatogenesis before the onset of autoimmune orchitis

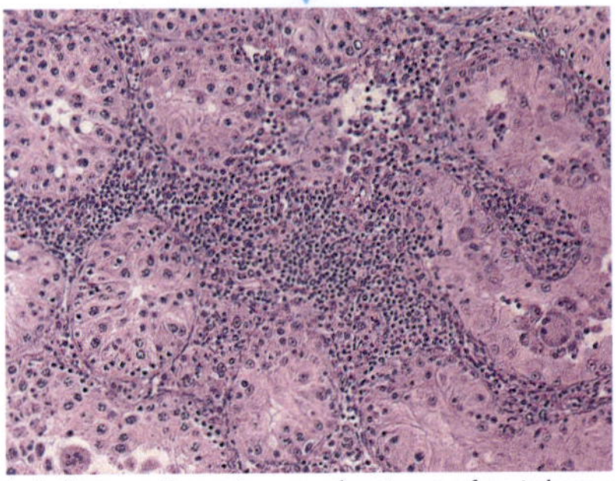

Lymphocytic inflammation at an early stage of autoimmune orchitis

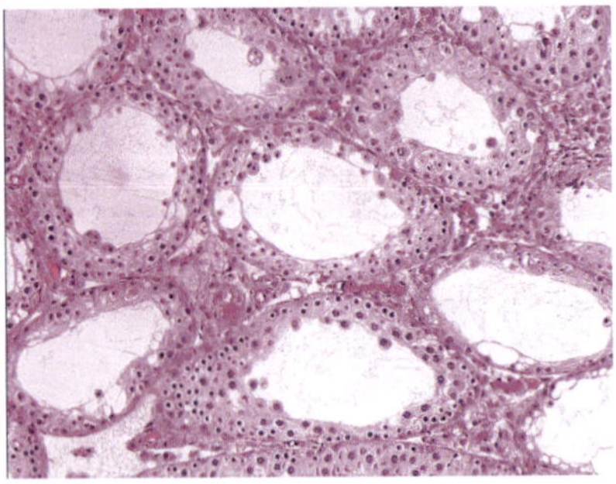

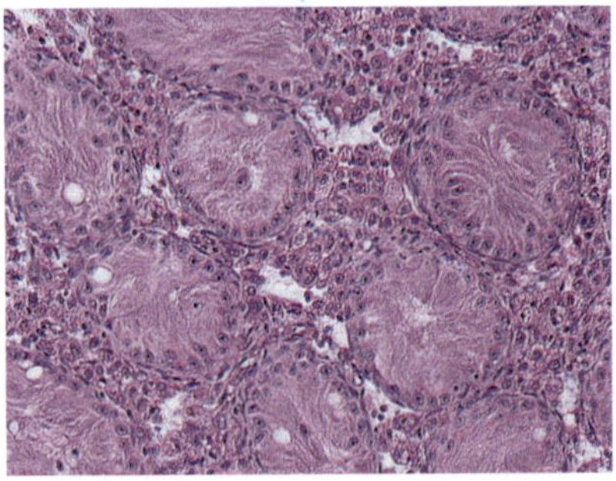

Maturation arrest (left) and Sertoli cell-only syndrome (right) at a late stage of autoimmune orchitis

Masahiro Itoh

Testicular Autoimmunity

A Cause of Male Infertility

Springer

Masahiro Itoh
Department of Anatomy
Tokyo Medical University
Shinjyuku-ku
Tokyo
Japan

ISBN 978-4-431-54459-3 ISBN 978-4-431-54460-9 (eBook)
DOI 10.1007/978-4-431-54460-9

Library of Congress Control Number: 2017946681

Printed on acid-free paper

This Springer imprint is published by Springer Nature
The registered company is Springer Japan KK
The registered company address is: Chiyoda First Bldg. East, 3-8-1 Nishi-Kanda, Chiyoda-ku, Tokyo 101-0065, Japan

This book is dedicated to
Professor Emeritus Kenji Hojo (1929–1998).

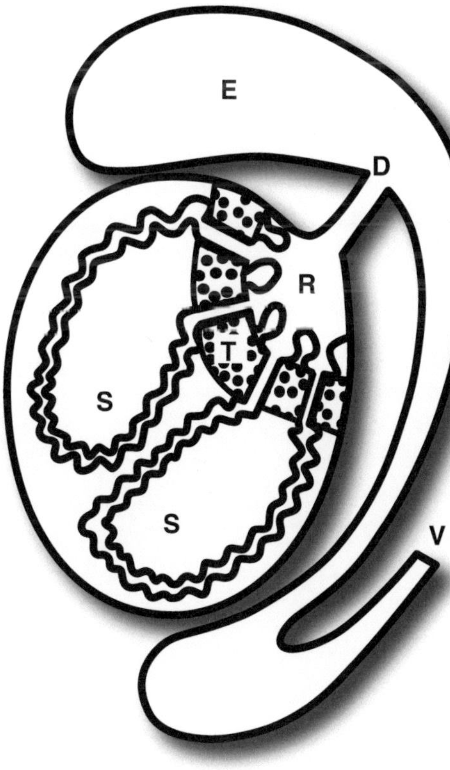

Preface

Approximately 120 years ago, Elia Metchinikoff suggested that the main destiny of immunity is not a battle against nonself, but rather a harmonization inside self. Although a prototype of the immune system seems to be for elimination of aliens such as viruses, bacteria, protozoa, parasites, and fungi, the system has originally evolved for clearance and utilization of emerging debris from lastingly dying cells of its own. Therefore, the immune functions are chiefly directed "inward" rather than "outward" and are based on the intrinsic recognizing components of the "self." That is why the immune system sometimes attacks its own organs and tissues, including the testis, under some abnormal conditions in mammals.

For living organisms, "growth and reproduction are basic," and the "self-defense system involving immunity" supports both. In medical schools, various practices in anatomy, physiology, biochemistry, pathology, and other important areas have been provided. Among these, practices in parasitology were most special and unique for the author. For medical students who are familiar with mammals, observing flatworms under a stereoscopic microscope may be an extraordinary experience. In the bodies of hermaphroditic animals, digestive and reproductive organs are closely compacted exactly as "growth and reproduction are basic for living organisms." However, in these parasites, the spermatozoa and ova are never rejected and damaged by the self-immune system. Therefore, autoimmune phenomena against gonads and gametes are considered a byproduct of biological evolution of far complexed immune system in mammals. Various relationships between the reproductive and immune systems in mammals have been explored in the field of "reproductive immunology."

In recent years, most publications in reproductive immunology have focused on the role of the uterus, fetus, placenta, and their combination; fewer papers have examined gonadal and gamete immunology. However, the gonads are core organs for the reproductive system. In this book, the author presented an idea that "the testis is an immunologically privileged but also immunologically fragile organ." Considering that idiopathic gonadal failure often involves the autoimmune responses, studies on the developmental association between the gonads and lymphoid organs must be more focused on. In particular, the testis is specific in that it produces spermatozoa of which differentiation antigens newly appear long after the establishment of immune tolerance and therefore contains strong and much autoimmunogenic antigens. In other words, spermatogenesis begins at puberty, at a time far after which the immune system recognized the body's own antigens as "self."

This book reviews various investigations on testicular autoimmunity and its biological background based on clinical and experimental approaches. In spite of the presence of highly autoimmunogenic antigens inside the testis, why do most men not develop testicular autoimmunity? Its aim is to attempt to understand the regulatory mechanisms that normally prevent testicular autoimmunity and the events that overcome the regulatory mechanisms. The author hopes that this book would be helpful for further investigation on inflammation of autoimmune or non-autoimmune origin in the testis.

Tokyo, Japan Masahiro Itoh, MD

The original version of this book was revised. An erratum to this chapter can be found at DOI 10.1007/978-4-431-54460-9_9

Acknowledgments

I express sincere gratitude to the following persons for experimental and secretarial support in completing this book: Dr. Akiko Matsuzaki (University of the Ryukus), Dr. Yo Tokunaga (Kawasaki Medical School), Dr. Yasuki Sakamoto (Kyushu University), Dr. Masahiro Koseto (Osaka University), Dr. Hayato Terayama and Dr. Ning Qu (Tokai University); Dr. Munekazu Naito, Dr. Shuichi Hirai and Dr. Naoyuki Hatayama (Aichi Medical School); Dr. Shogo Hayashi (International University of Health and Welfare); Dr. Yuki Ogawa, Dr. Ablake Maira, Dr. Yoshie Hirayanagi, Dr. Yumi Miura, Dr. Sachi Tainosho, Dr. Kuerban Maimaiti, Dr. Musha Muhetaerjiang, Dr. Takuya Omotehara, Dr. Hidenobu Miyaso, Dr. Zhong-Lian Li, Mrs. Miyuki Kuramasu, Mr. Shinichi Kawata, Mr. Kenta Nagahori, Mrs. Yuka Kobayashi, Mrs. Kazuyo Izawa, Mrs. Akiko Abo, and Mrs. Keiko Kuwana and Dr. Takayoshi Miyaki (Tokyo Medical University); and Dr. Shinji Soramoto, Dr. Kensaku Miyamoto, Mrs. Midori Miyawaki, Mr. Hiroshi Miyanaka, Mrs. Hiromi Sangawa, and Mrs. Mizue Fukutomi (Kagawa University). I also deeply appreciate Dr. Yoshiki Takeuchi (Kagawa University), Dr. Jinzo Yamada and Dr. Hiroshi Ito (Tokyo Medical University) who always supported the research environment for the completion of this book.

I take this opportunity to express a heartfelt respect for Dr. Chiharu Hiramine and the late Dr. Kenji Hojo (1929–1998, Kagawa University) and the late Dr. Shigeru Hatakeyama (1925–2007, Tokyo Medical and Dental University) who advanced testicular immunopathology.

Finally, I deeply wish to acknowledge the editorial assistance of Springer Japan. A particular note of gratitude goes to Mrs. Sachiko Hayakawa, Mrs. Kanako Homma, Mrs. Chieko Watanabe, Mrs. Chihiro Haraguchi whose guidance, advice and encouragement contributed significantly to the completion of this book. I also offer my thanks to Mr. Vignesh Iyyadurai and Mr. S. Deepak Kumar for their professionalism for the proofreading of this book.

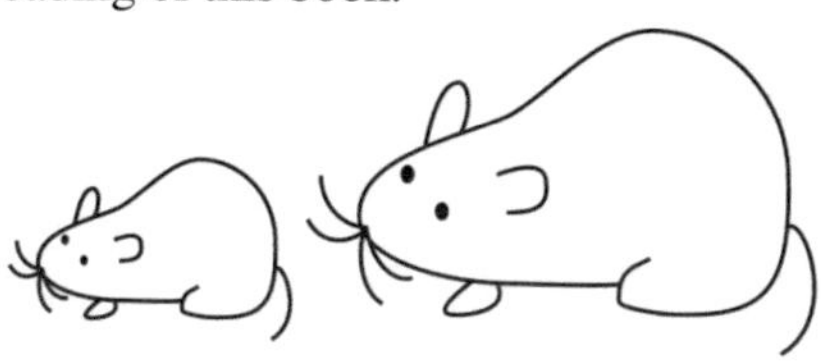

These animals have given us a lot of
information on testicular autoimmunity.

Contents

Abbreviations

BP	*Bordetella pertussis* antigens
BTB	Blood-testis barrier
CFA	Complete Freund's adjuvant
DTH	Delayed-type hypersensitivity
EAO	Experimental autoimmune orchitis
GVHD	Graft-versus-host disease
IFN	Interferon
IL	Interleukin
LPS	Lipopolysaccharide
MHC	Major histocompatibility
NK	Natural killer
TCR	T cell receptor
TGC	Testicular germ cells
TLR	Toll-like receptor
TNF	Tumor necrosis factor
Treg	Regulatory T cells

Biological Background of Testicular Autoimmunity

1

1.1 Introduction

The process of sperm formation can be divided into three separate components: (1) spermatogenesis, the formation of spermatids that have undergone first and second meiotic divisions but have remained round in shape; (2) spermiogenesis, the process for that spermatids to undergo a morphologic change in shape from round cells to potentially motile, tadpole-shaped cells; and (3) spermiation, the release of elongated spermatids into the seminiferous tubules' lumen from their relationship with Sertoli cells. The entire process of sperm production occurs over approximately 4 and 10 weeks in mice and men, respectively (Oakberg 1956; Heller and Clermont 1963). Spermatogenesis, spermiogenesis, and spermiation begin at puberty, at a time long after which the immune system recognizes the body's own antigens as "self." In particular, haploid cells (=spermatids and spermatozoa) are quite new typed for the body and express various new differentiation antigens that are not found in diploid cells such as spermatogonia and spermatocytes. Therefore, there is a risk that all men develop autoimmunity to their own spermatids and spermatozoa under some pathological condition.

The origin of infertility of many cases is now believed to be primarily in the male partner. Indeed, a considerable number of cases are characterized by idiopathic male infertility, a disturbance of spermatogenesis that is without obvious causes at the time of diagnosis. Recently, testicular autoimmunity is considered to be a significant cause of idiopathic male infertility (Naito et al. 2012). Many cases of the spermatogenic disturbance associated with male infertility may be the end stage of earlier episode of autoimmune orchitis. Experimentally, it is very easy to induce autoimmune orchitis by various protocols in mice, rats, and guinea pigs (Tung 1998; Itoh et al. 2005; Lustig and Tung 2006; Naito and Itoh 2008). This means that, among various autoantigens in the whole body, testicular ones may be highly autoimmunogenic.

The original version of this chapter was revised. An erratum to this chapter can be found at DOI 10.1007/978-4-431-54460-9_9

M. Itoh, *Testicular Autoimmunity*, DOI 10.1007/978-4-431-54460-9_1

1.2 Developmental Phase Differences Between Reproductive and Lymphoid Organs

All living organisms are subject to the principle of transience, i.e., they go through birth, growth (activity), and, after a peak is reached, regression and eventual death (extinction) (Fig. 1.1). This pattern applies not only to living organisms but also to everything in this world, including inanimate objects such as tools, cars, and buildings.

Miki (1983) noticed "phase alternation from growth to reproduction," which is common to plants and animals. He offered profound insight into the constant change that is characteristic of everything in the universe, the spiral of eternal circumnavigation, the rhythm of the universe, and cosmic rhythm (Fig. 1.2). Scammon (1930) also described "developmental phase in each organ system," demonstrating that each organ system has its own growth time course in an individual organism (Fig. 1.3). Based on Scammon's growth curves, the author created the developmental waves depicted in Fig. 1.4, illustrating only the lymphoid and reproductive organs. This figure shows that the lymphoid organs are the earliest to degenerate, and the reproductive organs are the slowest to mature.

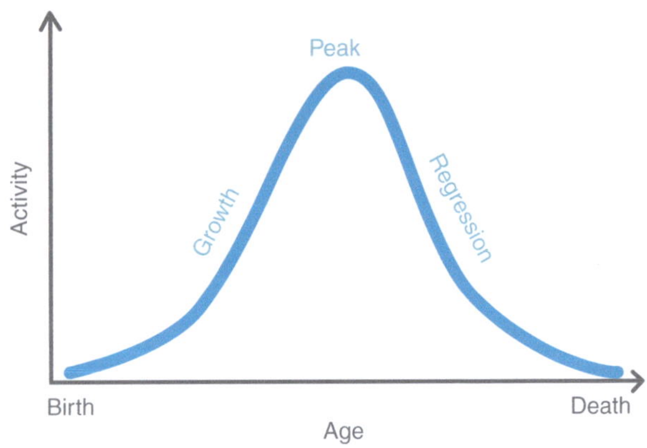

Fig. 1.1 A schema showing that all things flow and nothing is permanent

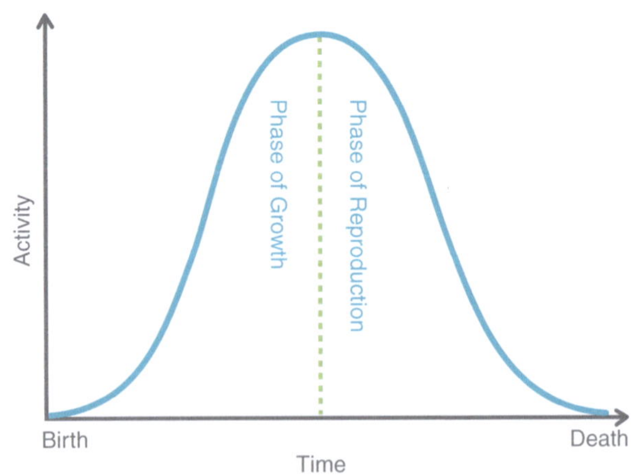

Fig. 1.2 A flow from the growth to the reproduction (Miki 1983; partly modified)

Fig. 1.3 Human growth curves (Scammon 1930; partly modified)

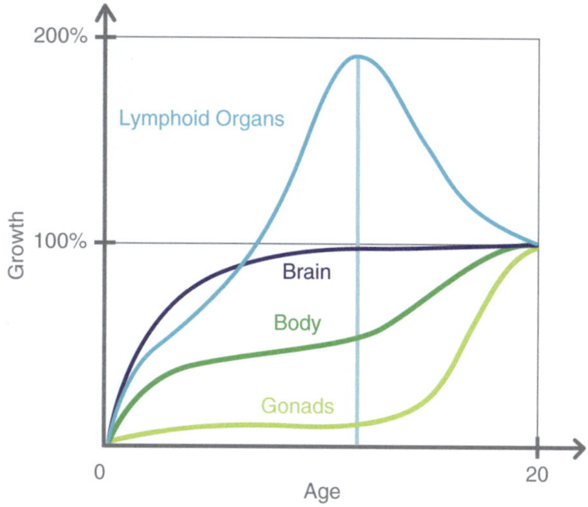

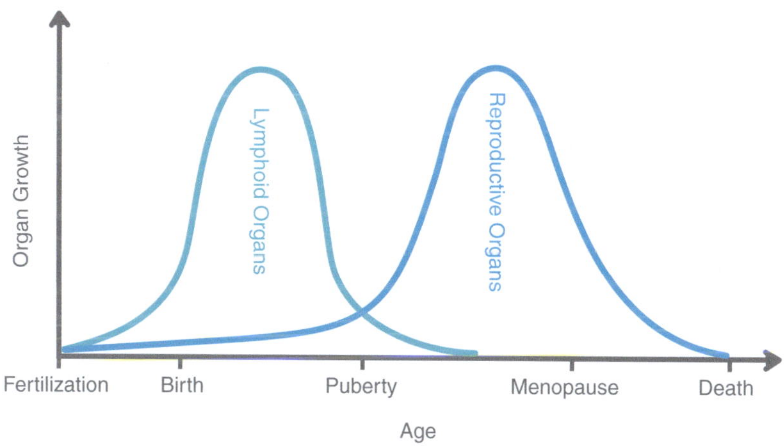

Fig. 1.4 The change from lymphoid phase to reproductive phase during pubertal period

1.3 Evolution of the Reproductive and Immune Systems

The reproductive system is responsible for maintaining species and connecting lives. The immune system, or the self-defense system, is responsible for preserving the individual. When considered from the perspective of the recognition system, which recognizes the distinction between self and nonself, immunity is also involved in maintaining species. For example, if tissues and organs from other animals could be easily transplanted with no immunological rejection, the very concept of species would be questionable. Therefore, both immune and reproductive systems provide support for the maintenance of species (Fig. 1.5).

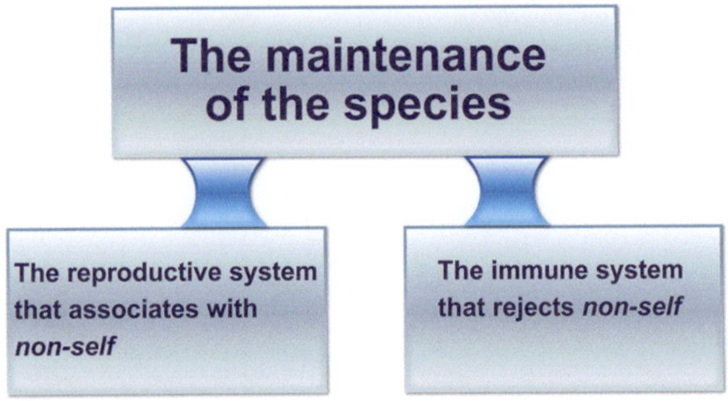

Fig. 1.5 The species supported by both reproductive and immune systems

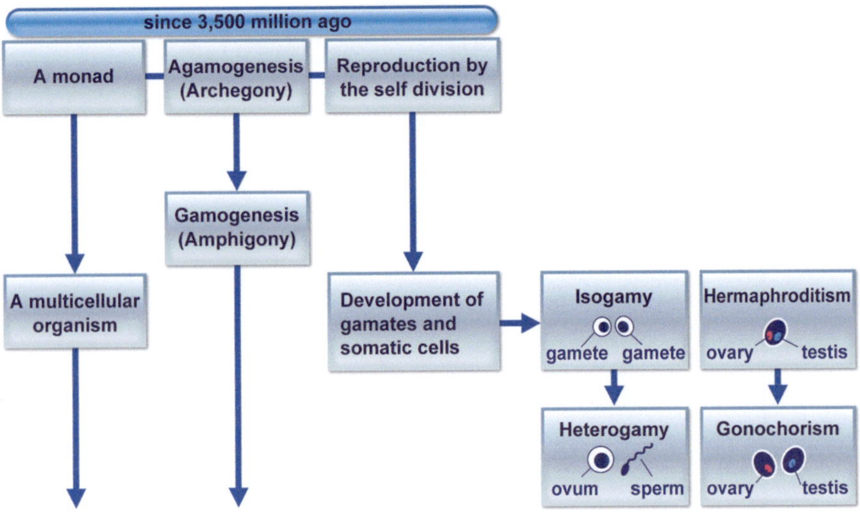

Fig. 1.6 The evolution of the reproductive system

It is known that life was born approximately 3500 million years ago. In the process of evolving from unicellular to multicellular organisms, living organisms also evolved from asexual to sexual reproduction (Fig. 1.6). If males are considered as DNA presenters and females as DNA receivers, sexual reproduction may be present at the unicellular level (Ramaley 1968; Sherwood et al. 2014). In addition, during the course of evolution, multicellular organisms acquired a system that allows classification of cells into two types: somatic and germ cells (gametes). Germ cells have further evolved from isomorphic gametes to heterogametes, and the mode of existence of the sexes has evolved from hermaphroditic to gonochoristic.

The Earth came into existence approximately 4500 million years ago, and unicellular organisms are believed to have emerged approximately 3500 million years ago. Multicellular organisms are believed to have emerged approximately 1000 billion years ago, and the appearance of spermatozoa and ova among multicellular organisms is believed to have occurred approximately 600 million years ago (Fig. 1.7). Spermatozoa and ova arose from porifera (sea sponges). By the coelenterate stage,

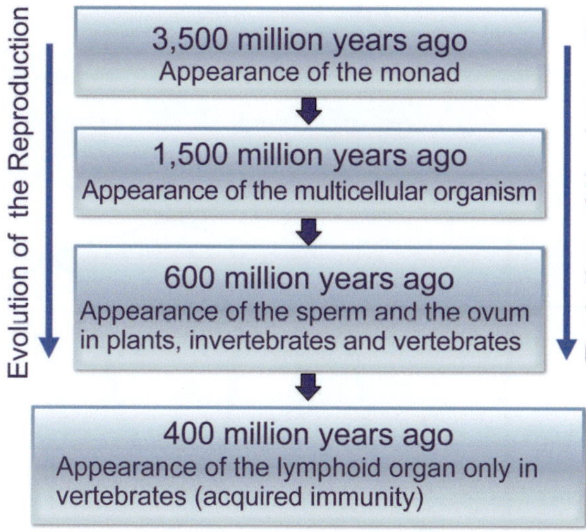

Fig. 1.7 Evolution of both reproductive and immune systems

animals were equipped with testes and ovaries. When platyhelminthes emerged, the reproductive system started to develop to the point that reproductive organs could be identified; however, no lymphoid organ-like structure had yet developed at this evolution stage. The development of immune system is another change during the evolution from unicellular to multicellular organisms. This system development was based on receptors that allowed for adherence (acceptance) between individual similar cells and rejection of foreign cell adherence. This possibly began when various humoral substances responsible for innate immunity were first produced, and then macrophages capable of phagocytozing foreign substances came into existence. Later, approximately 400 million years ago, the lymphocytes responsible for acquired immunity started to emerge (Fig. 1.7). However, only vertebrates have possessed highly evolved lymphoid organs such as thymus, spleen, tonsils, Peyer's patches, appendix, and lymph nodes. Lymph nodes therefore did not exist until the appearance of higher organisms such as mammals and some birds (Itoh 2009).

Collectively, spermatozoa and ova, which developed earlier in the process of evolution, appeared approximately 600 million years ago, and their existence was found to be widespread in plants, invertebrates, and vertebrates. Lymphocytes, on the other hand, which developed approximately 400 million years ago and therefore later than germ cells in the process of evolution, have been absent in invertebrates. Invertebrates thus have developed only innate immunity. Therefore, the emergence of lymphoid organs has been restricted to only in higher vertebrates and was approximately 0.2 million years later than that of spermatozoa and ova (Fig. 1.8). Meanwhile, a reverse phenomenon occurs during the development of individual mammals: the more newly evolved lymphoid organs containing lymphocytes now undergo maturation earlier than the appearance of differentiated germ cells, which arose earlier in the evolution process (Fig. 1.8). The physiological relationship between the regression of lymphoid organs and the maturation of gonads in an individual mammal is characterized by the fact that when the mammal is

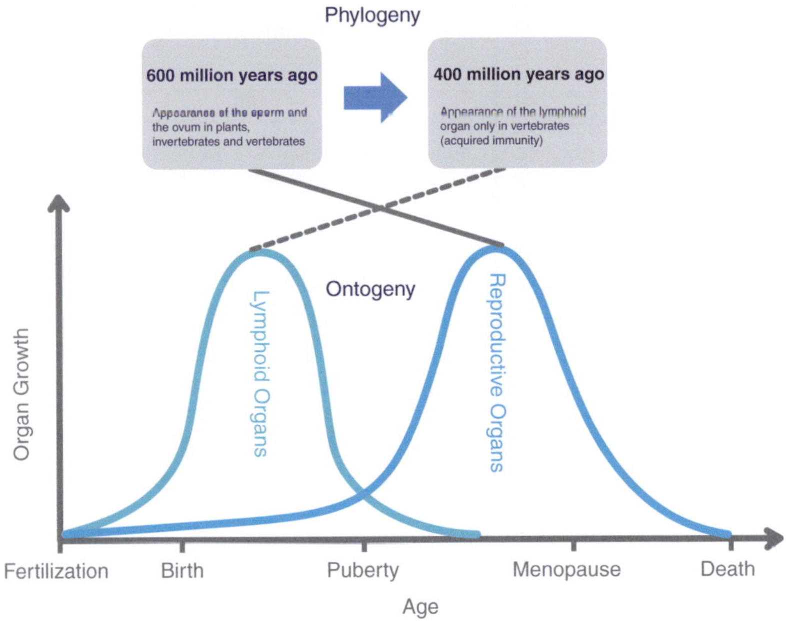

Fig. 1.8 The phylogeny of lymphoid and reproductive organs is reversed with the ontogeny

experimentally castrated during its sexual maturation period, the atrophied thymus and spleen become hypertrophic again (Dean et al. 1984; Utsuyama and Hirokawa 1989; Utsuyama et al. 1995).

1.4 Offensive Attack on Germ Cells by Acquired (Adoptive) Immunity

The reproductive system has evolved to allow individuals to interact with each other (i.e., fusion with the nonself), whereas immune system has evolved to make distinctions between self and nonself, thereby allowing the elimination of nonself. Therefore, while these two systems cooperate in maintaining species, they are also polar opposites (Fig. 1.9). This contradiction is especially pertinent in higher organisms because "after the immune system consisting of the exclusion of non-self has been established, mature germ cells containing new differentiation antigens (=self-antigens but recognized as non-self-like ones) appear and have a chance of their fusion (i.e., fertilization)." As a result, acquired immunity (which evolved later) may attack mature germ cells and fertilized eggs (which evoluted earlier). In fact, phenomena related to this issue include defects in the maturation of germ cells, failed fertilization, failed implantation, and miscarriages by autoimmune mechanisms (Itoh 2009).

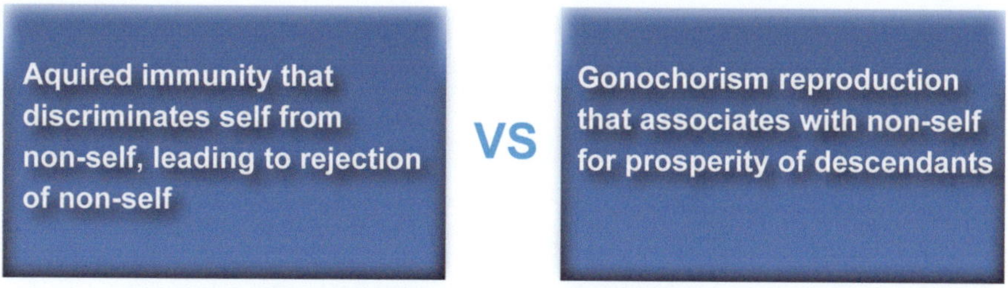

Fig. 1.9 Immunity and reproduction in terms of relation with nonself

1.5 Harsh Immunological Fate of Male Haploid Germ Cells (Spermatids/Spermatozoa)

Female reproductive organs are strongly influenced by changes in the endocrine environment such as menstruation, pregnancy, and menopause, whereas for male reproductive organs, the environment remains relatively constant after the drastic changes that take place during puberty. In the female reproductive organs, monthly ovulation and subsequent ovum transport occur, and also the entry of spermatozoa as allogeneic cells is permitted, and then the embryo and fetus as semi-allogeneic cells are nurtured. Therefore, spermatozoa, embryos, and fetuses are sometimes likely to be immunologically rejected in females. In contrast to female reproductive organs, male reproductive ones daily produce, transport, and excrete germ cells in a monotonous rhythm. Thus, the environment in the male reproductive organs seems more immunologically stable than that in the female reproductive organs. However, in the phase difference between lymphocytic differentiation and appearance of haploid cells, spermatids and spermatozoa are most likely to be targeted for immunological elimination not only in the female but also in the male (Fig. 1.10). It is noted that daily produced haploid spermatids are quite many in number compared to a monthly produced haploid ovum. Thus, males may daily present much autoimunogenic auto-antigens to the immune system. Moreover, an ovum is produced just after ovulation by dividing a diploid oocyte and survives only for 1 day, indicating that an ovum can pass through immune surveillance easily in females. In contrast, spermatids and spermatozoa that survive apparently longer than an ovum may easily stimulate immunity in both males and females. Figure 1.11 shows that the life cycles of germ cells are completely different between males and females. In humans, primordial germ cells of both males and females are ready in the form of immature cells inside the gonads by the eighth week of intrauterine life. However, the number of primordial follicles in the ovaries reaches a peak (approximately 7 million) at 5 months of intrauterine life and decreases to approximately 2 million at the time of birth, then to several tens of thousands by puberty, after which it continues to decrease rapidly. These primordial follicles disappear completely by the age of approximately

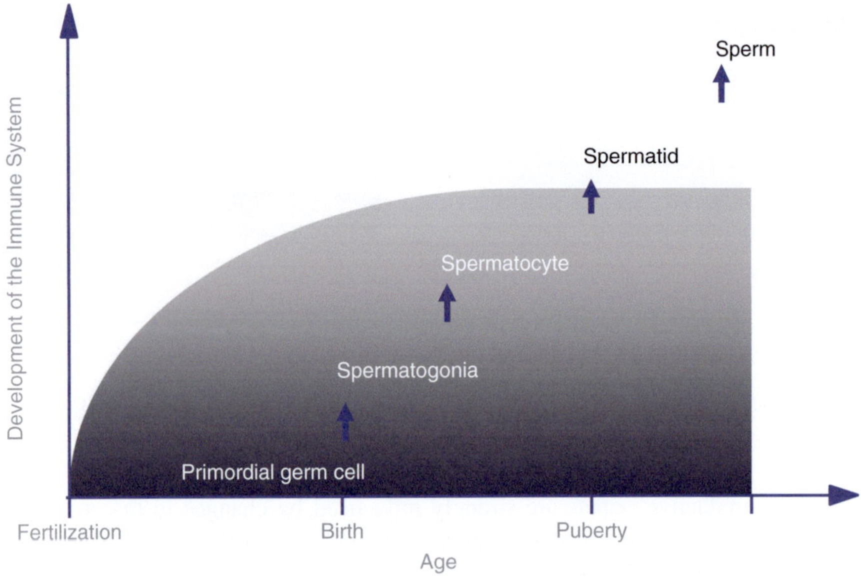

Fig. 1.10 Differentiation of male haploid germ cells after the establishment of immune tolerance

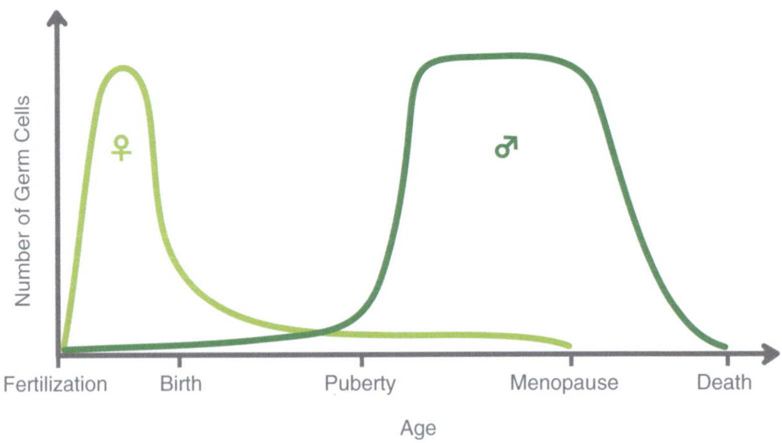

Fig. 1.11 Chronological changes of germ cell numbers in male and female gonads

50 years, at the time of menopause. On the other hand, only a small number of spermatogonia, which are the progenitors of spermatozoa, develop within the testis from the time of intrauterine life until puberty. Once puberty is reached and lymphoid organs regress, active spermatogenesis begins. Approximately 100 million spermatozoa are then produced on a daily basis. This process continues until old age.

Figure 1.12 is a combination of Figs. 1.4 and 1.11. In this figure, spermatids and spermatozoa are depicted as cells that are the last in the human body to mature.

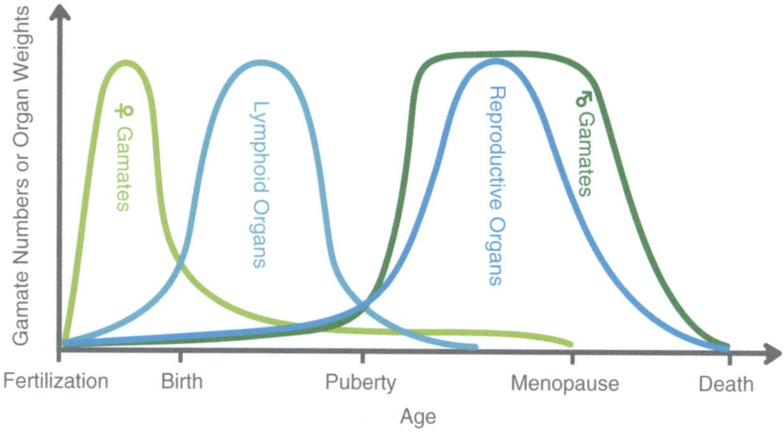

Fig. 1.12 The developmental relation among gametes, lymphoid organs, and reproductive organs

Spermatids are newcomers (=cells bearing new self-antigens and immunologically recognized as nonself-like ones) that emerge far later than the period of neonatal immune tolerance from fetal to infant period. According to previous studies, spermatids and spermatozoa on the adluminal side of the blood-testis barrier (BTB), which are composed of inter-Sertoli cell junctions in the seminiferous tubules, are believed to be protected from detrimental immune attacks (Fig. 1.13). However, based on the findings of several research groups, the BTB does not completely isolate spermatids and spermatozoa from immune system in mammals; instead, these cells are subtly maintained in a state of balance recognized by the individual's own immune system and are not rejected under normal circumstances (Taguchi and Nishizuka 1981; Itoh et al. 1991a, b, c, 1992, 1994; Yule and Tung 1993). If this balance is broken by any chance, the spermatogenic disturbance of autoimmune origin would be triggered immediately. In any case, haploid germ cells (having 23 chromosomes), which are at the apex of male germ cell differentiation, are completely different from diploid germ cells (having 46 chromosomes); therefore, they possess newly formed autoantigens that are recognized as nonself and are likely to be subjected to immunological rejection. This is an unacceptable risk in primitive animals.

In males, both spermatids and spermatozoa are autoimmunogenic; however, more vulnerable germ cells in autoimmune phenomena are spermatids (that have just completed meiosis) than spermatozoa (Itoh et al. 1991a, b, 1994). The male immune system may first perceive appearance of spermatids in the testis as completely different from any other previously encountered and tolerated diploid cells. Spermatids, which have more abundant cytoplasm than spermatozoa, should contain various types of autoimmunogenic differentiation antigens of large amounts. In contrast, spermatozoa are completed by sloughing off fragments of autoimmunogenic spermatid cytoplasm as residual bodies. Therefore, the elements most susceptible to autoimmune inflammation may be not the vas deferens and epididymis, which contain large amounts of mature spermatozoa in the lumen. Rather, the testes,

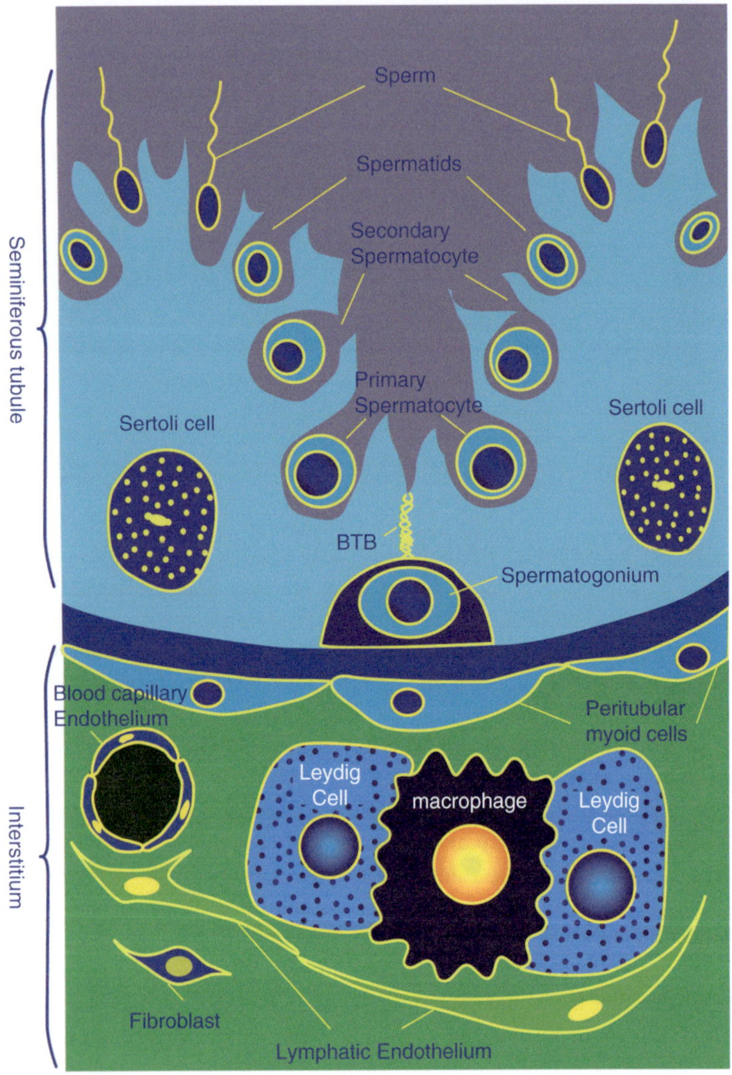

Fig. 1.13 Histology of the testis involving various cell kinds. *BTB* blood-testis barrier (composed of inter-Sertoli cell junctions)

where spermatids emerge from miosis, may be more susceptible. Factors likely to inhibit autoimmune responses to spermatids in the testis are summarized in Fig. 1.14. Although the actual contribution of each factor is unknown, a wide variety of inhibition mechanisms is estimated to be at work locally in the testes.

In female reproductive tracts, spermatozoa but not spermatids are transported to reach an ovum. Like spermatids, spermatozoa have acquired differentiation antigens unique to haploid cells as a result of meiosis, and the antigens will be recognized by female immune mechanisms as allogeneic antigens after ejaculation to the

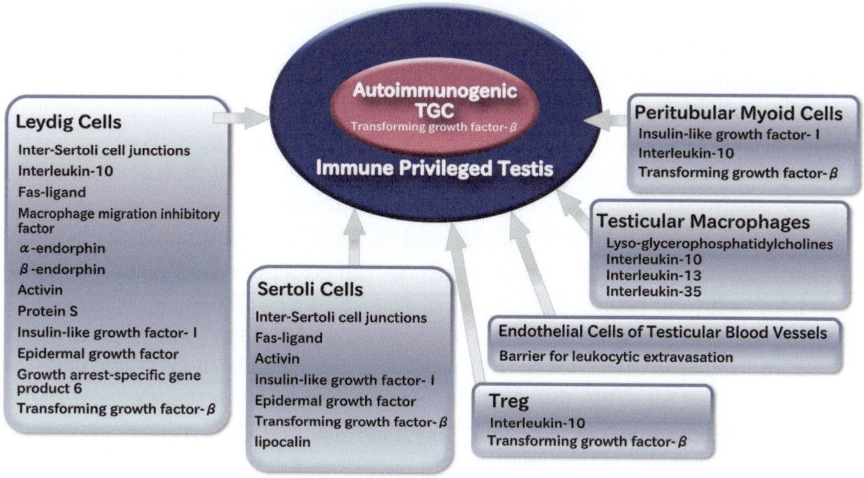

Fig. 1.14 Immunosuppressive factors in the testis. *TGC* testicular germ cells

female reproductive tracts. Therefore, they may be in serious danger on the way to the ovum. Even if they achieve fertilization and implantation of the blastocyst, both the embryo and the fetus which contain half the genes from a sperm may still be recognized as semi-allografts and be immunologically rejected. This is the pathetic fate of spermatozoa of higher organisms (Fig. 1.10).

1.6 Endocrinological Relation Between the Testicular and Immune Functions

The testis and systemic immunity are not only immunologically but also endocrinologically linked (Rebar et al. 1980, 1981a, b, 1982; Rebar 1982; Strich et al. 1985a; Suh et al. 1985; Farookhi et al. 1988; Hince et al. 2008). Many hormonal studies have demonstrated that the presence of thymic epithelial cells and thymic lymphocytes affects testicular function. A chromatographic fraction obtained from the acetone powder of prepubertal rat thymus increased secretion of luteinizing hormone and follicle-stimulating hormone from cultured pituitary cells stimulated with luteinizing hormone-releasing hormone. Thymosin beta-4, a product of thymic epithelial cells, stimulated the release of luteinizing hormone-releasing hormone from rat hypothalamus in vitro (Rebar et al. 1981a, Suh et al. 1985). Thymulin, another product of thymic epithelial cells, stimulated proliferation of spermatogonia in vitro (Prepin et al. 1994). In seminiferous tubules of congenitally athymic mice, degeneration of testicular germ cells (TGC) is focally found in athymic mice of CD1, BALB/c-nu/nu, LASAT, and KSN strains (Itoh et al. 1997). The degenerating morphology was characterized by karyopyknosis and karyolysis of immature TGC, multinuclear giant cell formation, and severe depletion of seminiferous epithelium with remaining Sertoli cells and/or some spermatogonia. The severity and the onset of spontaneous degeneration and depletion of TGC in congenitally athymic mice were different among the four strains examined. Plasma testosterone levels of neonatally thymectomized male rats were significantly lower than those of sham-operated animals. Congenitally athymic male mice had an insufficient secretion of both gonadotropin and testosterone compared to thymus-bearing normal mice (Pierpaoli and Besedovsky 1975; Rebar et al. 1980, 1982; Chesnokova et al. 1987). Human chorionic gonadotropin binding to rat testis receptors is inhibited by a thymus factor with the resultant reduction of testosterone secretion (Pedernera et al. 1986; Hiriart and Romano 1986; Reyes-Esparza and Romano 1989). Neonatally thymectomized animals at 4 weeks of age had a significantly higher concentration of plasma testosterone than did the sham-operated animals (Deschaux et al. 1979). Estradiol benzoate injected into 5-day-old male rats produced marked damage to the seminiferous epithelium, azoospermia, and decreased androgen production in later life. However, rats injected with a suspension of thymic cells within the first 24 h of life and then with estradiol benzoate at 5 days of age were fertile (Kincl et al. 1965). Therefore, male infertility induced by neonatal estradiol treatment could be prevented by adoptive transfer of thymocytes. These findings indicate that the thymus modulates testicular function and may affect testicular autoimmunity from both immunological and endocrinological aspects.

On the contrary, the testis affects the immune function involving the thymus. Testosterone impairs thymocyte proliferation in response to the mitogen (Yao and Shang 2005). Hypertrophy of the thymus is induced in mice and rats by gonadectomy (Dean et al. 1984; Utsuyama and Hirokawa 1989). In experiments using mice that were gonadectomized and grafted with thymus from irradiated newborn, 6-week-old, or 26-week-old syngeneic donors, gonadectomy appeared to promote immigration of thymocyte precursors into the grafted thymus and to enhance proliferation and differentiation of thymocytes toward $CD4^{+}CD8^{-}$ T cells, in an age-related manner (Utsuyama et al. 1995). The presence of androgen and estrogen receptors on macrophages, lymphocytes, and thymic stromal cells was noted (Cutolo et al. 1996; Hince et al. 2008). It was also demonstrated that orchiectomy induced electron microscopic changes of Kupffer cells. Gonadotropin-releasing hormone antagonists significantly reduce the percentage of Treg and increase the proportion of NK cells in human males (Page et al. 2006). This suggests that sex hormones directly act on lymphocytic function. Ovariectomy does not significantly affect activities of hepatic and splenic reticuloendothelial system. In contrast, orchidectomy results in significant enhancement of both hepatic and splenic reticuloendothelial system activities (Ooga et al. 2001). Furthermore, orchiectomy results in expansion in the numbers of B cells in the bone marrow and spleen (Viselli et al. 1997). B cell expansion in the bone marrow and the spleen was not altered by prior thymectomy, suggesting that thymic androgen receptors are not involved in the observed effects. Androgen receptors were also found to be present in both immature B cells and marrow stromal cells (Viselli et al. 1997). On the measurement of sex hormones, the serum concentrations of testosterone in control males (approximately 7000 pg/ml) were much higher than those of estradiol in control females (approximately 20 pg/ml) in mice (Ooga et al. 2001). In human, the serum concentrations of testosterone in males range from 250 to 1100 ng/dl, while those of estradiol in females range from 10 to 60 ng/dl. Therefore, changes in the sex steroid concentrations caused by gonadectomy more dramatically occur in males rather than in females. Moreover, in human, it was demonstrated that androgen receptor expression is greater in macrophages of males than of females (McCrohon et al. 2000). It was also reported that male mice have fewer epidermal Langerhans cells than females and that orchiectomy resulted in induction of their mitosis leading to an increase in their density (Koyama et al. 1990). This indicates that the presence of testosterone-secreting testis physiologically downregulates male immune system (Trigunaite et al. 2015). Therefore, testicular dysfunction induced by various causes may augment systemic immune responses and affect testicular autoimmunity.

More recently, Markle et al. (2013) studied a sex differences in the gut microbiome drive hormone-dependent regulation of autoimmunity and suggested that changing the gut microbial environment can change testosterone levels, thereby modifying progression to autoimmunity. They demonstrated that colonization by commensal microbes elevated serum testosterone and protected NOD males from type 1 diabetes. Transfer of gut microbiota from adult males to immature females altered the recipient's microbiota, resulting in elevated testosterone and metabolic changes, reduced islet inflammation and autoantibody production, and robust type 1 diabetes protection. These effects were dependent on androgen receptor activity.

References

Chesnokova VM, Grutenko EV, Ivanova LN, Ignatyeva EV. Evidence for thymus involvement in development of adrenal and gonadal endocrine functions in mice. Endocrine Exp. 1987;21:133–42.

Cutolo M, Accardo S, VillaggioB BA, Sulli A, Coviello DA, Carabbio C, Felli L, Miceli D, Farruggio R, Carruba G, Castagnetta L. Androgen and estrogen receptors are present in primary cultures of human synovial macrophages. J Clin Endocrinol Metab. 1996;81:820–7.

Dean DH, Hiramoto RN, Ghanta VK, Hiramoto NS, Wall CN. Effects of orchiectomy on spleen cell mitogen response and on the thymus of aged mice. Exp Aging Res. 1984;10:189–91.

Deschaux P, Massengo B, Fontanges R. Endocrine interaction of the thymus with the hypophysis, adrenals and testes: effects of two thymic extracts. Thymus. 1979;1:95–108.

Farookhi R, Wesolowski E, Trasler JM, Robaire B. Modulation by neonatal thymectomy of the reproductive axis in male and female rats during development. Biol Reprod. 1988;38:91–9.

Heller CG, Clermont Y. Spermatogenesis in man: an estimate of its duration. Science. 1963;140:184–6.

Hince M, Sakkal S, Vlahos K, Dudakov J, Boyd R, Chidgey A. The role of sex steroids and gonadectomy in the control of thymus involution. Cell Immunol. 2008;252:122–38.

Hiriart M, Romano MC. Human chorionic gonadotropin binding to rat testis receptors is inhibited by a thymus factor. Life Sci. 1986;38:789–95.

Itoh M, Hiramine C, Hojo K. A new murine model of autoimmune orchitis induced by immunization with viable syngeneic testicular germ cells alone. I. Immunological and histological studies. Clin Exp Immunol. 1991a;83:137–42.

Itoh M, Hiramine C, Tokunaga Y, Mukasa A, Hojo K. A new murine model of autoimmune orchitis induced by immunization with viable syngeneic testicular germ cells alone. II Immunohistochemical findings of fully-developed lesion. Autoimmunity. 1991b;10:89–97.

Itoh M, Mukasa A, Tokunaga Y, Hiramine C, Hojo K. New experimental model for adoptive transfer of murine autoimmune orchitis. Andrologia. 1991c;23:415–20.
Itoh M, Hiramine C, Mukasa A, Tokunaga Y, Fukui Y, Takeuchi Y, Hojo K. Establishment of an experimental model of autoimmune epididymo-orchitis mediated by T cell line in mice. Int J Androl. 1992;15:170–81.
Itoh M, Miyake M, Miki T, Takeuchi Y, de Rooij DG. Immunohistological localization of autoantigens detected by serum autoantibodies from mice with experimental autoimmune orchitis without using adjuvants. Arch Androl. 1994;32:45–52.
Itoh M, Kokudo Y, Sakamoto Y, Takeuchi Y. Spontaneous degeneration of testicular germ cells in congenitally athymic nude mice of four strains: a light microscopical observation. Int J Androl. 1997;18:672–80.
Itoh M, Terayama H, Naito M, Ogawa Y, Tainosho S. Tissue microcircumstances for leukocytic infiltration into the testis and epididymis in mice. J Reprod Immunol. 2005;67:57–67.
Itoh M. Developmental relation between the gonads and the lymphoid organs. Reprod Immunol Biol. 2009;24:63–9.
Kincl FA, Oriol A, Folch-Pi A, Maqueo M. Prevention of steroid-induced sterility in neonatal rats with thymic cell suspension. Proc Soc Exp Biol Med. 1965;120:252–5.
Koyama Y, Nagao S, Ohashi K, Takahashi H, Marunouchi T. Induction of Langerhans' cell mitosis in vivo after orchiectomy on mice. Acta Derm Venereol. 1990;70:505–8.
Lustig L, Tung KS. Orchitis and male Infertility. The autoimmune diseases. 4th ed. Amsterdam: Elsevier Acadcmic Press; 2006. 3rd ed. pp. 841–847.
Markle JG, Frank DN, Mortin-Toth S, Feazel LM RCE, Rolle-Kampczyk U, von-Bergen M, KD MC, Macpherson AJ, Danska JS. Sex differences in the gut microbiome drive hormone-dependent regulation of autoimmunity. Science. 2013;339:1085–8.
McCrohon JA, Death AK, Nakhla S, Jessup W, Handelsman DJ, Stanley KK, Celermajer DS. Androgen receptor expression is greater in macrophages from male than from female donors. A sex difference with implications for atherogenesis. Circulation. 2000;101:224–6.
Miki S. Taiji-no-sekai (in Japanese). Tokyo: Chuko-Shinsho; 1983. p. 1–226.
Naito M, Itoh M. Patterns of infiltration of lymphocytes into the testis under normal and pathological conditions in mice. Am J Reprod Immunol. 2008;59:55–61.
Naito M, Terayama H, Hirai S, Qu N, Lustig L, Itoh M. Experimental autoimmune orchitis as a model of immunological male infertility. Med Mol Morphol. 2012;45:185–9.
Oakberg EF. Duration of spermatogenesis in the mouse and timing of stages of the cycle of the seminiferous epithelium. Am J Anat. 1956;899:507–16.
Ooga T, Itoh M, Miyamoto K, Takeuchi Y, Nishioka M. Image analysis of the effects of gonadectomy on colloidal carbon uptake in vivo by sinusoidal cells in liver and spleen of the mouse. Am J Reprod Immunol. 2001;45:246–54.
Page ST, Plymate SR, Bremner WJ, Matsumoto AM, Hess DL, Lin DW, Amory JK, Nelson PS, Wu JD. Effect of medical castration on $CD4^{+}CD25^{+}$ T cells, $CD8^{+}$ T cell IFN-gamma expression, and NK cells: a physiological role for testosterone and/or its metabolites. Am J Physiol Endocrinol Metab. 2006;290:E856–63.
Pedernera E, Diaz-Osuna J, Calcago M. A thymus factor influences the in vitro testosterone secretion of Leydig cells in the rat. Life Sci. 1986;38:779–87.
Pierpaoli W, Besedovsky HO. Role of the thymus in programming of neuroendocrine functions. Clin Exp Immunol. 1975;20:323–38.
Prepin J, Le-Vigouroux P, Dadoune JP. Effects of thymulin on in vitro incorporation of ^{3}H-thymidine into gonocytes of newborn rat testes. Reprod Nutr Dev. 1994;34:289–94.
Ramaley AW. Sexuality in chodatella. Science. 1968;161:809–10.
Rebar RW, Morandini IC, Benirschke K, Petze JE. Reduced gonadotropins in athymic mice: prevention by thymic transplantation. Endocrinology. 1980;107:2130–2.
Rebar RW, Miyake A, Low TLK, Goldstein AL. Thymosin stimulates secretion luteinizing-hormone-releasing factor. Science. 1981a;214:669–71.

Rebar RW, Morandini IC, Erickson GF, Petze JE. The hormonal basis of reproductive defects in athymic mice: diminished gonadotropin concentrations in prepubertal females. Endocrinolgy. 1981b;108:120–6.

Rebar RW. The thymus gland and reproduction: do thymic peptides influence the reproductive lifespan in females? J Am Geriatr Soc. 1982;30:603–6.

Rebar RW, Morandini IC, Petze JE, Erickson GF. Hormonal basis of reproductive defects in athymic mice: reduced gonadotropins and testosterone in males. Biol Reprod. 1982;27:1267–76.

Reyes-Esparza JA, Romano MC. An age-dependent thymic secretion modulates testicular function. J Steroid Biochem. 1989;34:541–5.

Scammon RE. The measurement of the body in childhood. In: Harris JA, Jackson CM, Paterson DG, Scammon RE, editors. The measurement of man. Minnesota: University of Minnesota Press; 1930. p. 173–215.

Sherwood RK, Scaduto CM, Torres SE, Bennett RJ. Convergent evolution of a fused sexual cycle promotes the haploid lifestyle. Nature. 2014;506:387–90. doi:10.1038/nature 12891.

Strich G, Petze JE, Silva de Sa MF, Rebar RW. The effects of thymus-derived peptides on hypothalamic LRF and pituitary gonadotropin content in prepubertal congenitally athymic nude mice and their normal heterozygous littermates. J Reprod Immunol. 1985;7:351–9.

Suh BY, Naylor PH, Goldstein AL, Rebar RW. Modulation of thymosin beta 4 by estrogen. Am J Obstet Gynecol. 1985;151:544–9.

Taguchi O, Nishizuka Y. Experimental autoimmune orchitis after neonatal thymectomy in the mouse. Clin Exp Immunol. 1981;46:425–34.

Trigunaite A, Dimo J, Jorgensen TN. Suppressive effects of androgens on the immune system. Cell Immunol. 2015;294:87–94.

Tung KS. Autoimmune disease of the testis and the ovary. The Autoimmune Diseases. 3rd ed. Amsterdam: Academic Press; 1998. p. 687–704.

Utsuyama M, Hirokawa K. Hypertrophy of the thymus and restoration of immune functions in mice and rats by gonadectomy. Mech Ageing Dev. 1989;47:175–85.

Utsuyama M, Hirokawa K, Mancini C, Brunelli R, Leter G, Doria G. Differential effects of gonadectomy on thymic stromal cells in promoting T cell differentiation in mice. Mech Ageing Dev. 1995;81:107–17.

Viselli SM, Reese KR, Fan J, Kovacs WJ, Olsen NJ. Androgens alter B cell development in normal male mice. Cell Immunol. 1997;182:99–104.

Yao G, Shang XJ. A comparison of modulation of proliferation of thymocyte by testosterone, dehydroisoandrosterone and androstenedione in vitro. Arch Androl. 2005;51:257–65.

Yule TD, Tung KSK. Experimental autoimmune orchitis induced by testis and sperm antigen-specific T cell clones: an important pathogenic cytokines is tumor necrosis factor. Endocrinology. 1993;133:1098–107.

Microcircumstance for Induction and Prevention of Testicular Autoimmunity

2

2.1 Introduction

The major functions of the testis are spermatogenesis and steroidogenesis. The histological structure of the adult testis is organized by two distinct regions: the seminiferous tubules and the interstitial spaces between tubules. Spermatogenesis takes place within the convoluted seminiferous tubules, which originate from the peripheral testis, connect the tubuli recti, and then terminate at the rete testis (Fig. 2.1). Testicular germ cells (TGC) leave the testis from the rete testis. The seminiferous tubules, tubuli recti, rete testis, ductuli efferentes, epididymal ducts, and vas deferens form a functional unit and are in direct continuity for the transport of germ cells (Fig. 2.1). Steroidogenesis is fulfilled by Leydig cells in the interstitial spaces. The sex hormones, mainly testosterone, are critical for normal spermatogenesis by their paracrine action on the seminiferous epithelium. These histological structures for spermatogenesis and steroidogenesis are broken by local inflammation. Testicular autoimmunity is caused by immune responses against various testicular autoantigens, resulting in the lymphocytic infiltration and the spermatogenic disturbance. For induction or inhibition of testicular autoimmunity, controls of both systemic immune responses against testicular autoantigens and local immuno-circumstances inside the testis are important.

2.2 Autoimmunogenicity of Spermatids and Spermatozoa

The seminiferous epithelium is subdivided into two compartments. The first (basal) compartment, which is basal to the blood-testis barrier (BTB), contains spermatogonia and young spermatocytes that have free access to substances from the vascular compartment; the second (adluminal) compartment lies above the BTB and represents the microenvironment that is isolated from the vascular system, where meiosis, spermiogenesis, and spermiation occur.

M. Itoh, *Testicular Autoimmunity*, DOI 10.1007/978-4-431-54460-9_2

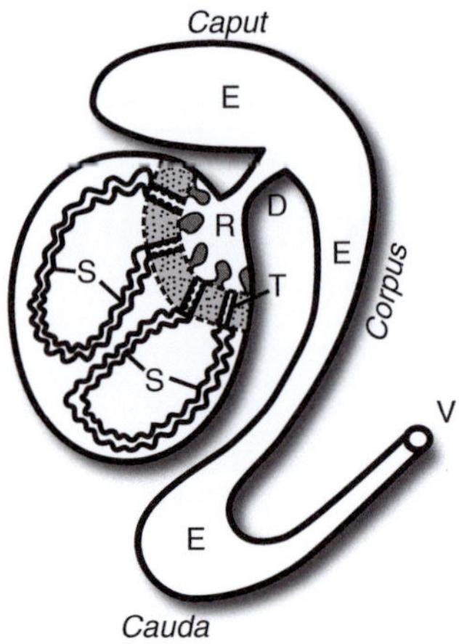

Fig. 2.1 Anatomy of germ cell duct system in males. *D* ductuli efferentes, *E* epididymis, *R* rete testis, *S* seminiferous tubule, *T* tubuli recti, *V* vas deferens

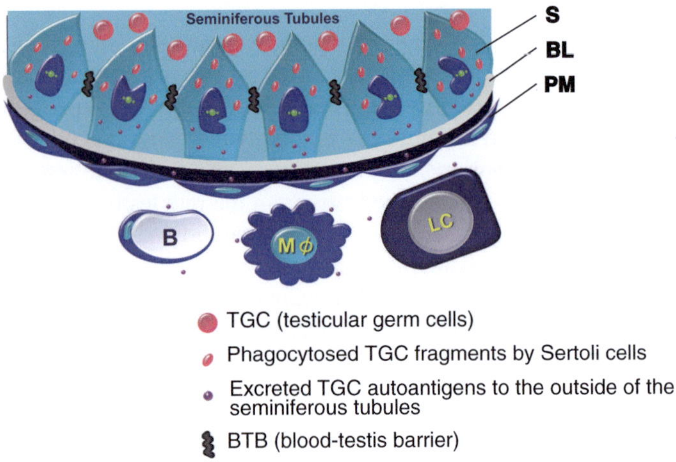

Fig. 2.2 A hypothesis of excretion of TGC autoantigens to the testicular interstitium under physiological condition. *B* blood capillary, *BL* basal lamina, *LC* Leydig cell, *Mφ* macrophage, *PM* peritubular myoid cell, *S* Sertoli cell

Spermatids and spermatozoa emerging from meiosis do not appear in the seminiferous epithelium until puberty, when immune tolerance has already been established. Different from spermatogonia and preleptotene spermatocytes having 46 chromosomes, spermatids and spermatozoa are quite new in that they have only 23 chromosomes and express various new developing antigens (Ike et al. 2007). A large number of novel proteins are expressed in developing TGC during spermatogenesis (Fig. 2.2). Hence, they contain various autoimmunogenic antigens which are recognized as foreign bodies, alien substances, nonself, or neo-self by self-immune system, leading to a challenge to the immune system. However, under normal conditions, the haploid cells are sequestered and preserved from the circulatory system by the BTB.

Localization of autoantigens detected by circulating autoantibodies in mice injected with syngeneic TGC alone was immunohistochemically studied by reaction of the immune sera with frozen sections of the testes from various aged mice (Itoh et al. 1994). The results showed that the reactivity of immune sera was detected in the testis sections of normal mice older than 24 days of age but not in those mice younger than 20 days of age. It is well known that the seminiferous tubules of mice contain spermatogonia at the day of birth, preleptotene spermatocytes at 1 week of age, pachytene spermatocytes at 2 weeks of age, round and oval spermatids at 3 weeks of age, the elongating spermatids at 4 weeks of age, and most mature (elongated) spermatids at 5 weeks of age (Vergouwen et al. 1995). Therefore, the immunostain was detected on spermatids of various stages, and immature TGC, such as spermatogonia, preleptotene spermatocytes, and pachytene spermatocytes, are not reactive with the immune sera. Using microarray analyses of 1315 testicular genes in adult and juvenile mice, 46% exhibited an increase of twofold or more in adults compared to juveniles and 22% decrease of twofold or more (Ike et al. 2007). On the basis of the fundamental difference in expression profiles, and molecular functions of the encoded products, the genes were classified into seven groups: the postmeiotically upregulated genes encoding various enzymes, structural proteins, regulatory proteins, chaperones, downregulated genes encoding hemoglobulins, oxidation-/reduction-related proteins, or machinery associated with protein synthesis, such as ribosomal proteins. Liu et al. (1992) have immunohistochemically demonstrated that mouse sperm antigen (MSA-63) detected by a monoclonal antibody (HS-63), which mainly recognizes proteins on the acrosomal region of the spermatozoa, was not expressed until 25 days after birth. This period is in accord with the time at which TGC initially acquire a delayed-type hypersensitivity (DTH)-eliciting capacity and lymphostimulatory activities for cytokine production in the immunized mice (Soramoto et al. 1993). In addition to the appearance of new autoantigens in mice older than 24 days of age, TNF-alpha, a potent pro-inflammatory cytokine, is endogenously synthesized by TGC within normal seminiferous tubules (De et al. 1993).

Severe inflammation is easily and locally induced by subcutaneous injection with prepared syngeneic spermatozoa without the use of any adjuvants in mice (Ball 1984). The lesion at the injection site developed in a characteristic sequence which is divided into four stages: acute inflammation, simple chronic inflammation, granuloma formation, and repair. The acute inflammation was seen at 6 and 24 h. Large numbers of neutrophils, many containing phagocytosed sperm heads, were present. The small number of macrophages was noted at 6 h, but they were more conspicuous by 24 h. Between 2 and 4 days, large numbers of spermatozoa persisted and were associated with an infiltrate of many macrophages. Neutrophils were rarely seen in such lesions. From 5 to 9 days, discrete masses of mononuclear inflammatory cells, predominantly macrophages but including some epithelioid cells and a few Langhans-type giant cells, were present. The lesions generally contained few spermatozoa. Some lymphocytes and eosinophils were seen at the periphery of the lesions, and there was a fibrous connective tissue at this site. By 14–21 days, small numbers of extracellular spermatozoa were associated with an infiltrate of macrophages surrounded by a zone of immature fibrous tissue. The acute inflammatory phase of the lesion appeared more severe and vigorous in the mice previously immunized against syngeneic spermatozoa than in its immunologically innocent counterparts. There is a sex difference in DTH reaction to syngeneic TGC. Both male and female mice were subcutaneously injected with TGC, and the DTH reaction was elicited with TGC 6 days after the immunization. The results showed that the DTH was detected in female mice, but not in male mice. A sex difference in the DTH reaction to sheep red blood cells was not detected. It is noted that the sex differences in the DTH against TGC were attributed to TGC other than spermatozoa because a sex difference was not detected against spermatozoa (Ball 1984; Yoshida et al. 1983).

2.3 Protection of Autoimmunogenic Spermatids and Spermatozoa by the Blood-Testis Barrier (BTB)

The functional meaning of the BTB can be referred to two main aspects: (1) the maintenance of a specific milieu for the differentiation of TGC and (2) their segregation from the immune system of the body. The BTB is created near the basal lamina by various junctions including tight junction, basal ectoplasmic specializations, gap junctions, and desmosome-like junctions between two adjacent Sertoli cells (Mruk and Yan Cheng 2015). The BTB function is to completely exclude all cellular and molecular traffic via the extracellular space between the Sertoli cells (Dym and Fawcett 1970). Basal to the tight junctions, the premeiotic spermatogonia are located near the basal lamina and the bloodstream. After the first step in meiosis, a new tight junction is formed below the developing spermatogonia, and the old tight junction above the new one will be lost (Bart et al. 2002). During spermatogenesis, maturing spermatogonia are transported toward the luminal side of the seminiferous tubules. The BTB must physically disassemble permitting the passage of preleptotene and leptotene spermatocytes. This dynamic process is regulated by transforming growth factor-beta-3 and TNF-alpha (Bronson 2010). It is absolutely essential for creating a highly specialized biochemical environment for the meiotic and postmeiotic cells, but the BTB also limits the access of systemic immunity and sequesters the majority of the autoimmunogenic TGC. The BTB, formed by Sertoli cells, primarily protects postmeiotic spermatids and spermatozoa from attack by the self-immune system. Most recently, transplantation of rat spermatogenesis inside the BTB of immunocompetent mice has succeeded (Qu et al. 2012; Hirayanagi et al. 2015). This indicates that the BTB protects not only autologous but also xenogeneic TGC from attack by self-immune system. However, if the BTB is functionally damaged, autoantigens of these haploid cells leak out beyond the BTB, leading to a continuous supply of the autoantigens to the immune system, with the resultant chronic inflammation in the testis for a prolonged length of time (Itoh et al. 2005; Naito and Itoh 2008). In particular, the BTB at the tubuli recti and the rete testis is not as strong as that in the peripheral testis. In a study of topographical uptake of blood-borne horseradish peroxidase in the testis, no horseradish peroxidase infiltrated into the lumen of the seminiferous tubules; however, some horseradish peroxidase was detected in tubular walls and epithelial cells lining the tubuli recti and the rete testis, indicating that these regions are permeable to horseradish peroxidase (Itoh et al. 1998a). IL-1, a pro-inflammatory cytokine, is expressed in the testis and regulates testicular functions under physiological conditions. IL-1 facilitates the BTB opening by affecting the actin cytoskeleton (Sarkar et al. 2008).

Under normal condition, the blood-epididymal barrier formed by epididymal epithelial cells also protects autoimmunogenic spermatozoa from attack by the self-immune system. However, the blood-epididymal barrier is less exclusive than the highly specialized tight junctions of the BTB (Hinton and Palladino 1995). Consequently, immune cells are common among the epithelial cells of the epididymal duct (Wang and Holstein 1983; Ritchie et al. 1984).

2.4 Protection of Autoimmunogenic Spermatids and Spermatozoa by Various Local Elements Other Than the BTB

There are certain areas in the body where immune responses are "forbidden." These sites are referred to as "immunologically privileged" sites. The mechanisms underlying immune privilege result from "immunologic ignorance" or "immunologic tolerance." Testicular immune privilege was once believed to be mainly based on the sequestration of autoantigens from the immune system by the BTB in the seminiferous tubules. However, recent evidence has suggested that the testicular interstitium represents the first line of testicular defense against pathogens from the bloodstream. The multiplex immunosuppressive mechanisms, involving various local elements of different origins, participate in the formation of an immunologically privileged area within the testis. Indeed, the testicular interstitium outside the BTB, where many resident macrophages and Leydig cells are normally present, is also protected from attack by the self-immune system.

All testicular cells, involving Sertoli cells, Leydig cells, testicular macrophages, peritubular myoid cells, endothelia of blood and lymph capillaries, lymphocytes, and TGC themselves, may modulate local immunity in the testis (Itoh et al. 1995a, 1999a, 2005). To maintain the testicular immune privilege, the testicular cells express and secrete numerous immunoregulatory molecules including androgens, macrophage migration inhibitory factor, activin, Fas ligand, protein S, IL-10, IL-35, transforming growth factor-beta, programmed death-ligand 1, toll-like receptors (TLR), and Tyro-3, Axl, and Mer (TAM) receptors, which play critical roles in regulating immune responses in the testis (Fijak and Meinhardt 2006; Sun et al. 2010; Meinhardt and Hedger 2011; Winnall et al. 2011a, b; Li et al. 2012; Terayama et al. 2014; Deng et al. 2016). Both activin A and activin B are abundantly expressed by Sertoli cells. Activin A inhibits the expression of pro-inflammatory cytokines, including IL-1 and IL-6, thus suppressing the testicular inflammatory responses (Phillips et al. 2009). The Fas/Fas ligand system suppresses immune responses by inducing the apoptosis of Fas-bearing activated lymphocytes. Fas ligand, also called CD95L, is abundantly expressed in the testis. Testicular immune privilege is maintained by inducing lymphocyte apoptosis via Fas ligand expressed mainly in Sertoli cells. Fas ligand is also expressed in TGC. It remains to be investigated whether Fas ligand that is expressed in the TGC induces lymphocyte apoptosis and contributes to immune privilege within the seminiferous tubules. Programmed death receptor-1/programmed death-ligand 1 is another T cell tolerance system. Programmed death-ligand 1 inhibits T cell activation through programmed death receptor-1. It is constitutively expressed mainly by spermatocytes and spermatids in the seminiferous tubules and involved in the survival of allogeneic islet allografts, suggesting that programmed death receptor-1/programmed death-ligand 1 system is also a mechanism that underlies testicular immune privilege (Cheng et al. 2009). Furthermore, the testis locally generates an efficient innate immune system against pathogens. TLRs are pattern recognition receptors that recognize pathogen-associated molecular patterns. Various TLRs are expressed in various testicular cells of different species (Bhushan et al. 2008, 2011; Fujita et al. 2011; Hedger 2011a, b). Therefore, TLR-mediated innate immune responses by nonimmune cells in the testis also play a critical role in the protection of the testis from infectious diseases. Tyro-3, Axl, and Mer (TAM) receptors are negative regulators of TLR-initiated systemic innate immunity and play critical roles in regulating immune responses (Sun et al. 2010). They are abundantly expressed in Sertoli cells and Leydig cells under normal state and therefore regulate the tissue homeostasis in immunoprivileged testis (Deng et al. 2016).

2.5 Cell Populations Involved in the Testicular Immunoregulation

2.5.1 Sertoli Cells

The testicular cells that appear to be central to maintain testicular immune privilege are the Sertoli cells. These columnar cells extend from the basal lamina to the lumen of the tubules. The Sertoli cells are responsible for physical support of TGC, providing them with essential nutrients and growth factors. Sertoli cells forming the BTB support TGC development and also secrete some proteins for the suppression of lymphocyte proliferation to the outside of the BTB (Wyatt et al. 1988; De Cesaris et al. 1992). Inhibin and activin produced by the Sertoli cells also, respectively, accentuate and reduce thymocyte proliferation in response to mitogen (Lee et al. 1989; Hedger et al. 1989). Sulfated glycoprotein 2, a major product of the Sertoli cell, has been shown to inhibit cell lysis by the complement attack complex, C5b6789 (Jenne and Tschopp 1989; Griswold et al. 1986; Law and Griswold 1994). Sertoli cells secrete inhibitors of granzyme B, which is part of the destructive arsenal of cytotoxic lymphocytes (Sipione et al. 2006). Transforming growth factor-beta secreted by Sertoli cells also contributes to testicular immune privilege through their immunosuppressive activities (Pollanen et al. 1993). It was demonstrated that transforming growth factor-beta facilitates Sertoli cells to support graft survival in co-transplantation experiments (Suarez-Pinzon et al. 2000). In cultured Sertoli cells, inflammatory cytokines such as TNF-alpha, IL-1, IFN-gamma, and lipopolysaccharide strongly enhance the surface expression of integrin ligands, intercellular adhesion molecules-1 (ICAM-1), and vascular cell adhesion molecule-1 (VCAM-1). These molecules are known to be specific for binding of lymphocytes (Riccioli et al. 1995). This suggests that both direct and paracrine mechanisms of interaction between Sertoli cells and lymphocytes are present for the control of immune reactions in the testis (Fillipini et al. 2001).

The Fas/Fas ligand system has been considered to be one of the central mechanisms in homeostasis of the immune response. Fas is a type I membrane protein that belongs to the TNF receptor family and is known to be a receptor for Fas ligand, a cytokine also belonging to the TNF family. Activated lymphocytes that express Fas undergo apoptosis on interaction with cells bearing the Fas ligand. In the testis, the Fas ligand has been mainly detected in the Sertoli cells of the rodent testis (Bellgrau and Selawry 1990; Bellgrau et al. 1995). A developmental study in men demonstrated that Fas ligand expression was found in Sertoli cells of adult testis but not in fetal testis (Francavilla et al. 2000). In rat testes, Fas ligand expression is present from the early postnatal days up to adult, and the Sertoli cells are the main Fas ligand-expressing cell within the seminiferous tubules (D'Abrizio et al. 2004). Importantly, seminiferous tubules of normal mice survived under the kidney capsule of an allogeneic host for much longer periods than seminiferous tubules from gld mutant mice that lack a functional Fas ligand (Bellgrau et al. 1995). Therefore, the constitutive expression of Fas ligand on Sertoli cells may contribute to the testicular immune privilege by inducing the apoptosis of infiltrating T cells that express Fas (Takeda et al. 1998; Koji 2001; Koji et al. 2001). The interaction of Sertoli cells expressing Fas ligand with Fas-bearing autoreactive lymphocytes, leading to the death of the latter by apoptosis, has been proposed as the mechanism responsible for the maintenance of immune tolerance in the testis. The Sertoli cells also express the negative costimulatory ligand CD274 antigen (also called B7-H1), which has the capacity to induce apoptosis in antigen-specific T cells (Dal Secco et al. 2008). That may be why isolated Sertoli cells can survive in both allogeneic and xenogeneic barriers and also provide localized immunoprotective environment for allografts and xenografts (Selawry and Cameron 1993; Sanberg et al. 1996; Korbutt et al. 1997; Suarez-Pinzon et al. 2000; Dufour et al. 2008).

Sertoli cells have a strong phagocytic activity in vivo, like macrophages. Cultured Sertoli cells are also active phagocytes in vitro but do not express constitutively MHC class II antigens or macrophage-specific markers (Kohno et al. 1983). Phagocytic removal of the apoptotic TGC and residual bodies by Sertoli cells is critical for intact TGC to differentiate. The uptake of residual bodies and apoptotic TGC may endow Sertoli cells with producing factors necessary for spermatogenesis. Phagocytosis of apoptotic TGC by Sertoli cells may be also a process that regulates immunity to TGC autoantigens and supports self-tolerance. Therefore, timely removal of apoptotic TGC and residual bodies by the Sertoli cells is important to avoid autoimmune responses. It is unclear how Sertoli cells phagocyting apoptotic TGC induce self-tolerance to TGC autoantigens; however, there is a possibility that Sertoli cells excrete some phagocytosed materials to the outside of BTB (Fig. 2.2). The latent leakage of small amount of TGC autoantigens into the testicular interstitium under normal condition may play a role on peripheral tolerance preventing testicular autoimmunity (Naito et al. 2008).

Differing from the study by Kohno et al. (1983), it was later reported that, in response to IFN-gamma, mouse Sertoli cells strongly upregulate expression of MHC class II antigens, indicating an antigen-presenting capability of Sertoli cells (Dal Secco et al. 2008). Dal Secco et al. (2008) also demonstrated that Sertoli cells upregulate the negative costimulatory ligand B7-H1(CD274) in response to IFN-gamma. Blockade of B7-H1 on the Sertoli cell surface resulted in enhanced proliferation of $CD8^+$ T cells co-cultured with Sertoli cells. Moreover, co-culturing T cells with Sertoli cells can induce an increase in $CD4^+CD25^+$ T cells and a decrease in $CD4^+CD25^-$ T cells, suggesting Sertoli cell-mediated Treg conversion; this process was found to be B7-H1 independent (Dal Secco et al. 2008). It implies that Sertoli cells are potentially capable of downregulating the local immune response, on the one hand by directly inhibiting $CD8^+$ T cell proliferation through B7-H1 and, on the other hand, by inducing an increase in Treg that might suppress other bystander T cells.

Testosterone produced by Leydig cells is not only one of immunosuppressive steroid hormones but also has an effect on the BTB composed of inter-Sertoli cell junctions. Sertoli cell-specific deletion of the androgen receptor in knockout mice disrupts testicular immune privilege (Meng et al. 2005), possibly because androgens regulate Sertoli cells' tight junctions (McCabe et al. 2010, 2012, 2016; Meng et al. 2011).

Sertoli cells participate in the testicular defense system against viruses and bacteria. Mouse and rat Sertoli cells express functional TLR from TLR1 to TLR6 for innate immunity (Riccioli et al. 2000, 2006; Starace et al. 2008; Wu et al. 2008; Hedger 2011b; Winnall et al. 2011b). Under stimulation of TLR with various invading pathogens, Sertoli cells produce the pro-inflammatory molecules. Therefore, TLR3 activation induces antiviral immune responses in mouse Sertoli cells (Starace et al. 2008). Sertoli cells may create an immune-privileged microenvironment that protects TGC from interstitial and/or ascending pathogens; however, there is a risk that innate immune responses through TLR activation breakdown of a milieu of the spermatogenesis will result in male infertility.

TAM receptors composed of Tyro-3, Axl, and Mer are negative regulators of TLR-initiated systemic innate immunity and play critical roles in regulating immune responses (Sun et al. 2010). Indeed, various TLRs are expressed and functional in Sertoli cells, and TAM receptors inhibit TLR-mediated inflammatory cytokine production by Sertoli cells. Moreover, TAM system facilitates phagocytic clearance of apoptotic TGC by Sertoli cells. The removal of apoptotic TGC by phagocytes facilitates the elimination of the autoantigens, which may reduce endogenous inflammation.

In regard to the modified Sertoli cells at the tubule recti, they normally phagocytose apoptotic TGC for the elimination of unwanted spermatozoa (Naito et al. 2008, 2009). This phenomenon is regarded as a normal mechanism for transport of normal spermatozoa to the ductuli efferentes. It may be that some TGC autoantigens are excreted from the modified Sertoli cells into the area of adjacent multilayered basal lamina and peritubular myoid cells for inducing self-tolerance to TGC antigens (Fig. 2.3). In particular, both the basal lamina and the cytoplasm of modified Sertoli cell intimately interconnect with each other, similar to the sagittal suture in the human skull (Tainosho et al. 2011). This suggests that the modified Sertoli cells

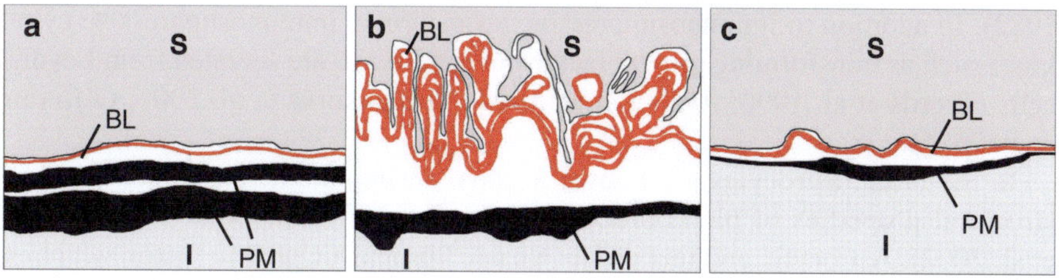

Fig. 2.3 Spaces among Sertoli cells, basal lamina, and peritubular myoid cells at seminiferous tubules (**a**), tubuli recti (**b**), and rete testis (**c**) in the mouse. *BL* basal lamina of the tuble (*red colored*), *I* interstitium, *PM* peritubular myoid cell cytoplasm, *S* Sertoli cell cytoplasm

have a wide surface area at their base and therefore can effectively excrete intratubular materials to the outside of tubuli recti or take various extra-tubular molecules into the tubuli recti. However, the modified Sertoli cells at the tubuli recti and epithelial cells at the rete testis may not directly present the autoantigens to lymphocytes because of a lack of class II MHC antigens, as seen in Sertoli cells in vivo (Itoh et al. 1991).

2.5.2 Leydig Cells

The normal testis is an organ packed compactly with seminiferous tubules, having little interstitium. However, many Leydig cells are compacted in its interstitium. Testosterone, an immunosuppressive steroid hormone, is produced by Leydig cells and suppresses lymphocyte proliferation. Testosterone also reduces TRL4 expression in macrophages (Rettew et al. 2008). Administration of testosterone suppresses autoimmune diseases (Cutolo et al. 2004; Gold and Voskuhl 2009). The intratesticular testosterone concentration is tenfold higher than the serum concentration and is far greater than necessary for the maintenance of normal spermatogenesis (Jarow et al. 2005).

Leydig cells exhibit high antiviral activities in response to viral infections (Dejucq et al. 1995, 1998; Melaine et al. 2003). TLR2, TLR3, and TLR4 are present in Leydig cells, and they trigger innate immunity in response to ligand stimulation (Shang et al. 2011). Although TLR activation of Leydig cells provides defense against invading pathogens, innate immune inflammation in testicular interstitium may also affect the spermatogenesis (Wu et al. 2016). It was also reported that Leydig cells regulate the expansion of testicular macrophages and lymphocyte numbers in the testis (Raburn et al. 1991, 1993; Hedger and Meinhardt 2000). Testosterone production by Leydig cells was stimulated by a conditioned medium from culture of testicular macrophages in a dose-dependent manner in vitro (Yee and Hutson 1985). It is also known that Leydig cells spontaneously adhere to lymphocytes and nonspecifically suppress the proliferation of lymphocytes in vitro without any dependence on testosterone (Born and Wekerle 1981,

1982). In addition to immunosuppressive testosterone, immunosuppressive cytokines such as transforming growth factor-beta and IL-10 are secreted from Leydig cells (Teerds et al. 1990; Avallet et al. 1994; Verajankorva et al. 2001; O'Bryan et al. 2005).

In the brain, astrocytes are known to have an important role in establishing structural properties of blood-brain barrier composed of endothelial cells (Bart et al. 2002). Astrocytic end feet produce basic fibroblastic growth factor, which is also produced by Leydig cells. Desert hedgehog gene is a signaling molecule expressed by Sertoli cells. Its receptor is localized to Leydig cells and also peritubular fibroblastoid cells (Clark et al. 2000). In mice lacking the desert hedgehog gene, adult-type Leydig cells were lacked, and numerous undifferentiated fibroblastic cells were in the testicular interstitium with production of abundant collagen. Moreover, the basal lamina, normally present between the peritubular myoid cells and Sertoli cells, was focally absent (Clark et al. 2000). This indicates that Leydig cells are also involved in maintaining the BTB. Fibroblastic cellular constituents exhibiting fibroblastoid morphology surrounding the seminiferous tubular wall are regarded as precursors of the functional Leydig cells (Hatakeyama 1965; Teerds et al. 1988, 1999). These peritubular precursor cells may support the BTB. Other studies demonstrated that testosterone regulates the permeability of the BTB by regulating the expression of a Sertoli cell tight junction protein, claudin-3 (Meng et al. 2005, 2011).

2.5.3 Testicular Leukocytes

In the normal testis, leukocytes are found almost exclusively within the interstitial tissue between the seminiferous tubules and under the tunica albuginea. These cells chiefly comprise of resident macrophages, dendritic cells, and circulating lymphocytes, although variable numbers of mast cells and eosinophils are also present, depending upon the species. For example, in the macaque, 42.7% of the testicular leukocytes were $CD163^+$ macrophages, while 4.5% were $CD14^+CD163^-$ monocyte-like macrophages. 30.8% of testicular leukocytes were $CD3^+$ T cells, with $CD4^+$ and $CD8^+$ cell proportions similar to those in the blood. B cells and granulocytes were 0.24% and 3.3% of testicular leukocytes, respectively. Small populations of dendritic cells, plasma cells, NK cells, and NKT cells were also detected (De Rose et al. 2013) (Table 2.1).

Table 2.1 Resident leukocytes in the testis

Macrophages ($CD163^+$/$CD68^+$)/dendritic cells
T lymphocytes ($CD4^+$/$CD8^+$) ($CD25^+$/$CD25^-$)
B lymphocytes/plasma cells
NK cells/NKT cells
Mast cells
Eosinophils

2.5.3.1 Macrophages

Not only Leydig cells but also macrophages are major components in testicular interstitium. Hume et al. (1984) were the first to identify testicular macrophages in the mouse by the use of the F4/80 marker and showed that approximately 20% of all interstitial cells in the normal testis were macrophages. There are many studies which demonstrate organ-specific features of testicular macrophages. The exposure to the testis-specific environment may give the testicular macrophages its unique functions. In the testicular interstitium, Leydig cells and testicular macrophages are coupled structurally by way of specialized membrane digitations in adult rats (Hutson 1990, 1992). The macrophages start to form these junctions with Leydig cells when the major increase in secretory activity of Leydig cells occurs during puberty. In vitro studies showed that co-culture of rat testicular macrophages and Leydig cells stimulates Leydig cell steroidogenesis when the macrophages are stimulated with lipopolysaccharide, while stimulated peritoneal macrophages had no such effect. Furthermore, conditioned medium from cultures of rat testicular macrophages but not of peritoneal macrophages stimulates testosterone production in a dose-dependent manner when added to Leydig cells in vitro (Yee and Hutson 1985; Lombard-Vignon et al. 1992). Another in vitro study demonstrated that follicle-stimulating hormone-treated testicular macrophages have a more potent effect on Leydig cell steroidogenesis when compared to untreated ones (Yee and Hutson 1983, 1985). Testicular macrophages but not peritoneal macrophages have specific receptors for follicle-stimulating hormone and respond to follicle-stimulating hormone in a dose-dependent manner by an increased secretion of lactate. An in vivo study showed that treatment of neonatal rats with human chorionic gonadotropin increases the numbers of macrophages in the testis but not in the liver (Yee and Hutson 1983, 1985). Therefore, testicular macrophages play endocrine and paracrine roles in the testis. Differences between macrophage populations from different tissues or organs are called "the inter-population heterogeneity" of macrophages. Local stimuli such as specific cell-cell interactions and production of organ-specific factors are likely to contribute to producing such heterogeneity.

Differing from the inter-population heterogeneity, differences between macrophage subpopulations obtained from one particular tissue or organ are called "the intrapopulation heterogeneity" of macrophages (Itoh et al. 1995b; Winnall and Hedger 2013). In the testis, there are resident macrophages and circulating macrophages. Rat testicular macrophages can be divided into two morphologically different types of cells: large round cell and small elongated cells (Pollanen and Maddocks 1988). In mice, macrophages in the testicular interstitium were various in shape, such as irregular-, elongate-, round-, or oval-shaped cytoplasm with short or elongate cytoplasmic protrusions (Itoh et al. 1995b). Much attention has been directed to a possible cell-cell interaction between macrophages and Leydig cells. However, macrophages are also closely associated with the seminiferous tubular walls or blood capillary walls, suggesting a functional coupling between macrophages and seminiferous tubules and blood capillaries (Itoh et al. 1995b). An immunohistochemical study showed that all testicular macrophages in the human fetus can be labeled by pan-myelomonocytic cell markers, but not all can be labeled by more mature myelomonocytic cell markers (Dechelotte et al. 1989). Examination of the staining pattern of the various antibodies against macrophage/dendritic cell antigens (F4/80, BM8, MP23, MOMA1, MOMA2, M5/114, BMDM1, and NLDC145) demonstrated that these cell antigens differed from each other in amount present and localization, indicating phenotypical heterogeneity of the testicular macrophages in mice. The intrapopulation heterogeneity of testicular macrophages might reflect diversities in their function, which may depend on their localization, differentiation stages, and degree of activation (Itoh et al. 1995b).

There is a speculation that testicular macrophages actively exert immunosuppressive activity. Allografts and xenografts have been shown to survive in the testes of rats for remarkably long times. However, the grafts were rejected from the testes of rams. Histochemical analysis of the testes revealed that the rat testicular interstitium contained approximately eight times as many macrophages/interstitial area as did ram testicular interstitium (Pollanen and Maddocks 1988). Moreover, large and round macrophages are rich in the rat but poor in the ram. Although the rat also contains some small and elongated macrophages, all testicular macrophages in the ram are small and elongated. This implies that round and large macrophages in the rat contribute to the immune privilege of this site by modifying directly or indirectly the activity of Leydig cells. Testicular macrophages are functionally classified into two populations, which are designated as "resident" and "newly arrived or circulating" according to the differential expression of surface scavenger receptor CD163. $CD163^+$ ($ED2^+$) macrophages, which are considered to be resident cells in the testis, represent the majority (approximately 80%) of testicular macrophages in rodents. They constitutively produce immuosuppressive IL-10 and are poor stimulators of T cell proliferation, indicating that they contribute to the maintenance of the testicular immune privilege. In mice, approximately 40% of testicular macrophages are constitutively IL-10 positive (Verajankorva et al. 2001). In cases of testicular inflammation, testicular macrophages produce more immunosuppressive transforming growth factor-beta and IL-10, which may contribute to the testicular immune privileged status. On the other hand, $CD68^+$ ($ED1^+$) macrophages, which are presumably derived from circulating monocytes/macrophages that have only recently arrived in the testis, represent a minor (approximately 20%) proportion of all testicular macrophages in rodents. They have a pro-inflammatory phenotype and express IL-1-beta, TNF-alpha, IL-6, activin A, inducible nitric oxide synthase, and other inflammatory factors (Terayama et al. 2014). However, TNF-alpha, which is synthesized by testicular macrophages, protects TGC from apoptosis at a physiologically low concentration in normal testis (Xiong and Hales 1993). What factors regulate the balance of $ED1^+$ pro-inflammatory cells and $ED2^+$-resident immunosuppressive macrophages in the testis under physiologic condition are still unknown. Systemic inflammation in response to lipopolysaccharide leads to an influx of $CD163^-$ monocyte-like "infiltrating" macrophages into the rodent testis in vivo. However, "newly arrived" $CD163^-$ testicular macrophages in the rat testis show very little response to lipopolysaccharide stimulation in vitro under normal homeostatic conditions. It indicates the presence of intrapopulation heterogeneity of $CD163^-$ testicular macrophages. "Newly arrived" testicular macrophages of the normal rat testis are derived from a monocyte subset that continuously repopulates the testis and distinct from the monocyte-like "infiltrating" subset, from which pro-inflammatory testicular macrophages may be derived during systemic inflammation (Winnall and Hedger 2013).

Testicular macrophages were purified and fractionated on discontinuous Percoll gradient in mice, and their antigen-presenting capacity in humoral and cell-mediated responses was tested in vitro (Mishell-Dutton cultures, proliferation assay) and in vivo (induction of contact sensitivity reaction) (Bryniarski et al. 2004). Heavier Percoll fractions produce little transforming growth factor-beta and are efficient antigen-presenting cells in humoral- and cell-mediated immune responses. Lighter fractions produce high amounts of transforming growth factor-beta and rather tolerogenic than immunogenic. Their immunosuppressive activity can be prevented by in vivo treatment of donor testicular macrophages with cyclophosphamide or in vitro treatment with anti-transforming growth-beta monoclonal antibodies. In non-separated testicular macrophage population, the immunosuppressive activity prevails. Therefore, subpopulation of testicular macrophages able to trigger specific immune responses is present in the testis but remains under control by other testicular macrophage populations which minimize the risk of development of autoimmune reactions.

IL-35 is another immunosuppressive and anti-inflammatory cytokine, which is produced by Foxp3^{+} Treg, suppresses cell proliferation, and downregulates Th17 cell development. IL-35 is a heterodimeric protein composed of two different subunits, Epstein-Barr virus-induced 3 (EBI3) and the p35 of IL-12. Intriguingly, EBI3- and p35-double-positive resident macrophages were found in the testicular interstitium (Terayama et al. 2014). They may produce IL-35 under physiological conditions as Treg. The lack of EBI3, p35, and IL-12 receptor caused significant infiltration of lymphocytes into the testicular interstitium with increased IFN-gamma expression and autoantibody production, resulting in spermatogenic disturbance (Terayama et al. 2014). Therefore, IL-35 may contribute to maintain the testicular immune privilege, and its lack develops autoimmune-like disorder in the testis.

Treatment of rats with human chorionic gonadotropin induces inflammation-like changes in the testicular microcirculation, and the gonadotropin-induced inflammation-like response is enhanced in macrophage-depleted rat testes (Bergh et al. 1987, 1993). Liposome-entrapped dichloromethylene diphosphonate was injected locally into the unilateral testes in order to deplete testicular macrophages. After the chorionic gonadotropin treatment, there was a large increase in the number of leukocytes in testicular blood vessels, and numerous leukocytes had migrated into the interstitial tissue of the unilateral testes. This response was greater than in the intact contralateral testis. This suggests that testicular macrophages are not the origin of the inflammatory mediator after the gonadotropin treatment. On the contrary, it appears that testicular macrophages secrete some factors inhibiting this type of inflammation.

The BTB at the tubuli recti and the rete testis is known to be incomplete. This implies that the testicular tissue around the tubuli recti is where autoreactive lymphocytes can gain access to autoimmunogenic TGC antigens. Many macrophages accumulate around the tubuli recti, and a few macrophages penetrate into the tubuli recti (Itoh et al. 1995a) (Fig. 2.4). Under normal condition, they may take materials leaked from the tubuli recti for prevention of inflammatory responses (Itoh et al. 1999b; Takahashi et al. 2007). However, when the testicular immune privilege is broken, the tubuli recti should be comprised of immunological-specific region, where lymphocytes are attracted.

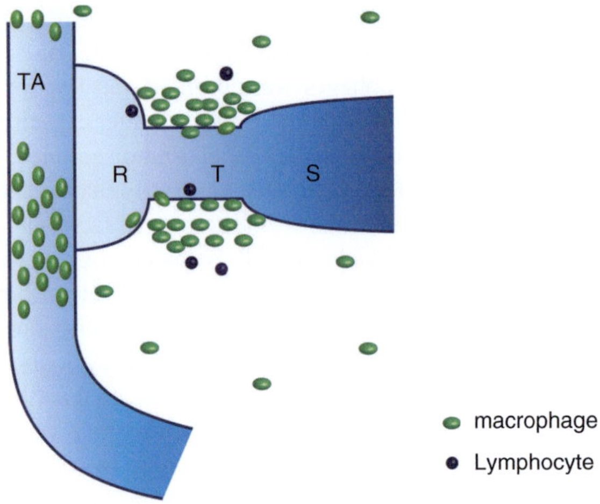

Fig. 2.4 Localization of lymphocytes and macrophages under normal condition. *R* rete testis, *S* seminiferous tuble, *T* tubuli recti, *TA* tunica albuginea

In summary, the testicular macrophages are the largest population of leukocytes in the immune-privileged testis, where both innate and acquired immune responses are effectively suppressed, and the testicular macrophages are predicted to be responsible for regulating this immunosuppression.

2.5.3.2 Dendritic Cells

Class II MHC antigen-bearing cells are known to be antigen-presenting cells for $CD4^{+}$T cells. Dendritic cells, the most powerful antigen-presenting cells, induce activation and differentiation of lymphocytes in response to alloantigens but also minimize the autoimmune response by tolerating T cells to autoantigens under physiological conditions (Banchereau and Steinman 1998). In human testis, no class II MHC antigens were identified on any cells within seminiferous tubules, and the antigens were found on dendritic-like cells between the seminiferous tubules and on vessel endothelium, although the expression was extremely limited (Pollanen and Niemi 1987). In a normal mouse testis, both the seminiferous tubules and the surrounding interstitium were negative for class II MHC antigens (Itoh et al. 1991). This indicates that antigen presentation to $CD4^{+}$T cells is not a common event inside the testis. In the rat, dendritic cells also represent a minor population of the interstitial cells, numbering about one-tenth of the macrophages (Rival et al. 2006). The dendritic cells of the normal testis have not yet been well physiologically characterized, but evidence from the rat suggests that the crucial antigen-presenting cells exert immunoregulatory functions in the testis under normal condition. However, in inflammatory condition, the number of class II MHC antigen-bearing cells increases in number (Tung et al. 1987; Itoh et al. 1991). Therefore, stimulated dendritic cells may convert immune privilege into expansion of autoreactive T cells (Rival et al. 2006, 2007; Fijak et al. 2011).

2.5.3.3 Lymphocytes

In the mouse, under normal conditions, it is noteworthy that the testis sections stain neither for T and B cell markers nor for immunoglobulins and complements; however, a small number of lymphocytes are observed in the epididymis (Itoh et al.

1991). Therefore, the presence of extremely limited number of lymphocytes in the testis may be derived from a poor microcircumstance for attraction of lymphocytes. By minute microscopic observation, only a few lymphocytes can be found in and around the tubuli recti and the rete testis of the mouse (Naito et al. 2008) (Fig. 2.4). Because of that, the tubuli recti and the rete testis are permeable to IgG and exogenously administered HRP; in the normal state, the presence of a few lymphocytes and macrophages penetrating the tubuli recti and the rete testis may be important for access to TGC autoantigens (Fig. 2.5). To investigate the function of the penetrating lymphocytes, the changes and distribution of these lymphocytes in some abnormal conditions, such as experimental cryptorchidism and experimental obstruction of TGC transport to the ductuli efferentes and epididymis, should be examined.

In the rat, intratesticular lymphocytes are consistently present under normal condition, and the population is skewed toward class I MHC antigen-restricted $CD8^+$ T cells, and $CD8^+$ T cell subset predominates over the $CD4^+$ T cell subset. Testicular $CD8^+$ T cell population also includes significant numbers of cytotoxic T cells (Tompkins et al. 1998; Hedger and Meinhardt 2000, 2003). In contrast to the peripheral blood, in which the $CD4^+$ T cell subset was the major lymphocyte subset, not only $CD8^+$ T cells but also NK cells were numerous in a normal rat testis (Tompkins et al. 1998). Destruction of the Leydig cells by the treatment with ethane dimethane sulfonate caused a rapid preferential increase in testicular $CD4^+$ T cells, which was followed by an increase in both $CD8^+$ T cell subset and T cell-inhibiting activity in the Leydig cell-deficient testis (Hedger et al. 1998). After Leydig cell recovery, there was a significant shift toward the $CD8^+$ T cell subset.

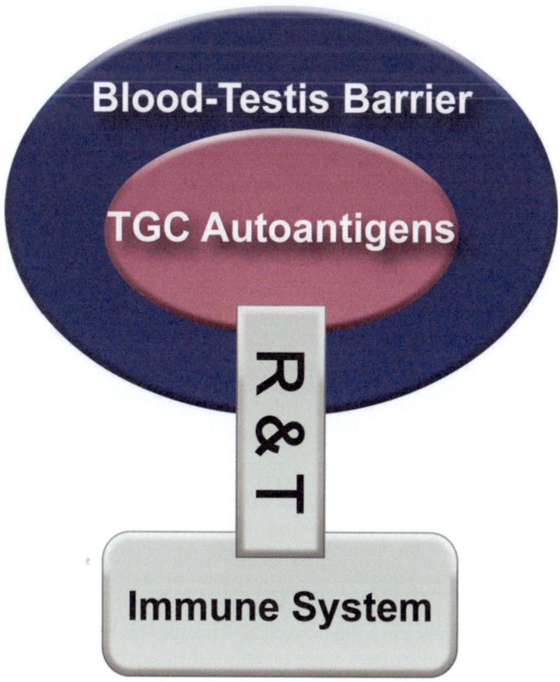

Fig. 2.5 Lymphocytes can gain access to autoimmunogenetic antigens of testicular germ cells (TGC) at the tubuli recti. *T* tubuli recti, *R & T* rete testis and tubuli recti

More recently, some $CD4^+CD25^+$ Treg are found within the testicular interstitium under physiological conditions (Jacobo et al. 2009). $Foxp3^+$ Treg are central to the maintenance of immunological homeostasis and tolerance. Recently, it was reported that a conditioned medium from primary mouse Sertoli cells may be able to induce Treg (Campese et al. 2014). Generation of $CD4^+CD25^+Foxp3^+$ Treg in Leydig cell-conditioned media was determined to investigate the influence of testosterone (Fijak et al. 2015). Leydig cell-conditioned media dose dependently stimulated expression of transcription factor Foxp3 and secretion of IL-10 in splenic $CD4^+$ T cells, an effect abolished by addition of the antiandrogen flutamide.

2.5.3.4 Other Leukocyte Populations

Distribution and numbers of mast cells or eosinophils were studied in the testes of 12 mammalian species (Anton et al. 1998). Mast cells were frequently found in horse and human testis, whereas eosinophils were nearly absent. On the contrary, eosinophils were abundant in the rabbit testis, while mast cells were lacking in the pig testis. Otherwise, mast cells and eosinophils were absent from the testicular interstitium proper in rats, dogs, cats, bulls, and deer, although they were present around blood vessels in the tunica albuginea. It remains unknown whether the presence of eosinophils in the testis plays a role in local immunoregulation. On the other hand, it is known that mast cells in the testis regulate steroidogenesis by Leydig cells (Aguilar et al. 1995). Mast cells secrete serine protease tryptase, which promotes the proliferation of fibroblasts and synthesis of collagen (Abe et al. 1998, 2000), leading to fibrosis, sclerosis, and thickening hyalinization of tissues. Mast cells also synthesize TNF-alpha, which protects TGC from apoptosis at a physiologically low concentration in normal testis (Xiong and Hales 1993). In human, mast cells in the interstitium, mediastinum, and tunica albuginea increase in number slightly during infancy, decrease during childhood, and then increase again at puberty, when active spermatogenesis starts. During adulthood, the number of mast cells progressively decreases in the testicular interstitium (Nistal et al. 1984, 1986). In the rat, mast cells in the testis were found almost exclusively around subcapsular blood vessels. In neonatally estrogen-treated rats, a greater number of mast cells were present in the testicular interstitium, whereas no significant increase in the number of mast cells was found for the epididymis, despite the induction of stromal proliferation. On the other hand, androgen-treated rats did not have increased mast cell numbers in any organ. These results indicate that the increase in mast cell numbers was estrogen dependent, specifically related to the testis, and did not seem to be a consequence of the increase in the connective interstitial tissue (Gaytan et al. 1989). By the treatment of rats with ethylene dimethane sulfonate, simultaneous proliferation and differentiation of mast cells and Leydig cells were found in the testis, indicating that Leydig cells and mast cells share some common regulatory factors (Gaytan et al. 1992). Clinically, in men with alcoholic and nonalcoholic cirrhosis, the testicular interstitium, consisting of small and poor collagen fiber bundles, was less developed than in normal testes. The appearance of connective tissue was associated with a decrease in the number of mast cells in the testes of cirrhotic males, suggesting the involvement of mast cells in the synthesis, packing, and organization of collagen fibers. The cause of the decrease in mast cell numbers may be related to hormone alterations, in particular testosterone deficiency (Nistal et al. 1986). Mast cells can be divided into two subtypes based on differences in their neutral serine protease content. MC_T contains only tryptase, whereas MC_{TC} contains both tryptase and chymase in addition to other proteases, including cathepsin G and carboxypeptidase (Yamanaka et al. 2000). In the normal testes, MCT are the predominant subtype. However, in male infertile patients, total number of mast cells increases, and the predominant subtype of mast cell is shifted to MCTC. Small populations of testicular leukocytes include B cells, plasma cells, NK cells, and NKT cells (De Rose et al. 2013).

2.5.4 Peritubular Myoid Cells and Basal Lamina

The seminiferous tubules are surrounded by peritubular myoid cells, which together with Sertoli cells secrete components of the basal lamina that encloses the seminiferous epithelium. Peritubular myoid cells are smooth muscle-like and surround the seminiferous tubules for autonomic contraction of the tubular walls to excrete immotile TGC to the epididymis. They may also contribute to the BTB. In an experimental study of permeation of administered lanthanum as a tracer on rats, electron microscopy showed that tight junctions between the peritubular myoid cells largely prevented permeation of the tracer to the seminiferous epithelium (Bart et al. 2002). Peritubular myoid cells also express androgen receptors and mediate androgen actions on fetal Sertoli cell proliferation. They support the inter-Sertoli cell junctions and also secrete some cytokines (Schuppe and Meinhardt 2005).

In regard to cytokines, peritubular myoid cells release transforming growth factor-beta-2, monocyte chemotactic protein-1, and leukemia inhibitory factor. Transforming growth factor-beta is an immuosuppressive protein, which is regulated by macrophage migration inhibitory factor secreted from Sertoli cells and Leydig cells (Muller et al. 2005). Monocyte chemotactic protein-1 should account for the recruitment of inflammatory monocytes and/or macrophages. Peritubular myoid cells also express TNF-alpha receptors 1 and 2, which mediate the expression of other inflammatory molecules, including IL-6 and cyclooxygenase-2 (Schell et al. 2008). Peritubular myoid cells are regulated by mast cell and macrophage products and produce factors that can fuel inflammatory changes (Mayerhofer 2013). Peritubular myoid cells were also able to markedly express IFNs and IFN-induced antiviral proteins after viral exposure (Dejucq et al. 1995, 1998). They possess a high degree of plasticity, which results in hypertrophy and loss of contractile abilities. Further studies should provide insights into the repertoire of the secretion products, contractile properties, and plasticity of peritubular myoid cells.

Basal lamina also provides a selective barrier and is an important component of the BTB. In general, the main components of basal lamina are type IV collagens, laminins, entactin/nidogen, and heparin sulfate proteoglycan, which are present on the basal surface of all epithelia. Morphological alterations of the basal lamina at the seminiferous tubules in various pathological conditions including a varicocele, cryptorchid testes, hypogonadotropic hypogonadism, and irradiated testes have been reported, suggesting the possibility that the basal lamina of the seminiferous tubules influences spermatogenic activity (Tainosho et al. 2011). The basal lamina of the modified Sertoli cells at the tubuli recti exhibited a wavy and multilayered structure, but the Sertoli cells of the seminiferous tubules and the epithelium of the rete testis had an almost flat and single-layered basal lamina (Tainosho et al. 2011) (Fig. 2.3). The wavy and multilayered basal lamina may function as a flexible and movable junction between the seminiferous tubules and the rete testis. Its structure may facilitate opening or closing of the valve-like structure formed by the modified Sertoli cells at the tubuli recti. It was also noted that wide gaps existed between the modified Sertoli cells, the basal lamina of the epithelial layer, and the peritubular myoid cell layer at the tubuli recti. The presence of the wide gaps might provide the microcircumstance in which lymphocytes can easily penetrate into the tubuli recti. Therefore, this characteristic structure of the basal lamina of the tubuli recti may be one of the factors for its incomplete BTB (Tainosho et al. 2011).

2.5.5 Blood Capillary Endothelium

Distribution of blood capillaries in the testis and the epididymis is quite regional (Hirai et al. 2010, 2012). In the epididymis, blood capillaries are dense in both the initial segment and cauda but not abundant in the caput and the corpus. In contrast, blood capillaries are relatively sparse throughout the testis.

Blood capillaries in the testis exist in its interstitium but never extend into the tubular walls of the seminiferous tubules, the tubuli recti, and the rete testis. In sharp contrast, some blood capillaries of the epididymis extend beyond the peritubular myoid cell layer and reach beneath the basal lamina of the epididymal ducts. Distinct from the epididymis and prostate, the testis is not vulnerable to nonspecific extravasation of polymorphonuclear leukocytes (Itoh et al. 1995a). Therefore, there is a possibility that a permeability of capillary blood vessels against leukocytes in the testis may first contribute to the immune-privileged status of the organ. Before the immunosuppressive actions by Leydig cells, testicular macrophages, peritubular myoid cells, and Sertoli cells, the testicular capillary vessels might primarily function as first BTB to protect the testis from inflammatory cell responses. Ultrastructural studies in rat testes showed that testicular capillaries share several properties with brain capillaries, such as the continuity and the rarity of fenestrations (Bart et al. 2002). Therefore, the mechanical BTB consists of tight junction not only between the Sertoli cells but also between the capillary endothelial cells as seen in the blood-brain barrier. Additionally, testicular blood capillaries are specific in that they are sensitive to the endothelial damage by cadmium and gonadotropin treatments (Bergh et al. 1987). Ogawa et al. (2012) demonstrated that the testicular capillary damage by low-dosed cadmium had broken down the immune privilege in the testis.

2.5.6 Lymphatic Capillary Endothelium

Testicular immune privilege had been proposed to be attributed to the absence of lymphatic drainage until evidence of the existence of afferent lymphatic vessels in the testis was obtained. Nowadays, it is known that the seminiferous tubules are bathed in a sea of lymph. There is a possibility that the sensitization of hosts with allograft antigens is failed due to anomalous lymph drainage due to anomalous lymph drainage whereby some lymphatic trunks from the testis bypassed regional lymph nodes and opened directly into the systemic blood circulation. Classic privileged sites such as the brain and anterior chamber of the eye owe their immunosuppressive status primarily to a deficient lymphatic drainage. Indeed, experimental interruption of lymphatic drainage or production of an alymphatic skin pedicle can create an immune-privileged site for a long graft survival. In contrast, reports of immune privilege in the testis are surprising, because its interstitial tissue is well endowed with abundant lymphatic sinusoids and capillaries. Head et al. (1990) revealed a consistent and very efficient lymphatic drainage involving primarily the iliac and renal lymph nodes and to a lesser extent the external lumbar, para-aortic, and posterior gastric nodes in the rat. It was demonstrated that the ligature occlusion of the testicular lymphatics induced retardation and disturbance of spermatogenesis with decreased testosterone secretion in the rat and rabbit (Kotani et al. 1974). This suggests that the integrity of the testicular function must be dependent at least partly on a free flow of the lymph from the testis. In horseradish peroxidase-administered mice, blood-borne horseradish peroxidase was seen in the lymphatic space under the tunica albuginea with the presence of many horseradish peroxidase-endocytosing macrophages (Itoh et al. 1998a). The tunica albuginea tissue filled with many lymphatic capillaries was rapidly loaded with blood-borne horseradish peroxidase that had drained from the testicular interstitium. In the tunica albuginea tissue adjacent to the mediastinum testis, large lymphatics contained much horseradish peroxidase. In mice that had received local injection of colloidal carbon into the testes, the carbon was rapidly excluded from the testis through the lymphatics (Itoh et al. 1998b, c). However, the carbon injected into the epididymis and vas deferens flowed into the lymphatics very slowly. In other experiments, spermatozoa that traumatically leaked from epididymal ducts to the surrounding interstitium consistently accumulated, followed by formation of granulomas; however, TGC that traumatically leaked from the seminiferous tubules to the surrounding interstitium quickly disappeared with no accumulation (Itoh et al. 1999a). Intratesticular injection of isolated epididymal spermatozoa also did not induce accumulation of the injected spermatozoa. This implies that lymph flow in the testicular interstitium is much faster than in the epididymal interstitium, and the rapid kinetics of lymph flow in the testis may be also one of the causes of prevention of leukocytic infiltration leading to granulomatous formation.

In deep testicular parenchyma, the peritubular lymphatic space surrounding the seminiferous tubules is present as polygonal piles (Hamasaki and Kumabe 1994). They are joined to the adjacent piles through fenestrae to form a loose spongiform structure. In the superficial parenchyma, the peritubular lymphatic spaces communicated to the lymphatic space under the tunica albuginea on one side. The lymphatic spaces under the tunica albuginea anastomosed each other through small bypasses to form a rich network. Near the mediastinum testis, the peritubular lymphatic spaces bifurcated and narrowed on another side. The abrupt narrowing of the lymphatic spaces should restrict the flux of the lymphatic fluids (Hamasaki and Kumabe 1994).

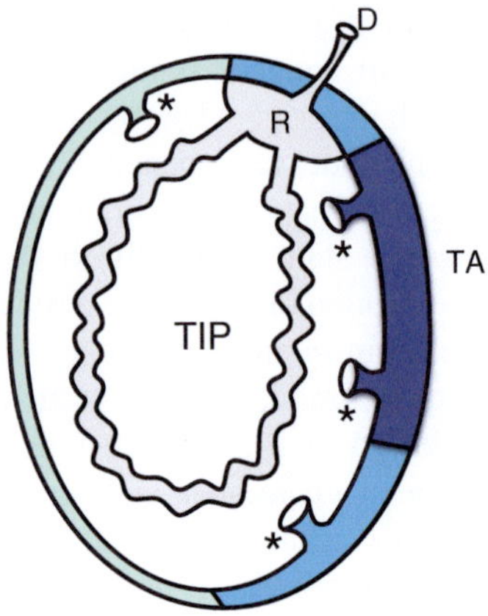

Fig. 2.6 Localization of lymphatic endothelial cells in the testis in the mouse. The abundance of lymphatic endothelial cells is represented by the intensity of the *blue color*. *D* ductuli efferentes, *R* rete testis, *TA* tunica albuginea, *TIP* testicular interstitium proper between the seminiferous tubules. *Asterisks* indicate lymphatic capillaries just beneath the tunica albuginea

Distribution of lymphatics in the testis and the epididymis is quite regional (Hirai et al. 2010, 2012). In the epididymis, lymphatic networks are quite scarce in the initial segment and strikingly dense in the cauda compared to the caput and the corpus. In the testis, lymphatic capillaries are in and just beneath the tunica albuginea but not in the interstitium between the seminiferous tubules (Fig. 2.6). Those lymphatic capillaries just beneath the tunica albuginea run into the tunica albuginea. It was also noted that lymphatic capillaries were abundant in the thickened tunica albuginea adjacent to the epididymis, but they were scarce in the thin tunica albuginea opposite the epididymis. When normal lymphocytes were locally injected into testes, the injected lymphocytes migrated between the seminiferous tubules and then drained into the lymphatic vessels in the tunica albuginea adjacent to the rete testis (Itoh et al. 1998b, c; Hirai et al. 2012).

2.5.7 Testicular Germ Cells (TGC)

In general, antigens of TGC are immunogenic to self. Moreover, TGC secrete various inflammatory cytokines, including IL-1 and TNF-alpha (De et al. 1993; Haugen et al. 1994). However, it was shown that human spermatozoa inhibited the in vitro proliferative responses of human peripheral blood leukocytes to mitogens such as phytohemagglutinin and concanavalin A (Shearer and Hurtenbach 1982). Hurtenbach and Shearer (1982) reported that in mice given intravenous injections with 1×10^7 syngeneic TGC taken from adult mice, antigen-nonspecific suppression of cell-mediated immunity was induced. Male mice injected intravenously with syngeneic TGC exhibited reduced NK cell activity, reduced mixed lymphocyte reactivity, enhanced auto-proliferation of spleen cells, and decreased potential to generate cytotoxic T lymphocyte responses. This indicates that TGC components also exert regulatory influences on immune potential. This suppressive effect was detected as early as 4 days after injection of TGC and persisted for at least 7 weeks. The reduction of cytotoxic T cell responses and NK cell function appeared to be antigen nonspecific, but the onset of the impairment of cytotoxic T cell function was detected earlier with hapten-modified cell autoantigens than with alloantigens. Moreover, suppressor-inducing properties of TGC from aged mice were stronger than those from young mice, showing the age-dependent potential. In addition, spermatozoa were much more effective than TGC, suggesting that more mature stages of germ cells induce significant suppression (Shearer and Hurtenbach 1982). The injection of allogeneic sperm into mice resulted in similar immunosuppression (Shearer and Hurtenbach 1982).

It was also shown that Treg for DTH to TGC were detected in the spleen cells of mice administered intravenously with 1×10^7 TGC (Sakamoto and Nomoto 1986). These Treg were sensitive to cyclophosphamide and suppress the generation of $CD4^+T$ cells for DTH. Therefore, TGC exhibit autoimmunogenicity when injected subcutaneously but exert immunosuppression when injected intravenously (Fig. 2.7). Also under in vitro conditions, lymphocyte proliferation was strongly reduced in the presence of TGC (Hurtenbach et al. 1980). This phenomenon may reflect mechanisms prevailing in vivo by which spermatogenesis proceeds normally in spite of the presence of the autoantigenicity of TGC and the incompleteness of BTB. In contrast, somatic cells of the testis stimulated lymphocytic proliferation under some experimental condition. Treg activated by autologous TGC in vitro were antigen nonspecific and capable of inhibiting lymphocyte proliferation against autologous and allogeneic somatic testicular cells as well as against allogeneic spleen cells. Therefore, autologous TGC are efficient inducers of tolerance by evoking Treg, whereas autologous somatic cells of the testis are immunogenic (Hurtenbach et al. 1980).

Furthermore, the seminiferous epithelium itself may participate in active immunosuppression with intra-seminiferous tubular fluid. In the fluid, proteins that inhibit complement activation exist, and they may reduce complement-mediated inflammation and complement-dependent cytolysis in the testis (Tarter and Alexander 1984). Moreover, spermatogonia produce antiviral proteins in response to IFN-alpha and IFN-gamma (Melaine et al. 2003).

Most intriguingly, Fas ligand is abundantly expressed in the meiotic and post-meiotic TGC (D'Alessio et al. 2001). Fas ligand-expressing cells may contribute to immune privilege by inducing apoptosis of Fas-bearing lymphocytes (Suda et al.

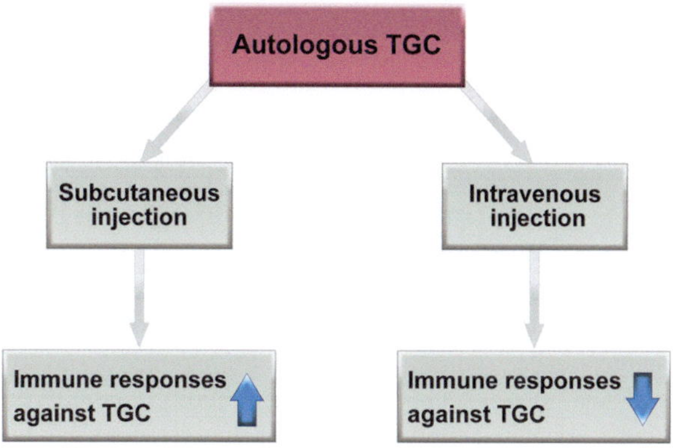

Fig. 2.7 Differences of specific immune responses between subcutaneous and intravenous injections with TGC

1993). However, it remains to be clarified whether TGC expressing Fas ligand contribute to the immune privileged status within the seminiferous tubules.

TLR2 and TLR4 on sperm recognize bacterial endotoxins and mediate apoptosis (Fujita et al. 2011). TLR3 and TRL11 in TGC also trigger innate immunity in response to ligand stimulation (Wang et al. 2012; Chen et al. 2014). Programmed death receptor-1 is a transmembrane protein, which is expressed on T cells. Programmed death ligand-1 is constitutively expressed in spermatocytes and spermatids in the seminiferous tubules and mediates T cell tolerance by activation of programmed death receptor-1 (Keir et al. 2006; Cheng et al. 2009).

2.5.8 Seminal Plasma

Seminal plasma, a mixture of aqueous extracts of prostate, seminal vesicle, Cowper's gland, vas deferens, and epididymis, exerts a potent immunosuppressive effect in vivo and in vitro (Anderson and Tarter 1982). The humoral immune responses to epididymal sperm were suppressed when sperms were incubated in the seminal plasma and then washed before immunization. Cell-mediated immunity and NK cell activity were also inhibited in the presence of the seminal plasma. Anticomplementary effects which inhibit the lytic effect of complement were also reported. Seminal plasma also suppressed mitogen-induced lymphocyte transformation. The seminal vesicle fluid and prostatic fluid can exert suppressive effects on lymphocytes independently (Saxena and Farroq 1987). Human seminal plasma at high concentrations is also lymphocytotoxic and inhibits the opsonization (Ig-mediated recognition and phagocytosis) of bacteria by phagocytic leukocytes (Alexander and Anderson (1987)). Components of human seminal plasma with well-established immunosuppressive effects include prostaglandins, polyamines, transglutaminase, proteases, opiates, transferrin, lactoferrin, macroglobulin, and microglobulin. The final product of spermatogenesis is the spermatozoon, which leaves the body of a male, travels through the reproductive tract of a female, and fuses with an oocyte. Therefore, the complex mechanisms underlying immune privilege in the testis can be regarded as a specialized microcircumstance, in which spermatozoa are adequately equipped, trained, and selected for their ability to survive as foreigners both in the males and females. Prevention of immune responses against testis-leaving spermatozoa by the seminal plasma may lead to inhibition of autoimmunity against elongated mature spermatids in the testis.

2.6 Resistance to Inflammatory Cell Responses of Various Types in the Testis

In general, the testis is resistant to induction of the interstitial inflammation. As documented earlier, sequestration of autoimmunogenic TGC by the BTB is important but not sufficient to prevent testicular autoimmunity. Lyso-glycerophosphatidylcholines in testicular interstitial fluid inhibit T cell activity, contributing to local immunosuppressive milieu (Foulds et al. (2008)). There should be other secretory materials in testicular fluid for immunosuppression. Sertoli cells, Leydig cells, testicular macrophages, peritubular myoid cells, and capillary endothelium are testicular somatic cells that should express or release some immunosuppressive proteins. Also, some inhibitory proteins derived from TGC may be delivered to the testicular interstitium through the medium of Sertoli cells.

2.6.1 Resistance to Rejection of Allografts in the Testis

The testicular interstitium is an immunologically suppressed space in which allogenic or xenogenic tissue grafts can survive for a long time. Allografts and xenografts, including parathyroid and pancreatic islets, which would be rapidly rejected under the renal capsule, survived for prolonged periods when engrafted inside the testis (Head and Billingham 1983, 1985; Selawry et al. 1987; Bellgrau and Selawry 1990). The intratesticular grafts are resistant to the adoptive transfer of lymphocytes from rat donors primed to xenograft antigens (Bellgrau and Selawry 1990). In fact, Sertoli cells display an inherent immunosuppressive role that supports the survival of cells from other tissues, such as pancreatic islet cells, when they were co-transplanted (Selawry and Cameron 1993; Suarez-Pinzon et al. 2000). Studies on pancreatic islet cell allografts in mouse testes showed that activated T cells are destroyed, and graft antigen-specific Treg are produced when they enter the testis environment (Dai et al. 2005; Nasr et al. 2005). A blockade of androgen production in Leydig cell rapidly rejects intratesticular allografts, suggesting the role of androgens in regulating immune privilege (Head and Billingham 1985).

2.6.2 Spontaneous Occurrence of Vasculitis-Like Lesions in the Male Reproductive System

In man, both systemic and isolated vasculitis in male reproductive tissues is often asymptomatic and subclinical. Therefore, many cases have been found at autopsy. In man, vasculitis involving the male reproductive tract has been described in polyarteritis nodosa, rheumatic arteritis, Goodpasture's syndrome, Henoch-Schönlein purpura, and dermatomyositis (Silva et al. 2012, 2014). However, in laboratory mice, spontaneous testicular vasculitis was detected in only 3 out of 66 (4.5%) genetically autoimmune MRL/lpr$^{+/+}$ mice that had systemic lupus erythematosus-like lesions, such as those in generalized lymphadenopathy, immune complex glomerulonephritis, and systemic vasculitis (Tokunaga et al. 1993). Isolated vasculitis lesions in the vas deferens and epididymis but not testis often occur in man without being a manifestation of systemic vasculitis lesions. Histological examination of normal Balb/c mice reared under specific pathogen-free conditions revealed that spontaneous vasculitis-like lesions comparable to those in man were significantly present in the epididymides and vasa deferentia of aged but not young mice (Itoh et al. 1999c). However, no significant lesions were found in the testes, ductuli efferentes, and other organs, such as salivary glands, thyroid glands, livers, pancreases, and kidneys. These results indicate that the epididymis and vas deferens but not testis are spontaneously apt to be affected by vasculitis-like lesions with advancing age but that the lesions are not due to a systemic vasculitis disease. It is conceivable that some exogenous agents, such as bacteria and virus, may preferably reach the epididymis and vas deferens and then evoke vasculitis-like lesions in man. It has also been postulated that endogenous agents, such as autoimmunogenic germ cell antigens, may leak from the epididymal duct and vas deferens under normal conditions. This possibility supports that spontaneous exposure to the leaked autoantigens leads to local inflammation without overt manifestation of a systemic inflammation.

2.6.3 Spermatic Granulomata by Local Trauma

The chronic inflammatory lesion induced by the interaction of extravasated autoimmunogenic spermatozoa with surrounding connective tissue is known as a spermatic granulomata (a mass of leaked germ cells surrounded by many epithelioid-type macrophages) (Lyons et al. 1967). When spermatozoa are experimentally leaked from the epididymal ducts to the surrounding interstitium, they induce inflammatory cell responses followed by the formation of a spermatic granuloma. However, such lesions cannot be induced in the testis in which TGC are traumatically leaked from the seminiferous tubules (Itoh et al. 1999a). To examine the possibility that epididymal spermatozoa have inherently greater ability to form spermatic granulomata than TGC, isolated epididymal spermatozoa or TGC were locally injected into the testes and epididymides of recipient mice (Itoh et al. 1999a). The results showed that spermatic granulomata were readily formed in the epididymides after local injection of either epididymal spermatozoa or TGC. In contrast, such lesions were not formed in the testes even when epididymal spermatozoa were locally injected. This indicates that the interstitial environment in the testis exhibits resistance to the formation of spermatic granulomata. In other words, the microcircumstance of the testicular interstitium, rather than the extravasated components from the ruptured seminiferous tubules, is the main factor determining the limited formation of spermatic granulomas in the testis. Indeed, spermatic granulomata are rarely seen in the human testis but are common in the epididymis and vas deferens (Nistal et al. 1997). It is known that testicular macrophages are less activated to pathogen stimulation, and they constitutively produced anti-inflammatory cytokines (Bhushan et al. 2008, 2011; Winnall et al. 2011a, b).

2.6.4 Spermatic Granulomata by Testosterone Treatment

Testosterone, a product of Leydig cells, is an important steroid hormone for the male reproductive system and also suppresses lymphocyte proliferation. Low or moderate doses of testosterone induce hypertrophy of the epididymides, vas deferens, prostates, seminal vesicles, and penis. However, high doses of testosterone exhibit various toxicities, such as salt and water retention leading to edema. In the reproductive system, spermatic granulomata were experimentally induced in the epididymides but not in testes of mice treated with high-dose testosterone (Itoh et al. 1999d). It is speculated that the testosterone-induced spermatic granulomata may be related to significant changes of degeneration of the epididymal rather than seminiferous epithelium, permitting spermatozoa to escape outside the epididymal ducts.

2.6.5 Reproductive Inflammation by Estrogen Treatment

Neonatal estrogen treatment in mice induced an inflammation in the ductuli efferentes, epididymis, and vas deferens, but not in the testis, provoking obstructive azoospermia in their postpubertal period (Naito et al. 2014). No morphological changes were observed until 4 weeks after the neonatal treatment. Some inflammatory cells were found in the epididymis and vas deferens after 6 weeks. Eight weeks after the treatment, inflammatory cells spread to the ductuli efferentes, and the inflammation became severe from 6 to 12 weeks after the treatment. Inflammatory cells were never seen in the testis, but cystic dilatation of the rete testis with spermatogenic disturbance was occasionally found around the mediastinum testis (Naito et al. 2014). Many inflammatory cells emigrated into the lumen of the epididymis, resulting in complete absence of spermatozoa in the vas deferens, although the spermatogenesis could be seen in the testis. Most of the inflammatory cells penetrating into the epithelial layers of epididymal ducts were neutrophils. Furthermore, many epithelioid-type macrophages and some $CD4^+$, $CD8^+$, or $B220^+$ lymphocytes were localized in the epididymal interstitium. In the estrogen-induced inflammation, it is speculated that neonatal estrogen treatment causes an increase in expression of estrogen receptor and decrease expression of testosterone receptor in the male reproductive organs. The changes of expression of these sex hormone receptors may cause stromal-epithelial degeneration of the epididymis and vas deferens rather than the testis, resulting in inflammatory cell infiltration into the epididymis and vas deferens. It remains unknown why the major populations of infiltrating cells are neutrophils and macrophages but not lymphocytes in spite of "chronic" inflammatory responses in the estrogen-treated mice. More recently, it was found that neonatal exposure to diethylstilbestrol, an artificial estrogenic compound, also induced epididymitis in mice with 100% incidence after 5 weeks of age. Furthermore, in approximately 20% of male mice treated with diethylstilbestrol, the epididymitis was accompanied by orchitis after 12 weeks of age (Miyaso et al. 2014). The epididymal inflammation was similar to that by estrogen treatment; however, the main testicular lesion is severe degeneration of the seminiferous epithelium and interstitial edema rather than inflammatory cell responses.

2.6.6 Reproductive Inflammation by Intravenous Administration of *Bordetella pertussis* (BP)

In mice that were intravenously injected with BP, systemic inflammation involving splenomegaly was induced. It was found that the ductuli efferentes, the epididymis, the vas deferens, and the accessory glands such as the prostate, the coagulating gland, and the seminal vesicle in BP-injected mice received extravasation of leukocytes into their interstitial tissues; however, the testicular interstitium was completely free from leukocyte infiltration (Itoh et al. 1995a). This indicates that the testis is resistant to leukocyte extravasation compared with the epididymis and the prostate. The BTB composed of blood capillary endothelium may prevent the testicular interstitium from inflammatory cell responses.

Recently, a new syndrome, namely, the "autoimmune/autoinflammatory syndrome induced by adjuvants" (ASIA) has been defined (Colafrancesco et al. 2014). In this syndrome, different conditions induced by various adjuvants such as infectious fragments, hormones, aluminum, silicone, and metal are included, and the syndrome is characterized by common signs and symptoms, resulting in boosting the immune response and triggering the development of autoinflammatory phenomena (Loyo et al. 2012; Cruz-Tapias et al. 2013; Lujan et al. 2013). Reproductive inflammation induced by BP or estrogen described above may be characterized by the ASIA syndrome.

2.6.7 Spontaneous Infiltration of Eosinophils and Macrophages in Reproductive Tissues of Congenitally Lymph Node-Lacked Mice

Mice with alymphoplasia (aly/aly) mutation are characterized by a lack of lymph nodes, Peyer's patches, and defined lymphoid follicles in the spleen (Wang et al. 2010). In male reproductive tissues, many eosinophils and macrophages spontaneously accumulate in the interstitial tissues of the epididymides and vasa deferentia, but not in the testes in this mutant mouse strain. Therefore, the testicular interstitium is resistant to infiltration of eosinophils and macrophages (Itoh et al. 1999e). In the liver and the pancreas, focal accumulation of lymphocytes and macrophages but not eosinophils was consistently found (Wang et al. 2010). It remains unclear why eosinophils specifically accumulated in the male reproductive tissues. It was noted that parenchymal and stromal injury to the epididymis and vas deferens, such as necrosis, fibrosis, granuloma, abscesses, edema, and congestion, was absent in aly/aly mice. This implies that the accumulation of eosinophils and macrophages is not an active inflammatory reaction. It might be that the systemic absence of lymph nodes may evoke abnormal lymph flow in the epididymis and vas deferens, resulting in a pool of leukocytes in their stromal tissues (Itoh et al. 1999e). In preliminary experiments involving normal mice, it was observed that locally injected colloidal carbon was rapidly excluded from the testis through the lymphatics; however, the injected carbon in the epididymis and vas deferens flowed into the lymphatics very slowly (personal observation). This indicates that the slow kinetics of lymph flow in the epididymis and vas deferens are one of the causes of leukocytic accumulation.

2.6.8 Multiple Organ-Localized Autoimmunity

In mice that had received thymectomy on day 3 after birth, multiple autoimmune diseases involving the retina, salivary glands, thyroid, stomach, prostate, and gonads were induced (Taguchi et al. 1990). In these neonatally thymectomized mice, the incidence of autoimmune oophoritis is more than 90%; however, that of autoimmune orchitis is only 25–30% (Taguchi et al. 1980; Taguchi and Nishizuka 1981). This suggests that the testis or males are apparently resistant to autoimmune disease compared with the ovary or females. Moreover, neonatal thymectomy initially causes epididymo-vasitis during the postpubertal period before the induction of orchitis, and the incidence of orchitis remains considerably lower than that of the epididymo-vasitis, even in mature adult mice. Therefore, the testis is relatively resistant to neonatal thymectomy-induced autoimmunity among various affected organs in multiple organ-localized autoimmunities.

There are many studies on sexual dimorphism in autoimmunity (Rubtsova et al. 2015). In general, autoimmune diseases affect 5–7% of the population, and females are more susceptible to the diseases than males (Dragin et al. 2016). It is generally accepted that androgens exert suppressive effects on both humoral and cellular immunity and seem to represent natural anti-inflammatory hormones; in contrast, estrogens exert immune-enhancing activities (Cutolo et al. 2002). The autoimmune regulator (Aire) is a gene of which mutation causes multiple organ-localized autoimmune diseases (Chan and Anderson 2015). In thymi in men and mice, females expressed less expression of mRNA and protein of Aire than males after puberty. In mice, Aire expression is related to sexual hormones, as male castration decreased Aire thymic expression and estrogen receptor-alpha-deficient mice did not show a sex disparity for Aire expression (Dragin et al. 2016). Moreover, estrogen treatment resulted in down-regulation of Aire expression in the thymus. Therefore, estrogen induces epigenetic changes in the Aire gene in females, leading to reduced Aire expression under a threshold that increases female susceptibility to autoimmune diseases.

2.6.9 Resistance to Rejection of Transplanted Allogeneic and Xenogeneic Testis

Ectopically transplanted xenografts of testicular tissues under the kidney capsule or subderma of immunodeficient recipient animals resist rejection and survive for a long time (Bellgrau et al. 1995; Oatley et al. 2004, 2005; Rathi et al. 2005). Testicular tissue from immature donors survives better as xenograft than tissue from mature adult donors, and complete spermatogenesis can occur albeit with species-specific differences (Arreguli et al. 2008). Testis grafts derived from mice that can express functional Fas ligand survived indefinitely when transplanted under the kidney capsule of allogeneic mice, whereas testis grafts derived from mutant gld mice, which express nonfunctional ligand, were surely rejected (Bellgrau et al. 1995). Fas ligand expression in the testis probably acts by inducing apoptotic cell death of Fas-expressing recipient T cells activated in response to the graft antigens. Crucially, there is little evidence for extended survival of the epididymal allograft or xenograft. Although immune privilege exists in the testis, the epididymis is much more susceptible to loss of immune tolerance (Hedger 2011b). Therefore, the ectopically transplanted epididymal graft might not be long until its rejection.

2.6.10 Successful Transplantation of Allografts and Xenografts by Co-transplantation with Sertoli Cells

Rat islet beta-cell grafts were co-transplanted with or without murine Sertoli cells in diabetic mice. Graft survival time increased when xenografts were combined with Sertoli cells (Dufour et al. 2003, 2008; Mital et al. 2010). As anti-inflammatory factor, transforming growth factor-beta-1 derived from Sertoli cells is implicated in the protection of islet beta-cell grafts after co-transplantation with Sertoli cells.

2.6.11 Successful Transplantation of Xenogeneic Spermatogenesis into the Recipient Testis

It has been demonstrated that rat spermatogenesis can occur in the seminiferous tubules of congenitally immunodeficient recipient mice after transplantation of rat spermatogonia (Clouthier et al. 1996). Experimentally immunosuppressed adult mice were also used as recipients. In other studies, the successful use of normal infant rats as recipients of hamster spermatogonia was demonstrated for xenogeneic spermatogenesis (Tanaka et al. 1997). The success of transplanting hamster spermatogonia into the infant rats may be due to that the immune function of the infants was still immature, as seen in the immunodeficient or immunosuppressed state. Later, transplantation of rat spermatogonia into immunocompetent adult mice has also succeeded (Qu et al. 2012). By this experimental system, it appeared that transplanted rat spermatogonia could undergo complete spermatogenesis in normal immune system of the recipient mice (Hirayanagi et al. 2015). This indicates that xenogeneic germ cells can be immunologically sequestered and nourished by recipient's seminiferous tubules formed by Sertoli cells, basal lamina, and peritubular myoid cells.

2.6.12 Immune Tolerance Induced by Intratesticular Antigen Priming

In a study of experimental autoimmune uveoretinitis induced by soluble retinal antigens emulsified in CFA, it was reported that an injection of the retinal antigens into the rat testes prior to immunization for induction of the autoimmune uveoretinitis resulted in systemic tolerance and protects the animals from the disease induction (Li et al. 1997). Similar protection was also demonstrated in experimental allergic encephalomyelitis (Verajankorva et al. 2002). This phenomenon is called testicular-associated immune deviation, which is antigen specific and transferable to naïve recipients with spleen cells from the tolerized animals. This immunotolerance could be transferrable to syngeneic naïve rats by both $CD4^+$ Treg and $CD8^+$ Treg (Yotsukura et al. 1997). Further analyses revealed that IL-4 and IL-10 are important cytokines for the immunosuppressive effect of $CD4^+$ Treg, and transforming growth factor-beta is an important immunosuppressive cytokine for $CD8^+$ Treg. A striking feature of the tolerance is that orchiectomy within a few hours after treatment of the testis with the retinal antigens does not fully abrogate the systemic tolerance. The tolerance induction was not affected by injuring or removing the lymphatic vessels from the testis. These results indicate that, upon the intratesticular injection with retinal antigens, a signal for retinal antigen-specific tolerance is generated quickly and migrates in blood circulation from the testis to the spleen where Treg are produced. This signal does not seem to be the retinal antigen itself because intravenous injection of the antigen is not as effective as intratesticular injection to induce the tolerance. Increased expression of transforming growth factor-beta and Fas ligand in MHC-positive interstitial cells in the testis may play an important role in the generation of the tolerance induction signal.

2.7 Five-Phased Immunoregulatory Barriers in the Testis

As described above, testicular blood capillary endothelia may function as the first barrier for inhibition of extravasation of leukocytes. Leydig cells, testicular macrophages, lymphocytes, and other leukocytes may function as the second barrier protecting the testis from inflammatory cell responses by expression and/or secretion of various anti-inflammatory materials or by cell-cell contact. Thirdly, both peritubular myoid cells and basal lamina of the seminiferous tubules may inhibit invasion of autoreactive lymphocytes by cell-cell interaction. The classic BTB formed by inter-Sertoli cell junctions functions as the fourth barrier protecting autoimmunogenic TGC from attack by autoreactive lymphocytes. Furthermore, as described above, there is a possibility that autoimmunogenic TGC themselves bathed in the seminiferous tubular fluid also exert final inhibitory effects on proliferation and activation of infiltrating lymphocytes.

2.8 Immunological Fragility of the Testicular Microcircumstance

Although multiple mechanisms and factors, including the physical structure, the local and active immunosuppressive milieu, and the systemic immune tolerance, coordinate to regulate the testicular immune-privileged state, the privileged state could be easily overcome, resulting from immunological weakness in the testis.

2.8.1 Regional Differences in the Integrity of the Immunological Shield by the BTB

The BTB at the tubuli recti and the rete testis is less complete than at the seminiferous tubules and is regarded as a susceptible site for inflammatory cell infiltration (Itoh et al. 1998a; Naito et al. 2009). The seminiferous tubules connect the tubuli recti, which opens to the rete testis (Dym and Fawcett 1970; Dym 1973, 1976; Dym and Cavicchia 1978). Three-dimensional analysis showed that 14–16 tubuli recti appeared to be connected to the rete testis in the mouse (Takahashi et al. 2007). More recently, high-performance three-dimensional reconstruction software analysis revealed the presence of 28 connection points to the rete testis in the mouse (Nakata et al. 2015). In horseradish peroxidase-administered mice, blood-borne horseradish peroxidase infiltrated into the tubuli recti and rete testis but never into the seminiferous tubules (Itoh et al. 1998a). The tubuli recti epithelial cells, which are called modified Sertoli cells, formed protruding cytoplasmic strings and actively phagocytosed degenerating spermatozoa and germ cell remnants under normal conditions (Naito et al. 2009; Tainosho et al. 2011). In general, the phagocytosis of TGC remnants within the tubuli recti is regarded as the normal mechanism for the elimination of unwanted spermatozoa (Dym and Fawcett 1970; Dym and Cavicchia 1977). However, from an immunological aspect, it should also be emphasized that the tubuli recti contains many autoantigens of TGC. Therefore, if the tubuli recti epithelial cells excrete some autoantigens to the outside of the tubuli recti latently under normal condition, the immune cells could encounter these autoantigens there (Fig. 2.5). Actually, previous studies dealt with the antigen-presenting capability of testicular macrophages and Sertoli cells in mice (Kohno et al. 1983; Housseau et al. 1997). However, it appears that class II MHC antigen-bearing testicular macrophages but not Sertoli cells at the tubuli recti could present antigens to $CD4^+$ T cells. It has been demonstrated that not only the Sertoli cell junction but also the basal lamina and the peritubular myoid cells provide a selective filtration barrier. The basal lamina is developmentally formed by products of both Sertoli cells and the peritubular myoid cells. Sertoli cells of the seminiferous tubules had an almost flat and single-layered basal lamina. In contrast, the basal lamina of the modified Sertoli cells at the tubuli recti exhibited wavy and multilayered structures (Tainosho et al. 2011) (Fig. 2.3). In particular, at the middle segment of the tubuli recti, both the basal lamina and cell membrane of the modified Sertoli cells intimately interconnect with each other, similar to the sagittal suture in the human skull. This finding suggests that the modified Sertoli cells have a wide surface area at their base and therefore can effectively excrete or absorb various molecules. It may be that some TGC autoantigens are excreted into the wide gaps around the modified Sertoli cells in the normal state. Therefore, the presence of wide gaps between the modified Sertoli cells, basal lamina, and peritubular myoid cell layer at the tubuli recti might provide the microcircumstances in which lymphocytes and macrophages can easily penetrate into the tubuli recti. Furthermore, the macrophages surrounding the tubuli recti and rete testis can easily pick up the leaked autoantigens and present them to lymphocytes. At the tubuli recti, the modified Sertoli cells form a valve-like structure, and contraction of the peritubular myoid cells prevents the reflux of spermatozoa from the rete testis into the seminiferous tubules. A few thick myoid layers were piled around the middle and terminal segments of the tubuli recti (Tainosho et al. 2011). Therefore, the wavy and multilayered structures of the basal lamina may facilitate opening or closing of the valve-like structure of the tubuli recti. This implies that a significant amount of intratubular fluid (containing TGC autoantigens) at the tubuli recti might be effectively absorbed by the modified Sertoli cells.

2.8.2 Pro-inflammatory Cytokines in the Testis Under Normal Condition

Pro-inflammatory cytokines are produced within the testis even in the absence of inflammation or immune activation events. Pro-inflammatory cytokines including IL-1 and IL-6 have direct effect on TGC differentiation and testicular steroidogenesis (Hedger and Meinhardt 2003). IL-1 is involved in the paracrine stimulation of Leydig cell steroidogenesis, and, on the contrary, IL-6 has been suggested to induce persistent testicular resistance to luteinizing hormone action and/or suppress Leydig cell steroidogenesis (Bornstein et al. 2004). IL-1 is constitutively secreted from not only testicular macrophages but also both Sertoli cells and TGC (Huleihel et al. 2001). The levels of IL-1 were increased in Sertoli cells when stimulated with lipopolysaccharide. IL-6 is expressed by TGC at different stages of differentiation, Leydig cells, and peritubular myoid cells under normal state (Potashnik et al. 2005). Both IFN-gamma and TNF-alpha are normally secreted from Sertoli cells (Terayama et al. 2011). Monocyte chemotactic protein-1, which is involved in macrophage and lymphocyte chemoattraction, was found to be expressed by peritubular myoid cells (Aubry et al. 2000). The expression was markedly stimulated by IL-1, TNF-alpha, IFN-gamma, and lipopolysaccharide. Leydig cells also expressed monocyte chemotactic protein-1 when stimulated by IL-1. Therefore, it is concluded that the pro-inflammatory cytokines in the testis could be involved in the mobilization and migration of leukocytes, leading to testicular inflammation, when the testicular immune-privileged status becomes weak under some pathological condition.

2.8.3 Specific Localization of Immune Cells in the Testis Under Normal Condition

While the testis is a remarkable immune-privileged site, it is well connected to afferent lymph nodes. Therefore, the testis has most types of immune cells, including macrophages, lymphocytes, dendritic cells, granulocytes, and mast cells. Many macrophages that are positive with F4/80, pan-macrophage antigens, preferentially accumulate around the tubuli recti under normal condition in mice (Itoh et al. 1995b, 1998a). In particular, F4/80$^+$ macrophages expressing class II MHC antigens are very sparse in normal interstitium between the seminiferous tubules but form a cuff around the tubuli recti (Tung et al. 1987). To determine whether the specific accumulation of macrophages around the tubuli recti and rete testis is a congenital or acquired phenomenon, the distribution of testicular macrophages obtained from various aged mice was investigated (Li et al. 1998; Itoh et al. 1999b). Macrophages were homogenously distributed throughout the testicular interstitium with no specific accumulation until 2 weeks of age. However, between 3 and 4 weeks of age in the mouse, macrophages rapidly accumulated around the tubuli recti and rete testis. The density of macrophages at 4 weeks of age reached the level of the mature testes of 8-week-old mice (Fig. 2.8). Therefore, the characteristic accumulation of macrophages is an acquired phenomenon that is completed when spermatids start to differentiate in the seminiferous tubules. Therefore, the accumulation of macrophages around the tubuli recti coincides with the time of the first appearance of autoimmunogenic spermatids in the seminiferous tubules. In the tunica albuginea, some stretched- or irregular-shaped macrophages were concentrated in two regions: the inferior portion of the testis near the cauda epididymis and the upper portion adjacent to the rete testis and the tubuli recti (Fig. 2.4). These two portions are important routes for testicular lymphatic drainage from the inside to the outside of the testis. This preferential accumulation of macrophages at the tunica albuginea was also found to be an acquired phenomenon, starting and completing before puberty. It is not yet known what attracts many macrophages around the tubuli recti. It should be important to clarify whether the specific accumulation of testicular macrophages is due to the cell proliferation in situ or extravasation and arrival from the blood capillaries. In general, it is accepted that a primary function of macrophages is in the host defense system against exogenous agents, such as bacteria and viruses. Therefore, it should not be excluded that macrophages accumulate at the tubuli recti and the rete testis to protect the seminiferous epithelium from genital tract infections involving the prostates, vas deferens, and epididymis.

In contrast to the wide lumen of the rete testis, the tubuli recti lumen is occluded by tall epithelial cells called the modified Sertoli cells. They appear to form protruding cytoplasmic strings, which may serve as sensors, possibly touching the spermatozoa and monitoring their presence and antigenic expression. In addition to many macrophages in the testicular interstitium proper, a few macrophages and lymphocytes were

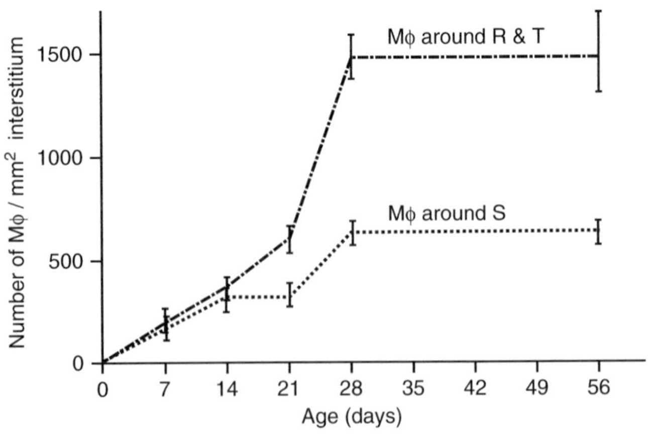

Fig. 2.8 Sequential changes in the density of F4/80-positive macrophages in the developing testes of the mouse. *Mφ* macrophages, *R & T* rete testis and tubuli recti, *S* seminiferous tubule

identified inside the tubuli recti but never inside the seminiferous tubules (Itoh et al. 1995b; Naito et al. 2008) (Fig. 2.4). A few cell bodies and many cell processes of the macrophages can be found in the lumen and wall of the tubuli recti in the mouse and the rabbit (Osman 1979; Itoh et al. 1995b, 1998a). The presence of phagocytosed spermatozoa within the modified Sertoli cells at the tubuli recti has been found in many species such as rat, rabbit, ram, goat, bull, and monkey (Sinowatz et al. 1979). Therefore, in the tubuli recti, a direct contact between immune cells and degradated TGC may be possible. Intratubular lymphocytes that are very close to both degradated TGC and their remnants could be occasionally found in the tubuli recti, rete testis, and epididymis, but not in the seminiferous tubules in mice and monkeys (Dym and Romrell 1975; Naito et al. 2008). Although the physiological function of these invading lymphocytes remains unknown, this microcircumstance provides a chance for evocation of autoimmune inflammation of the tubuli recti, rete testis, and epididymis under some pathological conditions. The appearance of lymphocytic infiltration around the tubuli recti was observed not only on immunological but also mechanical or chemical stimulations on the testis. In addition to the weak BTB at the tubuli recti and rete testis, the specific accumulation of many macrophages and occasional appearance of lymphocytes at the region might increase the chance of encountering testicular autoantigens.

2.8.4 Infiltration of Macrophages into the Testis in Secondary Biliary Cholestasis

Cholestasis can cause translocation of gut bacteria, endotoxemia, and systemic inflammation. The pathogenesis of hypogonadism in male patients with liver cirrhosis is complex and not well explained. In a rat biliary cholestasis model caused by common bile duct ligation, the magnitude of monocyte chemotactic protein-1 expression and $CD68^{+}$ macrophage infiltration within the testes was progressively upregulated along with increasing duration of common bile duct ligation (Shi et al. 2015a, b). In this model, testicular apoptosis was promoted with activation of mitophagy and autophagy.

2.8.5 Mononuclear Cell Responses to Primary Testicular Cancer

From the immunological point of view, an interesting finding is that inflammatory infiltrates are common in testicular seminomas (Lehmann et al. 1986; Lehmann and Muller 1987; Bart et al. 2002). Most of these cells consist of T cells, but whether T helper cells or cytotoxic T cells predominate is unclear. Furthermore, burnout lesions of primary testicular cancers have been described. In that case, patients had metachronous metastases of a testicular cancer, but only a scar is found in the testis instead of a primary tumor. This indicates that the testis permitted infiltration of lymphocytes with the resultant damage to the seminoma. These burnout lesions predominantly occur in disseminated seminoma and are rarely described in non-seminoma. The inflammatory T cell infiltrates can destroy the intratesticular tumor, which contradicts the opinion that cellular immune responses have less effect in the testis than in other tissues. A possible explanation could be that tumor expresses antigens that are foreign to the immune system or produce cytokines, thus inducing a cellular immune response, leading to an infiltration of lymphocytes.

Jahnukainen et al. (1995) evaluated the incidence of testicular mononuclear cell infiltrates in patients with carcinoma in situ and germ cell neoplasia. The results suggest that the incidence of mononuclear cell infiltration increases with increasing severity of testicular malignant changes. Moreover, the increased mononuclear cell infiltration is also evident in the contralateral testis where no malignant cells can be observed.

2.8.6 Frequent Involvement of Lymphocytic Leukemia in the Testis

Myelogenous, lymphocytic, and monocytic leukemia infiltration into the testis was confirmed at approximately 20% incidence, and a high-grade infiltration was most common in lymphocytic leukemia (Wakasa and Amano 1977). Blood capillaries were always increased in the area of dense infiltration of leukemic cells. Thin-walled canals located closely between the proper lamina of seminiferous tubules and the interstitial cell cluster were testicular lymphatics, which were extremely irregular in shape and occasionally did not have endothelium. Therefore, testicular lymphatics that are not a constant canal system but rather akin to narrow tissue space may allow lymphocytes to accumulate in the testis. Inhibition of testicular activity by estradiol treatment in rats that were injected intraperitoneally with rat T cell-leukemic lymphoblasts significantly decreased the proportion of the testis occupied by leukemic infiltrates (Jahnukainen et al. 1994). Daily treatment of pubertal rats with human chorionic gonadotropin did not have an effect on testicular leukemic infiltration (Jahnukainen et al. 1994). The proportion of the testis occupied by leukemic infiltrates was significantly higher in the abdominal testes of pubertal unilaterally cryptorchid rats than in the scrotal testes of leukemic control rats (Jahnukainen et al. 1994). In other experiments, it was found that mice inoculated by intramuscular route with lymphocytic leukemic cells recovered from the disseminated disease by cyclophosphamide, whereas mice inoculated by intratesticular route with the leukemic cells and then treated with cyclophosphamide died by the disseminated disease. This indicates that the testicular lymphatic sinusoidal system is equipped with a protected environment for leukemic cells against cyclophosphamide (Jackson et al. 1983).

2.8.7 Natural Autoantibodies to Testicular Antigens

It may be that some of the testicular autoantigens are physically released into the blood system and then encountered the immune system. Considering that TGC autoantigens are not immunologically sequestered but are linked to the immune system through the tubuli recti, the presence of natural autoantibodies against TGC autoantigens is possible under normal condition. Indeed, in enzyme-linked immunosorbent assay, titers of the autoantibodies in adult normal male mice were consistently higher than those in virgin normal female mice (Itoh et al. 1989). In rats, natural anti-sperm antibodies rose between 56 and 91 days of age and were significantly higher in 91- and 128-day-old rats than at earlier intervals (Flickinger et al. 1997). The rise in anti-sperm antibodies correlated temporally with events in the postnatal development of the male reproductive system. The increase in anti-sperm antibodies is most closely following the time when spermatozoa reach the epididymis and proximal vas deferens at approximately 56 days of age. The increased serum anti-sperm antibodies only after sexual maturation also suggest that some differentiation antigens of sperm are processed and presented the immune system under normal circumstances (Flickinger et al. 1997). However, there is a possibility that the titers detected by immunosorbent assay reflect not only amounts of anti-TGC antibodies but also nonspecific binding of immunoglobulin to Fc receptors on TGC (Sethi and Brandis 1980; Kamada et al. 1991). Autoantibodies to Sertoli cells were also detectable in healthy men (Hiyoshi et al. 1991). There is another possibility that antibodies against exogenous antigens such as ubiquitous microorganism cross-react with TGC and Sertoli cell antigens.

By using SDS-polyacrylamide gel electrophoresis and immunoblotting by reacting with the sera with normal murine testicular homogenates, two immunoreactive bands corresponding to approximately 45 and 100 kDa were definitely detected in normal sera, showing the biochemical presence of natural autoantibodies against these two testicular antigens (Qu et al. 2010; Musha et al. 2013). In rats, sera from normal postpubertal animals bound several testicular proteins, including bands of >100 kDa, 82–75 kDa, 78 kDa, 68 kDa, 65 kDa, 63 kDa, 54–55 kDa, 42 kDa, 37 kDa, 35 kDa, 26 kDa, and 20–22 kDa (Flickinger et al. 1997). The majority of these autoantibodies were sperm specific. Although this phenomenon is intriguing, at present, the true reason for the presence of the natural autoantibodies remains underdetermined. There is a possibility that the spermatogenic disturbance is easily induced by these natural autoantibodies under some particular conditions where the autoantibodies can be allowed to target TGC across the seminiferous tubular wall. On the contrary, these natural autoantibodies might protect the testis from its inflammation by means of action on some regulatory immune network. In spite of habitual ideas about immanently aggressive nature of any forms of autoimmunity, autoimmune phenomena involving natural autoantibodies are permanently present in any individual and may not always reflect the potentially self-destructive activity of the immune system (Poletaev 2014).

2.9 Relation Between Acquired (Adoptive) and Innate Immune Responses in the Testis

Historically, immunology emerged as a branch of applied microbiology in which a war against aliens is one of main subjects. Probably, one of the most important evolutionally archetypical functions of the immune system is "clearance," a prototype of the immune system eliminating viruses, bacteria, and fungi. However, it should be noted that the clearance of degenerated and dying self-cells is more critical for maintenance of the molecular homeodynamics of the whole body. Therefore, in the testis, clearance of both endogenous cells (apoptotic TGC) and exogenous cells (various microbes) contributes to normal spermatogenesis and testosterone production.

The testis possesses properties of both remarkable immune privilege and effective local innate immunity. Teleologically, testicular immune privilege protects immunogenic TGC from attack by self-immune system, and local innate immunity is important in preventing testicular microbial infections.

It is generally assumed that TGC sequestration by the BTB is important but not sufficient to protect TGC from inflammatory attack. The testicular interstitial space outside the BTB may also provide an immunosuppressive microcircumstance. The testicular interstitium in mice is resistant to rejection of allografts and also induction of vasculitis, lymphangitis, spermatic granuloma, and polymorphonuclear cell infiltration (Itoh et al. 2005). Lymphocyte response elicited was shown to be suppressed by proteins in fluids drained from the testicular interstitial space (Pollanen et al. 1988). Therefore, the testicular tissue outside the BTB is also protected from inflammatory cell infiltration, although many resident macrophages are normally present in the testis. Various testicular factors with the capacity to affect lymphocyte functions in vitro have been identified, although their physiological roles in vivo have not yet been fully evaluated. In local transplantation study, memory $CD8^{+}$T cells constitute a threat to the long-term survival of transplanted organs by mediating allograft rejection despite ongoing immunosuppression. However, $CD4^{+}CD25^{+}$ Treg play a key role in the maintenance of immunologic tolerance to both self and foreign antigens by suppressing aggressive T cell responses. Indeed, islet transplantation in the testis generates much less memory $CD8^{+}$ T cells but induces more antigen-specific $CD4^{+}CD25^{+}$ Treg than in a conventional site (Dai et al. 2005; Nasr et al. 2005). They may prevent allograft rejection and also prevent testicular autoimmunity. There is also a strong evidence for active immunoregulations by $CD4^{+}$ Treg on autoimmune response to testicular antigens (Teuscher et al. 1990; Itoh et al. 1992).

On the other hand, innate immunity for downregulation of infectious diseases has a capability to overcome the immune privilege. The testis can be infected by various microbial pathogens derived from the circulating blood or genitourinary tract. Testicular infection is followed by initiation of effective antimicrobial innate immune responses, in which the pattern recognition receptors are involved (Zhao et al. 2014). Several subfamilies of pattern recognition receptors have been identified, and TLRs are the best characterized pattern recognition receptors in the testis (Zhao et al. 2014). Thirteen TLR members have been found in mammals. The pattern recognition receptor-initiated innate responses would be important for testicular cells to overcome immune privilege and elicit an appropriate local response against pathogen invasion. In particular, testicular innate immunity is particularly critical when systemic immunity is reduced. Pattern recognition receptors can also be activated by endogenous autoantigens released from damaged tissues and necrotic cells, termed damaged-associated molecular patterns, for triggering endogenous inflammation. TLRs initiate the innate immune response in Sertoli cells by inducing immunoregulatory cytokines, including TNF-alpha, IL-1, IL-6, monocyte chemotactic protein-1, and type I IFNs (Zhao et al. 2014). Moreover, Leydig cells and TGC at different stages also express TLR. In *Chlamydia trachomatis* infection in the male genital tract such as the seminal vesicle, prostate, epididymis, and testis, chronic and mild inflammation often remains in most individuals (Mackern-Oberti et al. 2013). Recognition of chlamydial antigens is associated with TLR2 and TLR4, and *Chlamydia trachomatis* recognition by these TLR induces a local production of cytokines/chemokines, which, in turn, provoke chronic inflammation that might evolve in the onset of an autoimmune process. TAM receptors expressed on Sertoli cells are essential for phagocytic removal of apoptotic TGC, and the receptors expressed on macrophages, dendritic cells, and NK cells play critical roles in regulating innate immunity (Deng et al. 2016). It was found that TAM receptors negatively regulate TLR3 signaling in Sertoli cells. Actually, $TAM^{-/-}$-mutant mice exhibit an excessive activation of TLR3, resulting in the upregulation of inflammatory cytokines including IL-1-beta, IL-6, TNF alpha, and interferons alpha and beta (Sun et al. 2010).

In summary, testicular defense mechanisms have two aspects: protection of TGC autoantigens from detrimental immune response and counteraction of invading microbial pathogens in the testis. However, the latter may sometimes involve the chronic inflammation against resident bacteria or parasites, followed by autoimmune responses against testicular antigens.

References

Abe M, Kurosawa M, Ishikawa O, Miyachi Y, Kido H. Mast cell tryptase stimulates both human dermal fibroblast proliferation and type I collagen production. Clin Exp Allergy. 1998;28:1509–17.

Abe M, Kurosawa M, Ishikawa O, Miyachi Y. Effect of mast cell-derived mediators and mast cell-related neutral proteases on human dermal fibroblast proliferation and type I collagen production. J Allergy Clin Immunol. 2000;106:S78–84.

Aguilar R, Anton F, Bellido C, Aguilar E, Gaytan F. Testicular serotonin is related to mast cells but not Leydig cells in the rat. J Endocrinol. 1995;146:15–21.

Alexander NJ, Anderson DJ. Immunology of semen. Fertil Steril. 1987;47:192–205.

Anderson DJ, Tarter TH. Immunosuppressive effects of mouse seminal plasma components in vivo and in vitro. J Immunol. 1982;128:535–9.

Anton F, Morales C, Aguilar R, Bellido C, Aguilar E, Gaytan F. A comparative study of mast cells and eosinophils leukocytes in the mammalian testis. Zentbl Verterinarmed [A]. 1998;45:209–18.

Arreguli L, Rathi R, Zeng W, Honaranooz A, Gomendio M, Roldan ER, Dobrinski I. Xenografting of adult mammalian testis tissue. Anim Reprod Sci. 2008;106:65–76.

Aubry F, Habasque C, Satie AP, Jegou B, Samson M. Expression and regulation of the CC-chemokine monocyte chemoattractant protein-1 in the rat testicular cells in primary culture. Biol Reprod. 2000;62:1427–35.

Avallet O, Vigier M, Leduque P, Duois PM, Saez JM. Expression and regulation of transforming growth factors-beta 1 messenger ribonucleic acid and protein in cultured porcine Leydig and Sertoli cells. Endocrinology. 1994;134:2079–87.

Ball RY. Experimental production of spermatic granuloma in Balb/c mice. Andrologia. 1984;16:342–9.

Banchereau J, Steinman RM. Dendritic cells and the control of immunity. Nature. 1998;392:245–52.

Bart J, Groen JM, van der Graaf WTA, Hollema H, Hendrikse NH, Vaalburg W, Sleijfer DT, de Vries EGE. An oncological view on the blood-testis barrier. Lancet Oncol. 2002;3:357–63.

Bellgrau D, Selawry HP. Cyclosporine-induced tolerance to intratesticular islet xenografts. Transplantation. 1990;50:654–7.

Bellgrau D, Gold D, Selawry H, Moore J, Franzsoff A, Duke RC. A role of CD95 ligand in preventing graft rejection. Nature. 1995;377:630–2.

Bergh A, Rooth P, Widmark A, Damber JE. Treatment of rats with hCG induces inflammation-like changes in the testicular microcirculation. J Reprod Fertil. 1987;79:135–43.

Bergh A, Damber JE, van Rooijen N. The human chorionic gonadotrophin-induced inflammation-like response is enhanced in macrophage-depleted rat testes. J Endocrinol. 1993;136:415–20.

Bhushan S, Tchatalbachev S, Klug J, Fijak M, Pineau C, CHakraborty T, Meinhardt A. Uropathogenic *Escherichia coli* block MyD88-dependent and activate MyD88-independent signaling pathways in rat testicular cells. J Immunol. 2008;180:5537–47.

Bhushan S, Hossain H, Lu Y, Geisler A, Tchatalbachev S, Mikuiski Z, Schuler G, Klug J, Pilatz A, Wagenlehner F, Chakraborty T, Meinhardt A. Uropathogenic *E. coli* induce different immune response in testicular and peritoneal macrophages: implications for testicular immune privilege. PLoS One. 2011;6:e28452.

Born W, Wekerle H. Selective, immunologically nonspecific adherence of lymphoid and myeloid cells to Leydig cells. Eur J Cell Biol. 1981;25:76–81.

Born W, Wekerle H. Leydig cells nonspecifically suppress lymphoproliferation in vitro: Implications for the testis as an immunologically privileged site. Am J Reprod Immunol. 1982;2:291–5.

Bornstein SR, Rutkowski H, Vrezas I. Cytokines and steroidogenesis. Mol Cell Endocrinol. 2004;215:135–41.

Bryniarski K, Szczepanik M, Maresz K, Ptak M, Ptak W. Subpopulations of mouse testicular macrophages and their immunoregulatory function. Am J Reprod Immunol. 2004;52:27–35.

Bronson R. Biology of the male reproductive tract: its cellular and morphological considerations. Am J Reprod Immunol. 2010;65:212–9.

Campese AF, Graziolo P, de Cesaris P, RIcciolo A, Bellavia D, Pelullo M, Padula F, Noce C, Verkhovskaia S, Filippini A, Latella G, Screpanti I, Ziparo E, Starace D. Mouse Sertoli cells sustain de novo generation of regulatory T cells by triggering the notch pathway through soluble JAGGED1. Biol Reprod. 2014;90:53. doi:10.1095/biolreprod.113.113803.

Chan AY, Anderson MS. Central tolerance to self revealed by the autoimmune regulator. Ann N Y Acad Sci. 2015;1356:80–9.

Chen Q, Zhu W, Liu Z, Yan K, Zhao S, Han D. Toll-like receptor 11-initiated innate immune response in male mouse germ cells. Biol Reprod. 2014;90:38. doi:10.1095/biolreprod.113.114421.

Cheng X, Dai H, Wan N, Moore Y, Vankayalapati R, Dai Z. Interaction of programmed death 1 and programmed death-1 ligand-1 contributes to testicular immune privilege. Transplantation. 2009;87:1778–86.

Clark AM, Garland KK, Russell LD. Desert hedgehog (Dhh) gene is required in the mouse testis for formation of adult–type Leydig cells and normal development of peritubular cells and seminiferous tubules. Biol Reprod. 2000;63:1825–38.

Clouthier D, Avarbock M, Maika S, Hammer RE, Brinster RL. Rat spermatogenesis in mouse testis. Nature. 1996;381:418–21.

Colafrancesco S, Perricone C, Priori R, Valesini G, Shoenfeld Y. Sjogren's syndrome: another facet of the autoimmune/inflammatory syndrome induced by adjuvants (ASIA). J Autoimmun. 2014;51:10–6.

Cruz-Tapias P, Agmon-Levin N, Israeli E, Anaya JM, Shoenfeld Y. Autoimmune (auto-inflammatory) syndrome induced by adjuvants (ASIA)—animal models as a proof of concept. Curr Med Chem. 2013;20:4030–6.

Cutolo M, Seriolo B, VIllaggio B, Pizzorni C, Craviotto C, Sulli A. Androgens and estrogens modulate the immune and inflammatory response in rheumatoid arthritis. Ann N Y Acad Sci. 2002;966:131–42.

Cutolo M, Sulli A, Capellino S, Villaggio B, Montagna P, Seriolo B, Straub RH. Sex hormones influence on the immune system: basic and clinical aspects in autoimmunity. Lupus. 2004;13:635–8.

D'Abrizio P, Baldini E, Russo PF, Biordi L, Graziano FM, Rucci N, Properzi G, Francavilla S, Ulissie S. Ontogenesis and cell specific localization of Fas ligand expression in the rat testis. Int J Androl. 2004;27:304–10.

Dai Z, Nasr IW, Reel M, Deng S, Diggs L, Larsen CP, Rothstein DM, Lakkis FG. Impaired recall of CD8 memory T cells in an immunologically privileged tissue. J Immunol. 2005;174:1165–70.

D'Alessio A, Riccioli A, Lauretti P, Padula F, Muciaccia B, De Cesaris P, FIlippin A, Nagata S, Ziparo E. Testicular Fas ligand is expressed by sperm cells. Proc Natl Acad Sci U S A. 2001;98:3316–21.

Dal Secco V, Riccioli A, Padula F, ZIparo E, FIlippini A. Mouse Sertoli cells display phenotypical and functional traits of antigen-presenting cells in response to interferon gamma. Biol Reprod. 2008;78:234–42.

De SK, Chen HL, Pace JL, Hunt JS, Terranova PF, Enders GC. Expression of tumor necrosis factor-alpha in mouse spermatogenic cells. Endocrinology. 1993;133:389–96.

De Cesaris P, Filippin A, Cervelli C, Riccioli A, Muci S, Starace G, Stefanini M, Ziparo E. Immunosuppressive molecules produced by Sertoli cells cultured in vitro: biological effects on lymphocytes. Biochem Biophys Res Commun. 1992;186:1639–46.

Dechelotte P, Chassangne J, Labbe A, Afane M, Scheye T, de Leguillaumi B, Boucher D. Ultrastructural and immunohistochemical evidence of in situ differentiation of mononuclear phagocyte system in the interstitium of human fetal testis. Early Hum Dev. 1989;20:25–36.

Dejucq N, Dugast I, Ruffault A, van der Meide PH, Jegou B. Interferon-alpha and –gamma expression in the rat testis. Endocrinology. 1995;136:4925–31.

Dejucq N, Lienard MO, Guillaume E, Dorval I, Jegou B. Expression of interferons-alpha and -gamma in testicular interstitial tissue and spermatogonia of the rat. Endocrinology. 1998;139:3081–7.

De Rose R, Fernandez CS, Hedger MP, Kent SJ, Winnall WR. Characterization of macaque testicular leukocyte populations and T lymphocyte immunity. J Reprod Immunol. 2013;100:146–56.

Deng T, Chen Q, Han D. The role of TAM receptor tyrosine kinases in the mammalian testis and immunoprivileged sites. Front Biosci. 2016;21:316–27.

Dragin N, Bismuth J, Cizeron-Clairac G, Biferi MG, Berthault C, Serraf A, Nottin R, Klatzmann D, Cumano A, Barkats M, Le Panse R, Berrih-Aknin S. Estrogen-mediated downregulation of AIRE influences sexual dimorphism in autoimmune diseases. J Clin Invest. 2016;126:1525–37.

Dufour JM, Rajotte RV, Kin T, Korbutt GS. Immunoprotection of rat islet xenografts by cotransplantation with Sertoli cells and a single injection of antilymphocytic serum. Transplantation. 2003;75:1594–6.

Dufour JM, Lord SJ, Kin T, Rayat GR, Dixon DE, Bleackley RC, Korbutt GC, Rajotte RV. Comparison of successful and unsuccessful islet/Sertoli cell cotransplant grafts in streptozotocin-induced diabetic mice. Cell Transplant. 2008;16:1029–38.

Dym M, Fawcett DW. The blood-testis barrier in the rat and the physiological compartmentation of the seminiferous epithelium. Biol Reprod. 1970;3:308–26.

Dym M. The fine structure of the monkey (Macaca) Sertoli cell and its role in maintaining the blood-testis barrier. Anat Rec. 1973;175:639–56.

Dym M, Romrell LJ. Intraepithelial lymphocytes in the male reproductive tract of rats and rhesus monkeys. J Reprod Fertil. 1975;42:1–7.

Dym M. The mammalian rete testis—a morphological examination. Anat Rec. 1976;186:493–523.

Dym M, Cavicchia JC. Further observations on the blood-testis barrier in monkeys. Biol Reprod. 1977;17:390–403.

Dym M, Cavicchia JC. Functional morphology of the testis. Biol Reprod. 1978;18:1–15.

Fillipini A, Ricciolo A, Padula F, Lauretti P, D'Alessio A, de Cesaris P, Gandini L, Lenzi A, Ziparo E. Immunology and immunopathology of the male genital tract. Control and impairment of immune privilege in the testis and in semen. Hum Reprod Update. 2001;7:444–9.

Fijak M, Meinhardt A. The testis in immune privilege. Immunol Rev. 2006;213:66–81.

Fijak M, Schneider E, Klug J, Bhushan S, Hackstein H, Schuler G, Wygrecka M, Gromoll J, Meinhardt A. Testosterone Replacement Effectively Inhibits the Development of Experimental

Autoimmune Orchitis in Rats: Evidence for a Direct Role of Testosterone on Regulatory T Cell Expansion. The Journal of Immunology. 2011;186(9):5162–5172.
Fijak M, Damm LJ, Wenzel JP, Aslani F, Walecki M, Wahle E, Eisel F, Bhushan S, Hackstein H, Baal N, Shuler G, Konrad L, Rafiq A, O'Hara L, Smith LB, Meinhardt A. Influence of testosterone on inflammatory response in testicular cells and expression of transcription factor Foxp3 in T cells. Am J Reprod Immunol. 2015;74:12–25. doi:10.1111/aji.12363.
Flickinger CJ, Howards SS, Baran ML, Pessoa N, Herr JC. Appearance of 'natural' antisperm autoantibodies after sexual maturation of normal Lewis rats. J Reprod Immunol. 1997;33:127–45.
Foulds LM, Boysen RI, Crane M, Yang Y, Muir JA, Smith AI, De Kretser DM, Hearn MT, Hedger MP. Molecular identification of lysoglycerophosphocholines as endogenous immunosuppressives in bovine and rat gonadal fluids. Biol Reprod. 2008;79:525–36.
Francavilla S, D'abrizio P, Rucci N, Silvano G, Properzi G, Straface E, Cordeschi G, Necozione S, Gnessi L, Arizzi M, Ulisse S. Fas and Fas ligand expression in fetal and adult human testis with normal or deranged spermatogenesis. J Clin Endocrinol Metab. 2000;85:2692–700.
Fujita Y, Mihara T, Okazaki T, Shitanaka M, Kushino R, Ikeda C, Negishi H, Liu Z, Richards JS, Shimada M. Toll-like receptors (TLR) 2 and 4 on human sperm recognize bacterial endotoxins and mediate apoptosis. Hum Reprod. 2011;26:2799–806.
Gaytan F, Carrera G, Pinilla L, Aquilar R, Bellodo C. Mast cells in the testis, epididymis and accessory glands of the rat: effects of neonatal steroid treatment. J Androl. 1989;10:351–8.
Gaytan F, Aceitero J, Lucena C, Aguilar E, Pinilla L, Garnelo P, Bellido C. Simultaneous proliferation and differentiation of mast cells and Leydig cells in the rat testis. Are common regulatory factors involved? J Androl. 1992;13:387–97.
Gold SM, Voskuhl RR. Estrogen and testosterone therapies in multiple sclerosis. Prog Brain Res. 2009;175:239–51.
Griswold MD, Roberts K, Bishop P. Purification and characterization of a sulfated glycoprotein secreted by Sertoli cells. Biochemistry. 1986;25:7265–70.
Hamasaki M, Kumabe T. Three-dimensional structure of two different lymphatic spaces in rat testis, and the route of flow fluxes of their lymphatic fluids. Kaibogaku Zasshi. 1994;69:669–83.
Hatakeyama S. A study on the interstitial cells of the human testis, especially on their fine-structural pathology. Acta Pathol Jpn. 1965;15:155–96.
Haugen TB, Landmark BF, Josefsen GM, Hansson V, Hogset A. The mature form of interleukin-1 alpha is constitutively expressed in immature male germ cells from rat. Mol Cell Endocrinol. 1994;105:R19–23.
Head JR, Billingham RE. Immune privilege in the testis. I. Basic parameters of allograft survival. Transplantation. 1983;36:423–31.
Head JR, Billingham RE. Immune privilege in the testis. II. Evaluation of potential local factors. Transplantation. 1985;40:269–75.
Head JR, Neaves WB, Billingham RE. Reconsideration of the lymphatic drainage of the rat testis. Transplantation. 1990;35:91–5.
Hedger MP, Drummond AE, Robertson DM, Risbridger GP, de Kretser DM. Inhibin and activin regulate 3H-thymidine uptake by rat thymocytes and 3T3 cells in vitro. Mol Cell Endocrinol. 1989;61:133–8.
Hedger MP, Wang J, Lan HY, Atkins RC, Wreford NG. Immunoregulatory activity in adult rat testicular interstitial fluid: relationship with intratesticular $CD8^+$ lymphocytes following treatment with ethane dimethane sulfonate and testosterone implants. Biol Reprod. 1998;58:935–42.
Hedger MP, Meinhardt A. Local regulation of T cell numbers and lymphocyte-inhibiting activity in the interstitial tissue of the adult rat testis. J Reprod Immunol. 2000;48:69–80.
Hedger MP, Meinhardt A. Cytokines and the immune-testicular axis. J Reprod Immunol. 2003;58:1–26.
Hedger MP. Toll-like receptors and signaling in spermatogenesis and testicular responses to inflammation-a perspective. J Reprod Immunol. 2011a;88:130–41.
Hedger MP. Immunophysiology and pathology of inflammation in the testis and epididymis. J Androl. 2011b;32:625–40.
Hinton BT, Palladino MA. Epididymal epithelium: its contribution to the formation of a luminal fluid microenvironment. Microsc Res Tech. 1995;30:67–81.

Hirai S, Naito M, Terayama H, Qu N, Miura M, Shirakami G, Itoh M. Differences in abundance of blood and lymphatic capillaries in the murine epididymis. Med Mol Morphol. 2010;43:37–42.

Hirai S, Naito M, Terayama H, Qu N, Kuerban M, Musha M, Ikeda A, Miura M, Itoh M. The origin of lymphatic capillaries in murine testes. J Androl. 2012;33:745–51.

Hirayanagi Y, Qu N, Hirai S, Naito M, Terayama H, Hayashi S, Hatakeyama N, Kuramasu M, Ogawa Y, Itoh M. Busulfan pretreatment for transplantation of rat spermatogonia differentially affects immune and reproductive systems in male recipient mice. Anat Sci Int. 2015;90:264–74.

Hiyoshi T, Eishi Y, Hatakeyama S. Human autoantibody to Sertoli cells detected in healthy individuals. Acta Pathol Jpn. 1991;41:879–87.

Housseau F, Rouas-Freiss N, Roy M, Bidart JM. Antigen-presenting function of murine gonadal epithelial cell lines. Cell Immunol. 1997;177:93–101.

Hume DA, Halpin D, Charlton H, Gordon S. The mononuclear phagocyte system of the mouse defined by immunohistochemical localization of antigen F4/80: macrophages of endocrine organs. Proc Natl Acad Sci U S A. 1984;81:4174–7.

Huleihel M, Zeyse D, Lunenfeld E, Beck M, Prinsloo I, Potashnik G, Mazor M. Immunohistochemical staining of IL-1 alpha and IL-1 receptor antagonist but not IL-1 beta in cultures of Sertoli cells. Am J Reprod Immunol. 2001;45:135–41.

Hurtenbach U, Morgenstern F, Bennett D. Induction of tolerance in vitro by autologous murine testicular cells. J Exp Med. 1980;151:827–38.

Hurtenbach U, Shearer GM. Germ cell-induced immune suppression in mice. Effect of inoculation of syngeneic spermatozoa on cell-mediated immune responses. J Exp Med. 1982;155:1719–29.

Hutson JC. Changes in the concentration and size of testicular macrophages during development. Biol Reprod. 1990;43:885–90.

Hutson JC. Development of cytoplasmic digitations between Leydig cells and testicular macrophages of the rat. Cell Tissue Res. 1992;267:385–9.

Ike A, Tokuhiro K, Hirose M, Nozaki M, Nishimune Y, Tanaka H. Comprehensive analysis of gene expression in testes producing haploid germ cells using DNA microarray analysis. Int J Androl. 2007;30:462–75.

Itoh M, Hiramine C, Koseto M, Hojo K. Enzyme-linked immunosorbent assay (ELISA) for detecting antisperm antibodies in mice with testicular autoimmunity. Am J Reprod Immunol. 1989;21:9–15.

Itoh M, Hiramine C, Tokunaga Y, Mukasa A, Hojo K. A new murine model of autoimmune orchitis induced by immunization with viable syngeneic testicular germ cells alone. II. Immunohistochemical findings of fully-developed lesion. Autoimmunity. 1991;10:89–97.

Itoh M, Mukasa A, Tokunaga Y, Hiramine C, Hojo K. Suppression of efferent limb of testicular autoimmune response by a regulatory CD4+ T cell line in mice. Clin Exp Immunol. 1992;87:455–60.

Itoh M, Miyake M, Miki T, Takeuchi Y, de Rooij DG. Immunohistological localization of autoantigens detected by serum autoantibodies from mice with experimental autoimmune orchitis without using adjuvants. Arch Androl. 1994;32:45–52.

Itoh M, Chen XA, Takeuchi Y, Miki T. Morphological demonstration of the immune privilege in the testis using adjuvants: Tissue responses of male reproductive organs in mice injected with Bordetella pertussigens. Arch Histol Cytol. 1995a;58:575–9.

Itoh M, de-Rooij DG, Jansen A, Drexhage HA. Phenotypical heterogeneity of testicular macrophages/dendritic cells in normal adult mice; an immunohistochemical study. J Reprod Immunol. 1995b;28:217–32.

Itoh M, Ueno M, Li XQ, Satriotomo I, Takeuchi Y. Topographical uptake of blood-borne horseradish peroxidase (HRP) in the murine testis at the light microscopic level. Int J Androl. 1998a;21:74–80.

Itoh M, Moriyama H, Yano A, Li XQ, Takeuchi Y. Mode of migration of normal lymphocytes inside murine testis. Anat Rec. 1998b;251:152–60.

Itoh M, Li XQ, Yano A, Xie Q, Takeuchi Y. Patterns of efferent lymphatics of the mouse testis. Int J Androl. 1998c;19:466–72.

Itoh M, Xie Q, Miyamoto K, Takeuchi Y. Major differences between the testis and epididymis in the induction of granulomas in response to extravasated germ cells. I. A light microscopical study in mice. Int J Androl. 1999a;22:316–23.

Itoh M, Xie Q, Miyamoto K, Takeuchi Y. F4/80-positive cells rapidly accumulate around tubuli recti and rete testis between 3 and 4 weeks of age in the mouse: an immunohistochemical study. Am J Reprod Immunol. 1999b;42:321–6.

Itoh M, Miyamoto K, Ooga T, Takeuchi Y. Spontaneous occurrence of vasculitis-like lesions on male reproductive tissues in mice. a histological study. Arch Androl. 1999c;42:151–9.

Itoh M, Miyamoto K, Satriotomo I, Takeuchi Y. Spermatic granuloma are experimentally induced in epididymides of mice receiving high-dose testosterone implants. I. a light-microscopical study. Int J Androl. 1999d;20:551–8.

Itoh M, Miyamoto K, Ooga T, Iwahashi K, Takeuchi Y. Spontaneous accumulation of eosinophils and macrophages throughout the stroma of the epididymis and vas deferens in alymphoplasia (aly) mutant mice: I. a histological study. Am J Reprod Immunol. 1999e;42:246–53.

Itoh M, Terayama H, Naito M, Ogawa Y, Tainosho S. Tissue microcircumstances for leukocytic infiltration into the testis and epididymis in mice. J Reprod Immunol. 2005;67:57–67.

Jackson H, Bock M, Jackson NC, Lendon M. The testis. A protected environment for leukaemic cells against cyclophosphamide in a mouse model. Cancer Chemother Pharmacol. 1983;11:200–2.

Jacobo P, Guazzone VA, Jarazo-Dietrich S, Theas MS, Lustig L. Differential changes in $CD4^+$ and $CD8^+$ effector and regulatory T lymphocyte subsets in the testis of rats undergoing autoimmune orchitis. J Reprod Immunol. 2009;81:44–54.

Jahnukainen K, Saari T, Morris ID, Salmi TT, Pollanen P. Regulation of testicular infiltration in acute lymphoblastic leukemia of the rat. Leukemia. 1994;8:458–64.

Jahnukainen K, Jorgensen N, Pollanen P, Giwercman A, Skakebaek NE. Incidence of testicular mononuclear cell infiltrates in normal human males and in patients with germ cell neoplasia. Int J Androl. 1995;18:313–20.

Jarow JP, Wright WW, Brown TR, Yan X, Zirkin BR. Bioactivity of androgens within the testes and serum of normal men. J Androl. 2005;26:343–8.

Jenne DE, Tschopp J. Molecular structure and functional characterization of a human complement cytolysis inhibitor found in blood and seminal plasma: identity to sulfated glycoprotein 2, a constituent of rat testis fluid. Proc Natl Acad Sci U S A. 1989;86:7123–7.

Kamada M, Liang Z, Koide SS. Identification of IgG and Fc-binding proteins in human seminal plasma and sperm. Arch Androl. 1991;27:1–7.

Keir ME, Liang SC, Guleria I, Latchman YE, Qipo A, Albacker LA, Koulmanda M, Freeman GJ, Sayegh MH, Sharpe AH. Tissue expression of PD-L1 mediated peripheral T cell tolerance. J Exp Med. 2006;203:883–95.

Kohno S, Ziparo E, Marek LF, Yung KS. Murine Sertoli cells: major histocompatibility antigens and glycoconjugates. J Reprod Immunol. 1983;5:339–50.

Koji T, Hishikawa Y, Ando H, Nakanishi Y, Kobayashi N. Expression of Fas and Fas ligand in normal and ischemia-reperfusion testes: involvement of the Fas system in the induction of germ cell apoptosis in the damaged mouse testis. Biol Reprod. 2001;64:946–54.

Koji T. Male germ cell death in mouse testes: possible involvement of Fas and Fas ligand. Med Electron Microsc. 2001;34:213–22.

Korbutt GS, Elliott JF, Rajotte RV. Cotransplantation of allogeneic islets with allogeneic testicular cell aggregates allows long-term graft survival without systemic immunosuppression. Diabetes. 1997;46:317–22.

Kotani M, Seiki K, Hattori M. Retardation of spermatogenesis and testosterone secretion after ligature of lymphatics draining the testes of rabbits. Endocrinol Jpn. 1974;21:1–8.

Law GL, Griswold MD. Activity and form of sulfated glycoprotein 2 (clusterin) from cultured Sertoli cells, testis, and epididymis of the rat. Biol Reprod. 1994;50:669–79.

Lee W, Mason AJ, Schwall R, Szonyi E, Mather JP. Secretion of activin by interstitial cells in the testis. Science. 1989;243:396–8.

Lehmann D, Temminck B, Litmanen K, Leibundgut B, Hadziselimovic F, Muller HJ. Autoimmune phenomena and cytogenetic findings in a patient with carcinoma (seminoma) In situ. Cancer. 1986;58:2013–7.

Lehmann D, Muller H. Analysis of the autoimmune response in an 'in situ' carcinoma of the testis. Int J Androl. 1987;10:163–8.
Li H, Ren J, Dhabuwata CD, Shichi H. Immunotolerance induced by intratesticular antigen priming: expression of TGF-beta, Fas and Fas ligand. Ocul Immunol Inflamm. 1997;5:75–84.
Li N, Wang T, Han D. Structural, cellular and molecular aspects of immune privilege in the testis. Front Immunol. 2012;3:1–12.
Li XQ, Itoh M, Yano A, Xie Q, Miyamoto K, Takeuchi Y. Immunohistochemical detection of testicular macrophages during the period of postnatal maturation in the mouse. Int J Androl. 1998;21:370–6.
Liu MS, Aebersold R, Fann CH, Lee CY. Molecular and developmental studies of a sperm acrosome antigen recognized by HS-63 monoclonal antibody. Biol Reprod. 1992;46:937–48.
Lombard-Vignon N, Grizard G, Boucher D. Influence of rat testicular macrophages on Leydig cell function in vitro. Int J Androl. 1992;15:144–59.
Loyo E, Jara LJ, Lopez PD, Puig AC. Autoimmunity in connection with a metal implant: a case of autoimmune/autoinflammatory syndrome induced by adjuvants. Auto Immun Highlights. 2012;4:33–8.
Lujan L, Perez M, Salazar E, Alvarez N, GImeno M, Pincrowski P, Irusta S, Santamaria J, Insausti N, Cortes Y, Figueras L, Cuartielles I, Vila M, Fantova E, Chapulle JL. Autoimmune/autoinflammatory syndrome induced by adjuvants (ASIA syndrome) in commercial sheep. Immunol Res. 2013;56:317–24.
Lyons RC, Petre JH, Lee CN. Spermatic granuloma of the epididymis. J Urol. 1967;97:320–3.
Mackern-Oberti JP, Motrich RD, Breser ML, Sanchez LR, Cuffini C, Rivero VE. Chlamydia trachomatis infection of the male genital tract: an update. J Reprod Immunol. 2013;100:37–53.
McCabe MJ, Tarulli GA, Meachem SJ, Robertson DM, Smooker PM, Stanton PG. Gonadotropins regulate rat testicular tight junctions in vivo. Endocrinology. 2010;151:2911–22.
McCabe MJ, Allan CM, Foo CF, Nicholls PK, McTavish KJ, Stanton PG. Androgen initiates Sertoli cell tight junction formation in the hypogonadal (hpg) mouse. Biol Reprod. 2012;87:38. doi:10.1095/biolreprod.111.094318.
McCabe MJ, Tarulli GA, Laven-Law G, Matthiesson KL, Meachem SJ, McLachlan RI, Dinger ME, Stanton PG. Gonadotropin suppression in men leads to a reduction in claudin-11 at the Sertoli cell tight junction. Hum Reprod. 2016;31:875–86.
Mayerhofer A. Human testicular peritubular cells: more than meets the eye. Reproduction. 2013;145:107–16.
Meinhardt A, Hedger MP. Immunological, paracrine and endocrine aspects of testicular immune privilege. Mol Cell Endocrinol. 2011;335:60–8.
Melaine N, Ruffault A, Dejucq-Rainsford N, Jegou B. Experimental inoculation of the adult rat testis with Sendai virus: effect on testicular morphology and leukocyte population. Hum Reprod. 2003;18:1574–9.
Meng J, Holdcraft RW, Shima JE, Griswold MD, Braun RE. Androgens regulate the permeability of the blood-testis barrier. Proc Natl Acad Sci U S A. 2005;102:16696–700.
Meng J, Greenlee AR, Taub CJ, Braun RE. Sertoli cell-specific deletion of the androgen receptor compromises testicular immune privilege in mice. Biol Reprod. 2011;85:254–60.
Mital P, Kaur G, Dufour JM. Immunoprotective Sertoli cells: making allogeneic and xenogeneic transplantation feasible. Reproduction. 2010;139:495–504.
Miyaso H, Naito M, Hirai S, Matsuno Y, Komiyama M, Itoh M, Mori C. Neonatal exposure to diethylstilbestrol causes granulomatous orchitis via epididymal inflammation. Anat Sci Int. 2014;89:215–23.
Mruk DD, Yan Cheng C. The mammalian blood-testis barrier: its biology and regulation. Endocr Rev. 2015;36:564–91.
Muller R, Klug J, Rodewald M, Meinhardt A. Macrophage migration inhibitory factor suppresses transforming growth factor-beta2 secretion in cultured rat testicular peritubular cells. Reprod Fertil Dev. 2005;17:435–8.

Musha M, Hirai S, naito M, Terayama H, Qu N, Hatayama N, Itoh M. The effects of adjuvants on autoimmune responses against testicular antigens in mice. J Reprod Dev. 2013;59:139–44.
Naito M, Terayama H, Hirai S, Qu N, Moriyama H, Itoh M. The presence of intra-tubular lymphocytes in normal testis of the mouse. Okajimas Folia Anat Jpn. 2008;85:91–6.
Naito M, Itoh M. Patterns of infiltration of lymphocytes into the testis under normal and pathological conditions in mice. Am J Reprod Immunol. 2008;59:55–61.
Naito M, Terayama H, Hirai S, Qu N, Kawata S, Itoh M. Histopathology of the tubuli recti at the start of experimental autoimmune orchitis in mice. Med Mo Morphol. 2009;42:230–5.
Naito M, Hirai S, Terayama H, Qu N, Hayashi S, Hatayama N, Kawamura H, Nakano T, Itoh M. Neonatal estrogen treatment with beta-estradiol 17-cypionate induces in post-pubertal mice inflammation in the ductuli efferentes, epididymis and vas deferens, but not in the testis, provoking obstructive azoospermia. Med Mol Morphol. 2014;47:21–30.
Nakata H, Wakayama T, Sonomura T, Honma S, Hatta T, Iseki S. Three-dimensional structure of seminiferous tubules in the adult mouse. J Anat. 2015;227:686–94.
Nasr IW, Wang Y, Gao G, Deng S, Diggs L, Rothstein DM, Tellides G, Lakkis FG, Dai Z. Testicular immune privilege promotes transplantation tolerance by altering the balance between memory and regulatory T cells. J Immunol. 2005;174:6161–8.
Nistal M, Santamaria L, Paniagua R. Mast cells in the human testis and epididymis from birth to adulthood. Acta Anat. 1984;119:155–60.
Nistal M, Santamaria L, Paniagua R, Regadera J. Changes in the connective tissue and decrease in the number of mast cells in the testes of men with alcoholic and non-alcoholic cirrhosis. Acta Morphol Hung. 1986;34:107–15.
Nistal M, Mate A, Paniagua R. Granulomatous epididymal lesion of possible ischemic origin. Am J Surg Pathol. 1997;21:951–6.
Oatley JM, de Avila DM, Reeves JJ, McLean DJ. Spermatogenesis and germ cell transgene expression in xenografted bovine testicular tissue. Biol Reprod. 2004;71:494–501.
Oatley JM, Reeves JJ, McLean DJ. Establishment of spermatogenesis in neonatal bovine testicular tissue following ectopic xenografting varies with donor age. Biol Reprod. 2005;72:358–64.
O'Bryan MK, Gerdprasert O, Nikolic-Paterson DJ, Meinhardt A, Muir JA, Foulds LM, Phillips DJ, de Kretser DM, Hedger MP. Cytokine profiles in the testes of rats treated with lipopolysaccharide reveal localized suppression of inflammatory responses. Am J Phys Regul Integr Comp Phys. 2005;288:R1744–55.
Ogawa Y, Itoh M, Hirai S, Suna S, Naito M, Qu N, Terayama H, Ikeda A, Miyaso H, Matsuno Y, Komiyama M, Mori C. Cadmium exposure increases susceptibility to testicular autoimmunity in mice. J Appl Toxicol. 2012;33:652–60.
Osman DI. A comparative ultrastructural study on typical and modified Sertoli cells before and after ligation of the efferent ductules in the rabbit. Zbl Vet Med C Anat Histo Embryo. 1979;8:114–23.
Phillips DJ, de Kretser DM, Hedger MP. Activin and related proteins in inflammation: not just interested bystanders. Cyokine Growth Factor Rev. 2009;20:153–64.
Poletaev A. The natural autoimmunity: self-recognition, self-interaction, and self maintenance. J Autoimmun Res. 2014;1:1001.
Pollanen P, Niemi M. Immunohistochemical identification of macrophages, lymphoid cells and HLA antigens in the human testis. Int J Androl. 1987;10:37–42.
Pollanen P, Soder O, Uksia J. Testicular immunosuppressive protein. J Reprod Immunol. 1988;14:125–8.
Pollanen P, Maddocks S. Macrophages, lymphocytes and MHC II antigen in the ram and rat testis. J Reprod Fertil. 1988;82:437–45.
Pollanen P, Von Euler M, Jahnukainen K, Saari T, Parvinen M, Sainio-Pollanen S, Soder O. Role of transforming growth factor beta in testicular immunosuppression. J Reprod Immunol. 1993;24:123–37.
Potashnik H, Elhija MA, Lunenfeld E, Potashnik G, Schlatt S, Nieschlag E, Huleihel M. Interleukin-6 expression during normal maturation of the mouse testis. Eur Cytokine Netw. 2005;16:161–5.

Qu N, Naito M, terayama H, Hirai S, Li J, Ogawa Y, Kitaoka M, Itoh M. Developmental ontogeny of autoantigens associated with localized autoimmunity in murine testis and epididymis. J Reprod Immunol. 2010;87:45–51.

Qu N, Naito M, Li J, Terayama H, Hirai S, Itoh M. Xenogenic and endogenous spermatogenesis following transplantation of rat germ cells into testes of immunocompetent mice. Reprod Fertil Dev. 2012;24:337–43.

Raburn DJ, Coquelin A, Hutson JC. Human chorionic gonadotropin increases the concentration of macrophages in neonatal rat testis. Biol Reprod. 1991;45:172–7.

Raburn DJ, Coquelin A, Reinhart AJ, Hutson JC. Regulation of the macrophage population in postnatal rat testis. J Reprod Immunol. 1993;24:139–51.

Rathi R, Honaramooz A, Zeng W, Schlatt S, Dobrinski I. Germ cells fate and seminiferous tubule development in bovine testis xenografts. Reproduction. 2005;130:923–9.

Rettew JA, Huet-Hudson YM, Marriott I. Testosterone reduces macrophage expression in the mouse of toll-like receptor 4, a trigger for inflammation and innate immunity. Biol Reprod. 2008;78:432–7.

Riccioli A, Filippini A, De Cesaris P, Barbacci E, Stefanini M, Starace G, Ziparo E. Inflammatory mediators increase surface expression of integrin ligands, adhesion to lymphocytes, and secretion of interleukin 6 in mouse Sertoli cells. Proc Natl Acad Sci U S A. 1995;92:5809–12.

Riccioli A, Starace D, D'Alessio A, Starace G, Padula F, De Cesaris P, FIlippini A, Ziparo E. TNF-alpha and IFN-gamma regulate expression and function of the Fas system in the seminiferous epithelium. J Immunol. 2000;165:743–9.

Riccioli A, Starace D, Galli R, Fuso A, Scarpa S, Palombi F, De Cesaris P, Iparo E, FIlippini A. Sertoli cells initiate testicular innate immune responses through TLR activation. J Immunol. 2006;177:7122–30.

Ritchie AW, Hargreave TB, James K, Chisholm GD. Intra-epithelial lymphocytes in the normal epididymis. A mechanism for tolerance to sperm auto-antigens? Br J Urol. 1984;56:79–83.

Rival C, Lustig L, Iosub R, Guazzone VA, Schneider E, Meinhardt A, Fijak M. Identification of a dendritic cell population in normal testis and in chronically inflamed testis of rats with autoimmune orchitis. Cell Tissue Res. 2006;324:311–8.

Rival C, Guazzone VA, von Wulffen W, Hackstein H, Schneider E, Lustig L, Meinhardt A, Fijak M. Expression of co-stimulatory molecules, chemokine receptors and proinflammatory cytokines in dendritic cells from normal and chronically inflamed rat testis. Mol Hum Reprod. 2007;13:851–61.

Rubtsova K, Marrack P, Rubtsov AV. Sexual dimorphism in autoimmunity. J Clin Invest. 2015; 125:2187–93.

Sakamoto Y, Nomoto K. Suppression of delayed-type hypersensitivity to syngeneic testicular cells in mice: involvement of suppressor T cells which act at the induction stage. Cell Immunol. 1986;102:168–76.

Sanberg PR, Borlongan CV, Saporta S, Cameron DF. Testis-derived Sertoli cells survive and provide localized immunoprotection for xenografts in rat brain. Nat Biotechnol. 1996;14:1692–5.

Sarkar O, Mathur PP, Cheng CY, Mruk DD. Interleukin 1 alpha is a novel regulator of the blood-testis barrier in the rat. Biol Reprod. 2008;78:445–54.

Saxena S, Farroq A. Localization of source of immunosuppressive factor in the human male reproductive tract. J Reprod Immunol. 1987;12:149–53.

Schell C, Albrecht M, Mayer C, Schwarzer JU, Frungieri MB, Mayerhofer A. Exploring human testicular peritubular cell: identification of secretory products and regulation by tumor necrosis factor-alpha. Endocrinology. 2008;149:1678–86.

Schuppe HC, Meinhardt A. Immune privilege and inflammation of the testis. Chem Immunol Allergy. 2005;88:1–14.

Selawry H, Fojaco R, Whittington K. Extended survival of MHC-compatible islet grafts from diabetes-resistant donors in spontaneously diabetic BB/W rat. Diabetes. 1987;36:1061–7.

Selawry HP, Cameron DF. Sertoli cell-enriched fractions in successful islet cell transplantation. Cell Transplant. 1993;2:123–9.

Sethi KK, Brandis H. IgG Fc-binding receptors on spermatozoa. Eur J Immunol. 1980;10:964–5.
Shang T, Zhang X, Wang T, Sun B, Deng T, Han D. Toll-like receptor-initiated testicular innate immune responses in mouse Leydig cells. Endocrinology. 2011;152:2827–36.
Shearer GM, Hurtenbach U. Is sperm immunosuppressive in male homosexuals and vasectomized men? Immunol Today. 1982;3:153–4.
Shi SH, Jiang L, Xie HY, Xu J, Zhu YF, Zheng SS. The effect of secondary cholestasis on the CD68-positive and CD163-positive macrophage population, cellular proliferation, and apoptosis in rat testis. J Reprod Immunol. 2015a;110:36–47.
Shi SH, Jiang L, Xie HY, Zhu YF, Zhang WJ, Zheng SS. Secondary biliary cholestasis promotes testicular macrophage infiltration and autophagy in rats. Am J Reprod Immunol. 2015b;73:301–12.
Silva CA, Cocuzza M, Borba EF, Bonfa E. Cutting-edge issues in autoimmune orchitis. Clinic Rev Allerg Immunol. 2012;42:256–63.
Silva CA, Cocuzza M, Carvalho JF, Bonfa E. Diagnosis and classification of autoimmune orchitis. Autoimmun Rev. 2014;13:431–4.
Sinowatz F, Wrobel KH, Sinowatz S, Kugler P. Ultrastructural evidence for phagocytosis of spermatozoa in the bovine rete testis and testicular straight tubules. J Reprod Fertil. 1979;57:1–4.
Sipione S, Simmen KC, Lord SJ, Motyka B, Ewen C, Shostak I, Rayat GR, Dufour JM, Korbutt GS, Rajotte RV, Blrackley RC. Identification of a novel human granzyme B inhibitor secreted by cultured Sertoli cells. J Immunol. 2006;177:5051–8.
Soramoto S, Hiramine C, Takenaka I, Hojo K. Murine experimental autoimmune orchitis (EAO) induced by syngeneic testicular germ cells (TC) alone: orchitogenic and lymphostimulatory activities of TC from mice at various ages. Clin Immunol Immunopathol. 1993;69:292–9.
Starace D, Galli R, Paone A, De Cesaris P, Filippini A, Ziparo E, Ricciolo A. Toll-like receptors 3 activation induced antiviral immune responses in mouse Sertoli cells. Biol Reprod. 2008;79:766–75.
Suarez-Pinzon W, Korbutt GS, Power R, Hooton J, Rajotte RV, Rabinovitch A. Testicular Sertoli cells protect islet beta-cells from autoimmune destruction in NOD mice by a transforming growth factor-beta 1-dependent mechanisms. Diabetes. 2000;49:1810–8.
Suda T, Takahashi T, Goldstein P, Nagata S. Molecular cloning and expression of the Fas ligand, a novel member of the tumor necrosis factor family. Cell. 1993;75:1169–78.
Sun B, Qi N, Shang T, Wu H, Deng T, Han D. Sertoli cell-initiated testicular innate immune response through toll-like receptor-3 activation is negatively regulated by Tyro3, Axl, and Mer receptors. Endocrinology. 2010;151:2886–97.
Taguchi O, Nishizuka Y, Sakakura T, Kojima A. Autoimmune oophoritis in thymectomized mice: detection of circulating antibodies against oocytes. Clin Exp Immunol. 1980;40:540–3.
Taguchi O, Nishizuka Y. Experimental autoimmune orchitis after neonatal thymectomy in the mouse. Clin Exp Immunol. 1981;46:425–34.
Taguchi O, Takahashi T, Nishizuka Y. Self-tolerance and localized autoimmunity. Curr Opin Immunol. 1990;2:576–81.
Tainosho S, Naito M, Hirai S, Terayama H, Qu N, Itoh M. Multilayered structure of the basal lamina of tubuli recti in normal mice. Med Mol Morphol. 2011;44:34–8.
Takahashi K, Naito M, Terayama H, Qu N, Cheng L, Tainosho S, Itoh M. Immunomorphological aspects of the tubuli recti and the surrounding interstitium in normal mice. Int J Androl. 2007;30:21–7.
Takeda Y, Gotoh M, Dono K, Nishihara M, Grochowiecki T, Kimura F, Yoshida T, Ohta Y, Ota H, Ohzato H, Umechita K, Takeda T, Matsuura N, Sakon M, Kayagaki N, Yagita H, Okumura K, Miyasaka M, Monden M. Protection of islet allografts transplanted together with Fas ligand expressing testicular allografts. Diabetologia. 1998;41:315–21.
Tanaka A, Nagayoshi M, Awara M, Mawartari Y, Tanaka I, Sofkins N. Conclusions from the transplantation of human or hamster spermatogonia/primary spermatocytes to rat or mouse testis. Fertil Steril. 1997;68(Suppl):S61.
Tarter TH, Alexander NJ. Complement-inhibiting activity of seminal plasma. Am J Reprod Immunol. 1984;6:28–32.

Teerds KJ, de Rooij DG, Rommerts FF, Wensing CJ. The regulation of the proliferation and differentiation of rat Leydig cell precursor cells after EDS administration or daily HCG treatment. J Androl. 1988;9:343–51.

Teerds KJ, Rommerts FF, Dorrington JH. Immunohistochemical detection of transforming growth factor-alpha in Leydig cells during the development of the rat testis. Mol Cell Endocrinol. 1990;69:1–6.

Teerds KJ, de Boer-Brouwer M, Dorrington JH, Balvers M, Ivell R. Identification of markers for precursor and Leydig cell differentiation in the adult rat testis following ethane dimethyl sulphonate administration. Biol Reprod. 1999;60:1437–45.

Terayama H, Naito M, Qu N, Hirai S, Kitaoka M, Ogawa Y, Itoh M. Intra-testicular expression of mRNAs of both interferon gamma and tumor necrosis factor alpha is significantly increased in experimental autoimmune orchitis in mice. J Reprod Dev. 2011;57:296–302.

Terayama H, Yoshimoto T, Hirai S, Naito M, Qu N, Hatayama N, Hayashi S, Mitobe K, Furusawa J, Mizoguchi I, Kezuka T, Goto H, Suyama K, Sakabe K, Itoh M. Contribution of IL-12/IL-35 common subunit p35 to maintaining testicular immune privilege. PLoS One. 2014;9:e96120.

Teuscher C, Hickey WF, Korngold R. Experimental allergic orchitis in mice. V. Resistance to actively induced disease in Balb/cJ substrain mice is mediated by $CD4^{+}$ T cells. Immunogenetics. 1990;32:34–40.

Tokunaga Y, Hiramine C, Itoh M, Muaksa A, Hojo K. Genetic susceptibility to the induction of murine experimental autoimmune orchitis (EAO) without adjuvant. I. Comparison of pathology, delayed type hypersensitivity, and antibody. Clin Immunol Immunopathol. 1993;66:239–47.

Tompkins AB, Hutchinson P, de Kretser DM, Hedger MP. Characterization of lymphocytes in the adult rat testis by flow cytometry: effects of activin and transforming growth factor beta on lymphocyte subsets in vitro. Biol Reprod. 1998;58:943–51.

Tung KS, Yule TD, Mahi-Brown CA, Listrom MB. Distribution of histopathology and Ia positive cells in actively induced and passively transferred experimental autoimmune orchitis. J Immunol. 1987;138:752–9.

Verajankorva E, Martikainen M, Pollanen P. Cytokines in the BALB/c mouse testis in various conditions. Asian J Androl. 2001;3:9–19.

Verajankorva E, Setala N, Teros T, Salmi AA, Pollanen P. Testicular-associated immune deviation: flushing of the testicular lymph sinusoids induces immunosuppression and inhibits formation of EAE in SJL mice. Scand J Immunol. 2002;55:478–83.

Vergouwen RP, Huiskamp R, Bas RJ, Roepers-Gajadien HL, Davids JA, de Rooij DG. Radiosensitivity of testicular cells in the fetal mouse. Radiat Res. 1995;141:66–73.

Wakasa H, Amano S. Histopathology on testicular involvement of leukemia with an emphasis on lymphatics. Tohoku J Exp Med. 1977;123:147–59.

Wang HX, Yi SQ, Li J, Terayama H, Naito M, Hirai S, Qu N, Yi N, Itoh M. Effects of splenectomy on spontaneously chronic pancreatitis in aly/aly mice. Clin Dev Immunol. 2010;2010. Article ID 614890, 8 pages. doi:10.1155/2010/614890

Wang T, Zhang X, Chen Q, Deng T, Zhang Y, Li N, Shang T, Chen Y, Han D. Toll-like receptor 3-initiated antiviral responses in mouse male germ cells in vitro. Biol Reprod. 2012;86:1–10.

Wang YF, Holstein AF. Intraepithelial lymphocytes and macrophages in the human epididymis. Cell Tissue Res. 1983;233:517–21.

Winnall WR, Muir JA, Hedger MP. Rat resident testicular macrophages have an alternatively activated phenotype and constitutively produce interleukin-10 in vitro. J Leukoc Biol. 2011a;90:133–43.

Winnall WR, Muir JA, Hedger MP. Differential responses of epithelial Sertoli cells of the rat testis to Toll-like receptor 2 and 4 ligands: implications for studies of testicular inflammation using bacteria lipopolysaccharides. Innate Immun. 2011b;17:123–36.

Winnall WR, Hedger MP. Phenotypic and functional heterogeneity of the testicular macrophages population: a new regulatory model. J Reprod Immunol. 2013;97:147–58.

Wu H, Wang H, Xiong W, Chen S, Tang H, Han D. Expression patterns and functions of toll-like receptors in mouse Sertoli cells. Endocrinology. 2008;149:4402–12.

Wu H, Shi L, Wang Q, Cheng L, Zhao X, Chen Q, Jiang Q, Feng M, Li Q, Han D. Mumps virus-induced innate immune responses in mouse Sertoli and Leydig cells. Sci Rep. 2016;6:19507. doi:10.1038/srep19507.

Wyatt CR, Law L, Magnuson JA, Griswold MD, Magnuson NS. Suppression of lymphocyte proliferation by protein secreted by cultured Sertoli cells. J Reprod Immunol. 1988;14:27–40.

Xiong Y, Hales DB. Expression, regulation, and production of tumor necrosis factor-alpha in mouse testicular interstitial macrophages in vitro. Endocrinology. 1993;133:2568–73.

Yamanaka K, Fujisawa M, Tanaka H, Okada H, Arakawa S, Kamidono S. Significance of human testicular mast cells and their subtypes in male infertility. Hum Reprod. 2000;15:1543–7.

Yee JB, Hutson JC. Testicular macrophages: Isolation, characterization and hormonal responsiveness. Biol Reprod. 1983;29:1319–26.

Yee JB, Hutson JC. Effects of testicular macrophages-conditioned medium on Leydig cells in culture. Endocrinology. 1985;116:2682–4.

Yoshida S, Ohhara R, Sanui H, Nomoto K. Sex difference in delayed footpad reaction to syngenesis TGC in C3H/He mice. Immunology. 1983;48:537–42.

Yotsukura J, Huang H, Singh AK, Shichi H. Regulatory cells generated by testicular tolerization to retinal S-antigen: possible involvement of IL-4, IL-10, and TGF-beta in the suppression of experimental autoimmune uveoretinitis. Cell Immunol. 1997;182:89–98.

Zhao S, Zhu W, Xue S, Han D. Testicular defense systems: immune privilege and innate immunity. Cell Mol Immunol. 2014;11:428–37.

Human Testicular Autoimmunity as a Result of Breakdown of Testicular Immune Privilege

3

3.1 Introduction

The BTB physically divides the seminiferous epithelium into basal and adluminal compartments. Besides its function as an immunologic barrier to segregate post-meiotic TGC from the systemic circulation, it creates a microenvironment for TGC development and confers cell polarity (Fig. 3.1). At puberty, when immune competence is already established, TGC commence a new program which leads to the formation of mature spermatozoa. During this process, an array of new surface molecules is expressed on the differentiating spermatids and spermatozoa (Ike et al. 2007). Such autoantigens, therefore, do not belong to the "family" of those considered as "self" by the immune system. Therefore, under some condition in which the testicular immune privilege is broken, immune responses against the testicular autoantigens should be evoked.

Clinically, in human male infertility of immunologic origin, the presence of anti-sperm antibodies is a well-known cause of male infertility (Jodot-van de Casseye et al. 1980), and measurement and analysis of anti-sperm antibodies have been extensive. The six most common serological tests used for antibody detection include sperm agglutination, complement-dependent sperm immobilization, indirect immunofluorescence, the enzyme-linked immunosorbent assay, mixed antiglobulin reaction test, and immunobead test (Shibahara et al. 2005). Actually, male subfertile patients with significant titers of anti-sperm antibodies could be treated with steroid regimens (Hendry et al. 1979), and treatment of male autoimmune infertility with cyclosporine A has been clinically attempted (Bouloux et al. 1986). Moreover, autoantibodies against Sertoli cells, Leydig cells, and basement membrane of the seminiferous tubules were also detected in male infertility (Wall et al. 1974; Zanchetta et al. 1984; Silva et al. 2012). However, detection of the autoantibodies on sera and/or semen is not sufficient to diagnose testicular autoimmunity. The characteristic features of testicular autoimmunity include the detection of (1) inflammatory cell

---

The original version of this chapter was revised. An erratum to this chapter can be found at DOI 10.1007/978-4-431-54460-9_9

M. Itoh, *Testicular Autoimmunity*, DOI 10.1007/978-4-431-54460-9_3

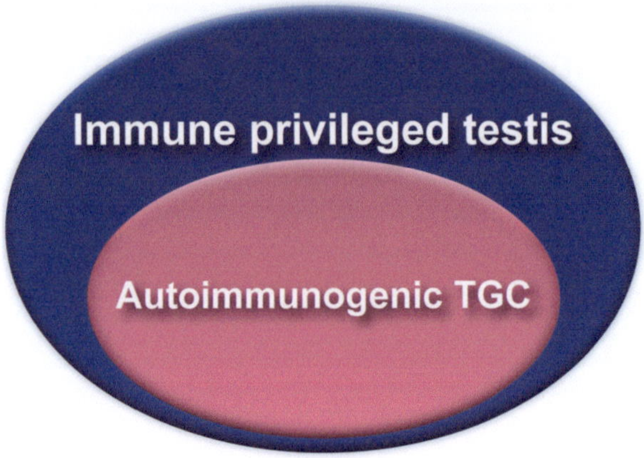

Fig. 3.1 Immuno-environment for the development of testicular germ cells (TGC)

infiltration into the testis (=orchitis), (2) spermatogenic disturbance, (3) T cell response against target testicular autoantigens, (4) serum autoantibodies against the target antigens, and (5) binding of the autoantibodies to the target antigen-bearing cells inside the testis. Clinically, it is quite difficult to detect all these features. Therefore, immunoreactions at the level of testicular tissue have been less well studied in humans. However, there is increasing evidence that autoimmune orchitis may be an etiological factor in human reproductive failure, perhaps even more often than expected.

3.2 Classification of Testicular Autoimmunity in Men

Testicular autoimmunity can be classified into primary and secondary ones. Primary testicular autoimmunity is defined by asymptomatic orchitis associated with anti-sperm antibodies without any evidence of systemic or local causes in infertile men. Secondary testicular autoimmunity is characterized by symptomatic orchitis and/or testicular vasculitis associated with local or systemic inflammatory disease (Silva et al. 2012, 2014). The patients suffering from secondary testicular autoimmunity typically demonstrate testicular pain, erythema, and/or swelling. Systemic autoimmunity, vasectomy, infection, tumor, or trauma may induce T cell response with pro-inflammatory cytokine production with a consequent BTB permeability alteration, anti-sperm antibody production, and apoptosis of TGC. Although the testicular autoimmunity can be classified into the two categories, the etiologies of both primary and secondary autoimmune orchitis are likely to be multifactorial and overlapped.

3.3 Histological Findings from Biopsy Specimens of Infertile Men

Of all cases of infertility, approximately 50% of cases occur in men. Although the literatures reported many causes of male infertility, approximately 65% of the cases are categorized as idiopathic spermatogenic disturbance (Fig. 3.2). The

Fig. 3.2 The causes of male infertility

① Obstruction of excurrent ducts for epididymal spermatozoa
② Damage to accessory sex organs
③ Dysfunction of ejaculation
} 10%

④ Disturbance of spermatogenesis
a) Varicocele
b) Cryptorchidism
c) Irradiation
d) Infection
e) Klinefelter syndrome
f) Other abnormality
} 25%
g) Idiopathic (unknown origin) 65%
} 90%

histopathology of idiopathic spermatogenic disturbance is characterized by seminiferous tubules showing Sertoli cell-only syndrome or TGC maturation arrest. In a study of patients with idiopathic male infertility, testicular biopsies showed that approximately 20% of patients had Sertoli cell-only syndrome, and approximately 50% of patients had maturation arrest (Hatakeyama 1984; Terada and Hatakeyama 1991). These features of spermatogenic disturbance were often accompanied by thickening and hyalinization of the seminiferous tubular wall (De Kretser et al. 1975; Terada and Hatakeyama 1991). Furthermore, fibrosis, sclerosis, and thickening and hyalinization of testicular interstitium are the features frequently found in the testis of infertile patients (Agarwal et al. 1987; Apa et al. 2002).

There have been some reports which showed lymphocytic infiltration and immune deposits in specimens of testicular biopsies from infertile men (Taylor et al. 1978; Suominen and Soderstrom 1982; Salomon et al. 1982; Salomon and Hedinger 1982; Hatakeyama 1984; Lehmann et al. 1987; Aitchison et al. 1990; Agarwal et al. 1990; Hassanin and Ayad 2016). Suominen (1995) reported a case, where a surgical operation for an inguinal hernia caused an orchitis first in the ipsilateral, and few weeks later also in the contralateral testis and which finally led to an atrophy of both testes, resulting from autoimmune sympathetic orchitis. The testicular biopsy revealed that the interstitial tissue contained numerous lymphocytes and macrophages. A typical feature was characterized by disturbed spermatogenesis in the seminiferous tubules that were surrounded by lymphocytic infiltration. Occasionally, intra-tubular lymphocytes were also found in both testes (Hussein et al. 2005). Nistal et al. (2002) evaluated the focal orchitis present in cryptorchid testes of men not previously treated for cryptorchidism or antecedents of infectious diseases and detected focal lymphocytic infiltration in the interstitium and/or seminiferous tubules associated with spermatogenic disturbance in 44% of examined patients. A picture resembling autoimmune orchitis can be found in unilateral testicular obstruction (Hendry et al. 1985, 1990). Mononuclear cell infiltration around the seminiferous tubules and the rete testis with anti-sperm antibodies was noted in men with unilateral testicular obstruction. Approximately 5% of testicular biopsies from men with azoospermia or oligozoospermia had focal or general leukocyte infiltration (Suominen and Soderstrom 1982). Jahnukainen et al. (1995) evaluated the incidence of testicular mononuclear cell infiltrates in patients with carcinoma in situ and germ cell neoplasia. The results suggest that the incidence of mononuclear cell infiltration increases with increasing severity of testicular malignant changes and also that increased mononuclear cell infiltration is evident in the contralateral testis where no malignant cells can be observed. Testicular lymphocyte numbers are increased in infertile patients with sperm autoimmunity, and the predominance of $CD8^+$ T cells was immunohistochemically demonstrated in the interstitium between the seminiferous tubules in them (El-Demiry et al. 1985, 1987). In infertile men with maturation arrest, Sertoli cell only, or mixed atrophy syndromes, and with cases of idiopathic infertility showing normal spermatogenesis, diagnostic testicular biopsy revealed the significant presence of $CD68^+$ macrophages in the testes of all patients (Frungieri et al. 2002). These macrophages expressed the genes for IL-1 and TNF-alpha and were located in the testicular interstitium and in/around the seminiferous tubules. In Sertoli cell only and germ cell arrest syndrome, the overall macrophage number was increased over twofold. A study of phenotypical characterization of testicular leukocytes demonstrated that cell counts of all examined populations (T cells, B cells, $CD68^+$ macrophages, and mast cells) in Sertoli cell-only syndrome and germ cell arrest were increased when compared with those in normal spermatogenesis (Hussein et al. 2005).

Aitchison et al. (1990) also reported several cases of granulomatous orchitis with chronic inflammation in humans. In idiopathic granulomatous orchitis, there is extensive destruction of the seminiferous tubules with tubular or interstitial pattern of granulomatous inflammation and prominent collagen fibrosis (Roy et al. 2011). Finally, the seminiferous epithelium was replaced by an admixture of large epithelioid cells, lymphocytes, plasma cells, and occasionally giant cells (Perimenis et al. 1991). Granulomatous orchitis is sometimes accompanied by inguinal or retroperitoneal lymphadenitis (Matsumura et al. 2016). Trauma and the following autoimmune responses against TGC have been postulated to be the underlying mechanism of the disease (Sporer and Seebode 1982; Wegner et al. 1994). Ischemia or preceded infection in the testis may be other origins of granulomatous orchitis (Kahn and Mcaninch 1980; Tarabuta-Cordun 1983; Rosi et al. 1984; Klein et al. 1985).

The increased number of mast cells in the testis is also associated with male infertility (Maseki et al. 1981; Nistal et al. 1984; Agarwal et al. 1987). With regard to their characteristic location within testicular tissue, two groups of mast cells could be distinguished, in both control and infertile patients: interstitial mast cells (located between Leydig and other interstitial cells as well as in the vicinity of blood vessels) and peritubular mast cells (located in the close proximity of the tubular lamina propria or incorporated in the lamina propria itself) (Jezek et al. 1999). It appeared that peritubular mast cells increased at a higher rate than interstitial mast cells in infertile patients when compared with controls. The increase in testicular mast cells in close contact to the seminiferous tubules indicates a relationship between mast cell proliferation and a dysfunction of the BTB (Haidl et al. 2011). The mast cells have been known to play a key role in the pathophysiology of various allergic, inflammatory, or fibrotic disorders, perhaps because of their chemical mediators such as biogenic amines, prostaglandins, neutral proteases, and proteoglycans (Schwartz and Austen 1984). There are two distinct subpopulations of mast cells, the connective tissue and mucosal mast cell (Irani and Schwartz 1989). Nearly all the mast cells in the normal human testes contain heparin and correspond to "connective tissue mast cells." In the infertile patients, chondroitin sulfate containing mast cells was substantial in number, and these cells correspond to "mucosal mast cells" (Nagai et al. 1992). Therefore, in male infertility, mast cells were increased in total number, and the degree of the increase in mucosal mast cells was greater than that in the connective tissue mast cells. Actually, a mast cell blocker is clinically useful for the treatment of idiopathic oligozoospermic men (Yamamoto et al. 1995; Matsuki et al. 2000).

Other studies have provided evidence of immune deposits in testis biopsies from male patients with impaired fertility (Vu Van et al. 1978; Lehmann et al. 1987). Salomon et al. (1982) and Salomon and Hedinger (1982) reported the presence of immune complex orchitis in infertile men. In the specimens, linear deposits of IgG and complement on the basement membrane of the seminiferous tubules were found. In other biopsy specimens from infertile patients, immune complexes were found to be localized not only on seminiferous tubule walls but also on Leydig cells and various staged TGC (Morgan 1976). A case of testis biopsy from a patient with oligospermia and a large varicocele in the left testis showed carcinoma in situ with atypical spermatogonia in the right testis. This lesion was immunologically characterized by the deposit of IgG restricted to the atypical cells and the presence of circulating anti-sperm antibodies (Lehmann et al. 1986, 1987; Lehmann and Muller 1987). In immune complex orchitis, at least two different immunological mechanisms, induced locally in the testis, may be involved: an immunoglobulin deposit, in a manner specifically against TGC, and the seminiferous tubular basement membrane, in a manner nonspecifically directed to them (Lehmann et al. 1987; Lehmann and Emmons 1989). Hence, the circulating autoantibodies could specifically react with various testicular cells and tissues, but the immune deposits to the seminiferous tubule walls, blood capillary walls, and other testicular tissues could be accounted for aggregation of not only the specific antibodies but also irrelevant serum immunoglobulins in an antigen-nonspecific manner.

Collectively, the detection of lymphocytic infiltration, deposits of IgG, and deposits of complements in testis biopsy specimens indicates that inflammatory or immunological factors contribute to the occurrence of some idiopathic male infertility. However, it is quite difficult to diagnose it, because testicular autoimmune inflammation may progress chronically, torpidly, and asymptomatically. Therefore, involvement of lymphocytic infiltration and immune deposits may be no longer detectable when Sertoli cell-only syndrome and maturation arrest of some immunologic origin are completely established.

Additionally, in recent study on testicular biopsy specimens from male patients with Sertoli cell-only syndrome and maturation arrest, increased apoptosis of TGC and Sertoli cells was observed. In maturation arrest, mRNA expression of Fas ligand was upregulated in Sertoli cells and Leydig cells, while intense expression of Fas was observed in primary degenerating spermatocytes, and active mRNA expression of caspase 3 was detected in cytoplasm of both Sertoli cells and TGC. In Sertoli cell-only syndrome, mRNA expression of Fas, Fas ligand, and active caspase 3 was detected both in Sertoli cells and in hyperplastic interstitial cells (Kim et al. 2007). It indicates that upregulation of the Fas system and caspase 3 activity in the testis may result in enhanced TGC apoptosis, which is involved in the spermatogenic disturbance (Eid et al. 2002).

More recently, human testicular biopsies from infertile men with focal lymphocytic infiltrates were probed with antibodies against high-mobility group box protein 1 (HMGB1), and it was found that HMGB1 was translocated from the nuclei in the testes of infertile men with spermatogenic disturbance and lymphocytic infiltrates (Aslani et al. 2014). Klune et al. (2008) reported that activated macrophages and monocytes secrete HMGB1 as a cytokine mediator of inflammation. HMGB1 is among the most important chromatin proteins, and the presence of HMGB1 in the nucleus depends on post-translational modifications. When the protein is not acetylated, it stays in the nucleus, but hyper-acetylation on lysine residues causes it to translocate into the cytosol. Furthermore, interaction of HMGB1 and TLR-4 results in upregulation of NF-kappa B, which leads to increased production and a release of cytokines in macrophages. Therefore, the binding of HMGB1 to TLR-4, which mediates HMGB1-dependent activation of macrophage cytokine release, may play an important role in the onset and progression of autoimmune diseases, involving human orchitis (Aslani et al. 2014).

Therefore, testicular biopsy has provided various information of immunological aspects on the spermatogenic disturbance; however, it must be kept in mind that testicular biopsy itself may injure BTB focally, leading to testicular autoimmunity (Hjort et al. 1974, 1982).

3.4 Anti-sperm and Anti-testis Autoantibodies in Men

Many studies suggest the involvement of humoral immunity in male infertility. Anti-sperm antibodies have been the center of attention in immunology and immunopathology of reproduction. Indeed, the presence of anti-sperm antibodies has been observed in approximately 5–12% of infertile male partners, compared to 0–2% of the general male population (Silva et al. 2012). Circulating anti-sperm antibodies detected in other studies ranged from 8 to 30% in unselected men with infertile marriages (Francavilla et al. 1999, 2007). Moreover, circulating antibodies against immature TGC, Sertoli cells, Leydig cells, and basal lamina of the seminiferous tubules were detected in serum samples from infertile patients (Wall et al. 1974; Hatakeyama 1984; Zanchetta et al. 1984; Silva et al. 2012).

Patients with high titers of anti-sperm antibodies had evidence of testicular damage with decreased testicular volumes, elevated serum FSH and LH levels, and reduced sperm density and motility, indicating the induction of the spermatogenic disturbance (Handelsman et al. 1983). *Chlamydia trachomatis*, *Ureaplasma urealyticum*, and *Mycoplasma hominis* compared to other sexually transmitted diseases cause statistically significant increase of anti-sperm antibodies concentration in blood serum, as well as in ejaculate. Local infection by them may induce orchitis and epididymitis, which results in inflammatory and toxic damage to the seminiferous epithelium, which in turn plays significant role in development of testicular autoimmunity (Tchiokadze and Galdava 2015).

The anti-sperm antibodies in males have been shown to have an inhibitory effect on fertilization. There is a possibility that fertilization-related antigens may be the targets of these anti-sperm antibodies. Such antigens are consisted of sperm surface antigens and acrosomal antigens. The former include PH-20, PH-30, fertilization antigen-1 (FA-1), sperm agglutination antigen-1, and lactate dehydrogenase-C_4, and the latter include SP-10 (Hall et al. 1994; Shibahara et al. 2005). Acrosin, hyaluronidase, RSA-1, MA-29, FA-1, SO3, S37, S61, S20, and YLP_{12} are also human sperm autoantigens presumably involved in anti-sperm immune response (Ishidori et al. 1988; Naz 2004). In particular, treatment with FA-1 was demonstrated to remove anti-sperm autoantibodies from spermatozoa of infertile men and results in increased rates of acrosome reaction (Menge et al. 1999). Seminal autoantibodies against laminin-1 are also important in infertile men (Ulcova-Gallova et al. 2008). In males, laminin is found on not only the surface of spermatozoa but also basal lamina of the seminiferous tubules. Sperm agglutination antigen-1 (SAGA-1) was characterized as a polymorphic, highly acidic, glycophosphatidylinositol-anchored glycoprotein on the surface of human spermatozoa (Diekman et al. 2000). It is unique in that SAGA-1 core peptide is identical to CD52, a glycoprotein on the surface of human lymphocytes. Therefore, autoimmunity to CD52 may be an important factor in the etiology of immunologic male infertility.

The incidence of epididymitis is greater than that of orchitis in humans, and susceptibility to anti-sperm antibody formation after damage to the epididymis or vas deferens increases with increasing distance of the damage from the testis. One important consideration must be the very different immunological environments of the testis, where sperms develop, and the epididymis, where sperms mature and are stored. Compared with the elaborate BTB, the tight junctions of the epididymal ducts are much less effective. Unlike the seminiferous epithelium, immune cells are commonly observed within the epididymal epithelium and can even be found within the lumen of the epididymis (Hedger 2011). Therefore, epididymal sperm autoantigens tend to be easily accessible to immune cells, resulting in anti-sperm antibody production.

It is noted that naturally occurring human anti-sperm autoantibodies, detectable by immunofluorescence, had a peak incidence of 90% in both sexes before puberty (Tung et al. 1976). Thereafter, the incidence declined to approximately 60% and persisted through life. Actually, it remains vague whether production of anti-TGC or anti-sperm autoantibodies is a cause or a result of testicular autoimmunity. In other words, it can be said that these autoantibodies become the cause, the result, or the both in each case. There is another possibility that those natural anti-sperm autoantibodies may down-regulate the specific autoimmune responses through some immune network system based on "idiotypic network theory," proposed by Jerne (1974). The BTB damage in testicular autoimmunity results in production of anti-TGC autoantibodies, and male infertility may result from the binding of anti-TGC or anti-sperm autoantibodies (Tung 1998; Lustig and Tung 2006). These autoantibodies present in local secretions of the germ cell tract rather than serum are associated with this type of male infertility. Primary testicular autoimmunity can be defined by isolated and asymptomatic orchitis with the autoantibodies but without evidence of local or systemic disease or injury. Most cases of the primary disease are torpidly and chronically advanced. On the other hand, secondary testicular autoimmunity accompanied by the autoantibodies involves orchitis associated with endogenous factors such as cryptorchidism, varicocele, torsion, tumor, or systemic autoimmune diseases and orchitis associated with exogenous factors such as trauma, biopsy, vasectomy, and infection. These are testicular autoimmunity associated with identified pro-inflammatory causes. Obstruction or injury of the male reproductive tract is associated with anti-TGC or anti-sperm antibody formation, since leakage of large quantities of TGC or sperm antigens from the tract can induce the antibody production. Anti-sperm antibodies attendant to vasectomy may be responsible for infertility in some patients following vasovastomy (Witkin et al. 1982; Lee et al. 2009). Anti-sperm antibodies are common in patients with congenital absence of the vas deferens associated with cystic fibrosis (D'Cruz et al. 1991; Lustig and Tung 2006). The role of anti-sperm antibodies in the pathogenesis of varicocele-related male infertility has been also noted. The prevalence of varicocele-related immune infertility is about 15% male subjects from infertile couples (Bozhedomov et al. 2014). Varicocele is not an immediate cause of autoimmune reactions against spermatozoa but is a cofactor increasing a risk of anti-sperm antibody formation. These disorders correlate with the level of sperm oxidative stress; reactive oxygen species production in anti-sperm antibody-positive varicocele patients is 2.8 and 3.5 times higher than in anti-sperm antibody-negative varicocele patients and control fertile men, respectively.

In general, anti-TGC and anti-sperm antibodies of IgG class are regarded as an important factor for male infertility; however, those of IgE class might also participate in the male infertility. The increased number of mast cells in the testis was found in cases of male infertility (Maseki et al. 1981; Agarwal et al. 1987; Hussein et al. 2005; Welter et al. 2011). Activated mast cells secrete enzymes, e.g., hyaluronidase, protease, cytochrome oxidase, phosphatases, histamine, serotonin, and heparin. Considering that these substances are important in the laying down of collagen, proliferation of mast cells may result in increasing fibrosis and hyalinization of seminiferous tubular wall and the surrounding interstitium, leading to the spermatogenic disturbance. Mathur et al. (1981) suggested that there may be a local IgE antibody response in the idiopathic infertile males. In response to seminal antigens, mucosal plasma cells are triggered to produce IgE antibodies locally in the male reproductive tracts. This possibility is supported by the elevated levels of IgE in the serum and the semen samples of infertile males with high anti-sperm antibody titer. The high affinity of these antibodies for mast cells induces release of various substances from mast cells described above. Intra-testicular T cells may stimulate mast cells, with the resultant increase of their cell number and stimulation of their secretion in the testis. However, it is yet unclear whether mastocytosis in the testis is a cause, or a result, of the testicular fibrosis in infertile male patients. Altogether, the analysis of epidemiological and prognostic studies may support the opinion that anti-sperm and/or anti-testis autoantibodies are a relative, rather than absolute, cause of immunologic male infertility (Francavilla et al. 1999, 2007).

3.5 Systemic Inflammatory Diseases and Orchitis in Men

Systemic inflammatory diseases causing male infertility include primary vasculitis such as polyarteritis nodosa, Behcet's disease, and Henoch-Schönlein purpura (Dahl et al. 1960; Lie 1988; Pannek and Haupt 1997; Silva et al. 2012, 2014). The overall frequencies of orchitis and anti-sperm antibodies in rheumatic diseases are 2–31% and 0–50%, respectively. The presence of anti-sperm antibodies was reported to be present in 13–50% of systemic lupus erythematosus patients (Silva et al. 2012). Orchitis occurs in 2–18% of patients with polyarteritis nodosa. Epididymo-orchitis was also observed in 4–31% of Behcet's disease patients. Orchitis was evidenced in 7–21% of Henoch-Schönlein purpura patients. Testicular vasculitis may be a part of systemic vasculitis or may exist as isolated testicular vasculitis. A study of patients with testicular vasculitis demonstrated that 51% of patients had isolated testicular vasculitis and 49% had systemic testicular vasculitis (Hernandez-Rodriguez et al. 2012). Non-granulomatous inflammation affecting medium-sized testicular vessels occurred in most patients with both isolated and systemic testicular vasculitis. Among systemic testicular vasculitis, polyarteritis nodosa was the most frequently diagnosed (63%), followed by Wegener's granulomatosis (17%) (Shurbaji and Epstein 1988). Focal non-granulomatous orchitis was also reported in a patient with Crohn's disease (Piton et al. 2015). Pathological examination of the testis revealed a focal inflammatory infiltrate predominantly composed of lymphocytes accompanied by few plasma cells, lacking giant cells or granulomata. Granulomatosis with polyangiitis is a systemic necrotizing granulomatous vasculitis, which predominantly affects small-sized blood vessels in the upper/lower respiratory tract and kidneys. In the patients, orchitis is also found but rare, reported in <1% of cases in large cohorts (Alba et al. 2015).

Humans who have inherited the human class I MHC allele HLA-B27 have a markedly increased risk of developing the multi-organ system diseases termed HLA-B27 syndromes. Clinical features in HLA-B27 syndromes include anterior uveitis, ankylosing spondylitis, reactive arthritis, psoriatic arthritis, and inflammatory bowel disease such as ulcerative colitis and Crohn's disease. Although autoimmune orchitis has not been reported in men with spondyloarthritis, these patients showed reduced sperm motility, higher plasma luteinizing hormone and follicle-stimulating hormone, and lower testosterone levels compared with control subjects (Villiger et al. 2010; Ramonda et al. 2014).

Autoimmune polyendocrine syndrome, also called autoimmune polyendocrinopathy, is a heterogeneous group of rare diseases characterized by autoimmune activity against multiple endocrine organs, although non-endocrine organs can be also affected. The skin and nails, ovary and testis, eyes, thyroid, and digestive system are affected. In regard to the male hypogonadism, anti-sperm autoantibodies and autoantibodies against steroidogenic enzymes and other antigens expressed in the Leydig cells were detected (Tsatsoulis and Shalet 1991. Maclaren et al. 2001). In the sera of patients, anti-testis-specific protein 10 antibodies were also detected (Reimand et al. 2008; Smith et al. 2011). The testis-specific protein 10 is a highly expressed protein in the testis and plays a key role in spermatogenesis. Therefore, autoimmune responses against these antigens may affect the spermatogenesis in the patients. Actually, the immunosuppressive action of cyclical intermediate-dose steroid therapy led to a significant improvement in semen parameters (Tsatsoulis and Shalet 1991).

More recently, some cases of orchitis were also reported in patients with multi-organ IgG4-related disease involving a broad range of organs and tissues such as the pancreas, biliary tract, liver, breast, thyroid gland, lymph nodes, skin, aorta, pituitary gland, meninges, lacrimal gland, lung, and reproductive organs (De Buy Wenniger et al. 2013; Karram et al. 2014; Migita et al. 2014; Lin et al. 2015). In these cases, dense interstitial lymphoplasmacytic infiltrate composed of IgG4-positive plasma cells and epithelioid histiocytes (macrophages) was observed around the seminiferous tubules and in the epididymis, and prominent interstitial fibrosis was also found.

In regard to infectious diseases, the best-known orchitogenic viruses in humans are the mumps virus and human immunodeficiency virus (HIV) (Aiman et al. 1980; Chabon et al. 1987; De Paepe and Waxman 1989; Jala et al. 2004; Chandrashekar et al. 2015). Anti-sperm antibodies have been detected in both mumps and acquired immune deficiency syndrome (AIDS) patients. In AIDS patients, marked spermatogenic disturbance was noted with Sertoli cells predominantly lining the hyalinized seminiferous tubular wall. Furthermore, the testicular blood vessels were thickened, and mononuclear inflammatory infiltration composed of lymphocytes and macrophages was seen, and the many lymphocytes were $CD4^+$ (Pudney and Anderson 1991). Five to 37% of adults with mumps infection develop orchitis. In mumps virus-affected testis, lymphocytic infiltration was followed by the spermatogenic disturbance with atrophy and fibrosis of the seminiferous tubules with the resultant transient or permanent infertility. The mumps virus does not appear to induce TGC transformation and may not be directly injure TGC. Actually, in the mouse, it was demonstrated that mumps virus induced innate immune responses in Sertoli and Leydig cells through TLR 2 and retinoic acid-inducible gene I signaling, resulting in the production of proinflammatory cytokines, including TNF-alpha, IL-6, monocyte chemotactic protein-1, IFN-alpha, and IFN-beta (Wu et al. 2016). By contrast, mumps virus did not induce the cytokine production in TGC. Clinically, serum IL-6 and IFN-gamma levels were elevated in severe mumps cases. Additionally, serum IL-10 level was also elevated in almost all patients with mumps (Wang et al. 2014). AIDS patients often suffer from orchitis, hypogonadism, oligozoospermia, or azoospermia. Lymphocytic infiltration, loss of TGC, and interstitial fibrosis were observed in AIDS patients (Rogers and Klatt 1988; Yoshikawa et al. 1989). It is speculated that the perivascular accumulation of $CD4^+/HIV^+$ cells and cytokine production could affect the integrity of the BTB and favor the development of autoimmune orchitis (Lustig and Tung 2006). Hepatitis B and C viruses and herpes simplex virus have been also found in the interstitial tissue and/or seminiferous tubules in men (Melaine et al. 2003). Granulomatous reactions in the testis have been ascribed to bacterial infections, including tuberculosis, syphilis, leprosy, and brucellosis (Kahn and Mcaninch 1980; Kumar et al. 1982; Roy et al. 2011; Bosilkovski et al. 2016). In most of these cases, the epididymis is primarily and predominantly involved and the testis is secondarily affected. Granulomatous inflammation involves other conditions such as sarcoidosis, malakoplakia, and granulomatous seminoma and lymphoma (Kleinman et al. 1983; Eyselbergs et al. 2011; Bosilkovski et al. 2016). Although these infectious diseases elicit specific immune responses against target virus or bacteria in the testis in early stage, the induced inflammation may break the BTB later and be followed by autoimmune responses in the testis, supporting a diagnosis of autoimmune orchitis.

Shiraishi et al. (2009) examined anti-sperm antibody in the sera of 70 males with systemic autoimmune disease and 80 healthy controls by usage of the indirect immunobead test and the sperm immobilization test. Among 70 males with systemic autoimmune diseases, five were positives, with incidence of 7.1%. However, no positives existed in 80 healthy males. Therefore, systemic autoimmune diseases may be one of the risk factors for developing anti-sperm antibody in men.

3.6 Cellular Immunity in Men

Although anti-sperm antibodies have been noted in testicular autoimmunity in men for long years, the occurrence of delayed-type hypersensitivity (DTH) responses against testicular antigens can be observed in cases of human immunologic infertility (Anderson and Hill 1998), indicating that cellular immunity against the testicular antigens may be also critical for testicular autoimmunity. Leukocyte migration inhibition was positive in infertile males with cryptorchidism, varicocele, genital tract infections, idiopathic oligozospermia, and vasectomy (Nagarkatti and Shanta 1976; Polidori et al. 1980). Recently, clinical studies have shown that macrophage numbers increased in the testes of patients with the spermatogenic disturbance of different etiologies (Frungieri et al. 2002). Previously, patients suffering from prostatic cancer received intra-testicular injection of BCG bilaterally instead of orchidectomy (Frick et al. 1983). Testicular biopsy of the patients revealed that the seminiferous tubules were partially or completely atrophied with hyalinization. Sertoli cells were vacuolated, and mononuclear infiltration was evident in the testicular interstitium. However, tuberculous structures were not seen. It was also reported that immune deviation toward a Th17 immune response was associated with testicular damage in azoospermic men (Duan et al. 2011). Th17 cells are a subset of T helper cells producing IL-17 and create inflammation and tissue injury in autoimmune disease. This indicates that control of not only humoral but also cellular immunity against testicular antigens is important for studying developmental pathways of orchitis and immunotherapeutic approaches for the disease.

A crucial role of Treg-mediated tolerance on prevention of orchitis was indicated by the autoimmune polyendocrinopathy, a condition of spontaneous autoimmunity in a number of endocrine glands, which is characterized by defective $CD4^{+}CD25^{+}$ Treg function (Kriegel et al. 2004). In patients with autoimmune polyendocrinopathy, expression of mRNA and protein of Foxp3 was significantly decreased (Kekalainen

① Active spermatogenesis in normal seminiferous tubules.

↓

② Spermatogenic disturbance in the seminiferous tubules surrounded by lymphocytic inflammation.

↓

③ Severe spermatogenic disturbance in the seminiferous tubules around which lymphocytic inflammation has subsided.

↓

④ Sertoli cell only syndrome and / or maturation arrest in the seminiferous tubules of which basal lamina walls have been thickened, hyalinized and distorted with or without immune complexes.

Fig. 3.3 Sequential changes of the seminiferous epithelium during autoimmune orchitis involved in idiopathic disturbance of spermatogenesis in men

et al. 2007). This suggests that loss of active suppression in the periphery could be a hallmark of this syndrome.

However, there is still little evidence regarding the role of cellular immunity in male infertility in men. In the majority of patients with testicular autoimmunity, there is a chronic and asymptomatic development of the inflammatory reaction. Therefore, this disease is very difficult to be diagnosed at the ongoing stage, and it is possible that many clinical findings of histopathology of idiopathic spermatogenic disturbance are those of the post-active inflammation stage of autoimmune orchitis. In other words, the biopsies from infertile men represent the final stage of the pathological process, and thus the reactive changes such as lymphocytic infiltration might be no longer detectable and only the spermatogenic disturbance remains (Fig. 3.3). Therefore, cellular immune responses may be more critical for male infertility than has been suspected in the past in cases of idiopathic spermatogenic disturbance.

3.7 Histopathology in Autopsy Cases in Men

Hatakeyama (1984) observed the human testes more thoroughly than anyone else previously and reported on the autopsy findings of approximately 400 independently examined patients with or without male infertility, out of which death resulting from some disease occurred in approximately 160 cases, and sudden deaths determined by medical examiners occurred in approximately 240 cases. He documented that autoimmune inflammation should occur in the testes and the epididymides more frequently than in any other organ and that approximately 70% of idiopathic spermatogenic failure is associated with autoimmune phenomena. Here, the immunological fragility of the testes will be discussed using the findings from Hatakeyama's autopsy reports and those from animal experiments.

Approximately 65% cases of male infertility in humans are due to idiopathic spermatogenetic failure (Fig. 3.2). In most cases, however, patients seek medical attention after becoming infertile; as a result, clinical laboratory testing to explore the process leading up to infertility cannot be conducted. In addition, although testicular biopsy is examined in clinical laboratory tests to detect spermatogenic state, the biopsy specimens provide a histological picture of only a very small part of the testis, not allowing the observation of whole testicular tissue. Therefore, Hatakeyama (1984) attempted to determine the pathological mechanism leading to spermatogenetic failure by conducting detailed laboratory examinations of cadaver testes. His review article included notes from the observations of the testes of 159 patients who had died from various diseases and 238 patients in whom sudden death had occurred (Oshima et al. 1984; Hatakeyama 1984). While examining a large number of specimens, a high incidence of "arteriolar hyalinosis in the testes" was found (Fig. 3.4). The incidence was particularly high in patients between 20 and 40 years old, during the period of active spermatogenesis (Fig. 3.4). Though the cause of this "arteriolar hyalinosis" remains unknown, four stressors against testicular arterioles are rapidly activated or increased after puberty. The four stressors are as follows: (1) the requirement of much blood flow for active spermatogenesis after puberty, (2) the rheological change of blood flow by the characteristic meandering of testicular arterioles, (3) the refrigeration of testicular arterioles by the adjacent pampiniform venous plexus in which the venous blood is cooled down in the scrotum, and (4) the permeation of the testosterone to testicular arterioles from the adjacent pampiniform plexus including much testosterone (Fig. 3.5). In particular, these stressors are directed to vascular endothelia of the testicular arterioles and their branches (Takizawa and Hatakeyama 1978). These physiological stressors against the testicular arteriolar endothelium may be a possible cause of induction of focal ischemia due to the vascular endothelial damage. In addition, a harmful effect of this ischemia on the germ cell ducts composed of seminiferous tubules, the tubuli recti, the rete testis, the ductuli efferentes, and epididymal ducts is presumed. At the ischemic area in the testicular interstitium, adjacent germ cell ducts may be damaged, and subsequent inflammation may develop due to leakage of highly autoimmunogenic TGC or epididymal spermatozoa outside the injured germ cell ducts (Fig. 3.5). Lymphocytic infiltration of the ductuli efferentes with ensued peritubular sclerosis has been found in approximately 50% of men in their third decade, which is an extremely high incidence (Hatakeyama 1984; Oshima et al. 1984) (Fig. 3.6). The incidence of inflammatory changes of the epididymis was about 15%, which was much lower than the one in the area of the ductuli efferentes (Oshima et al. 1984). In addition, the incidence of lymphocytic infiltration at various sites in the testicular interstitium has been found to increase gradually with aging (Fig. 3.6). Thus, the ductuli efferentes was described as the "immunological Achilles tendon" by Hatakeyama (1984).

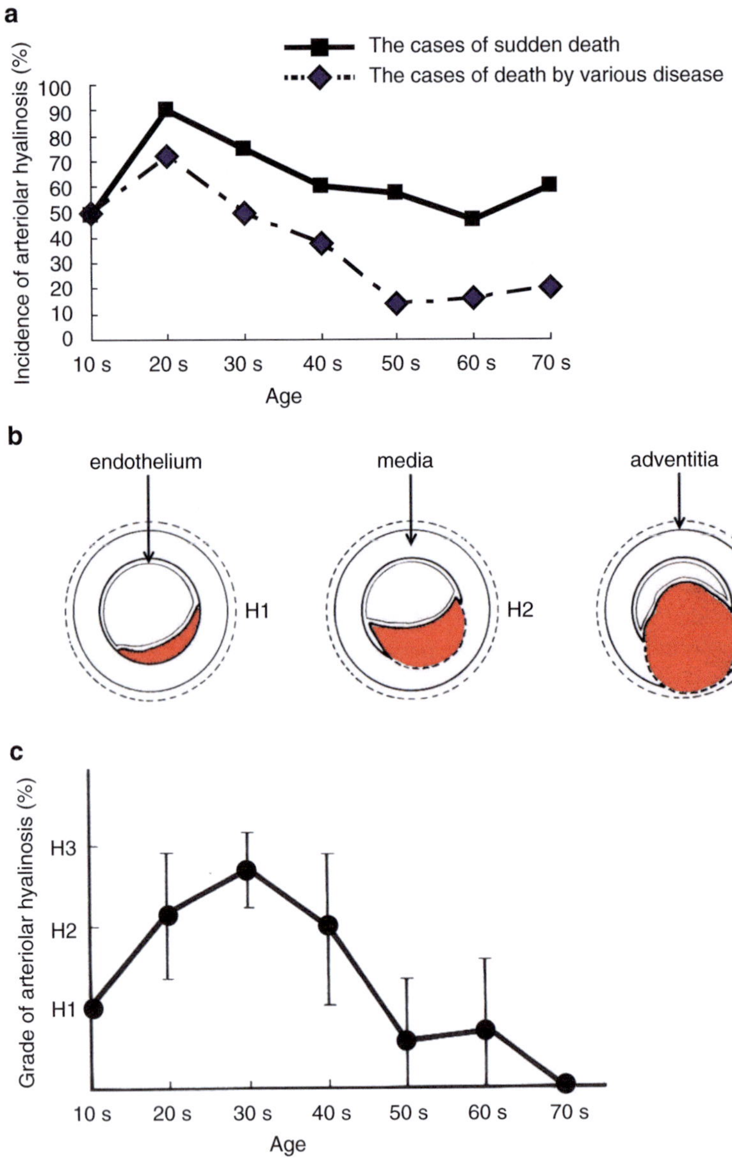

Fig. 3.4 Incidence, classification, and scoring of the arteriolar hyalinosis (H) (Hatakeyama 1984; partly modified). (**a**) The incidence of arteriolar hyalinosis in case of sudden death and death by various diseases. (**b**) The classification of arteriolar hyalinosis based on the extent of pinocytotic vesicle (*red colored*). The pinocytotic vesicles invading subendothelium, media, and adventitia are graded as H1, H2, and H3, respectively. (**c**) The scoring of arteriolar hyalinosis (H1–H3) in case of sudden death

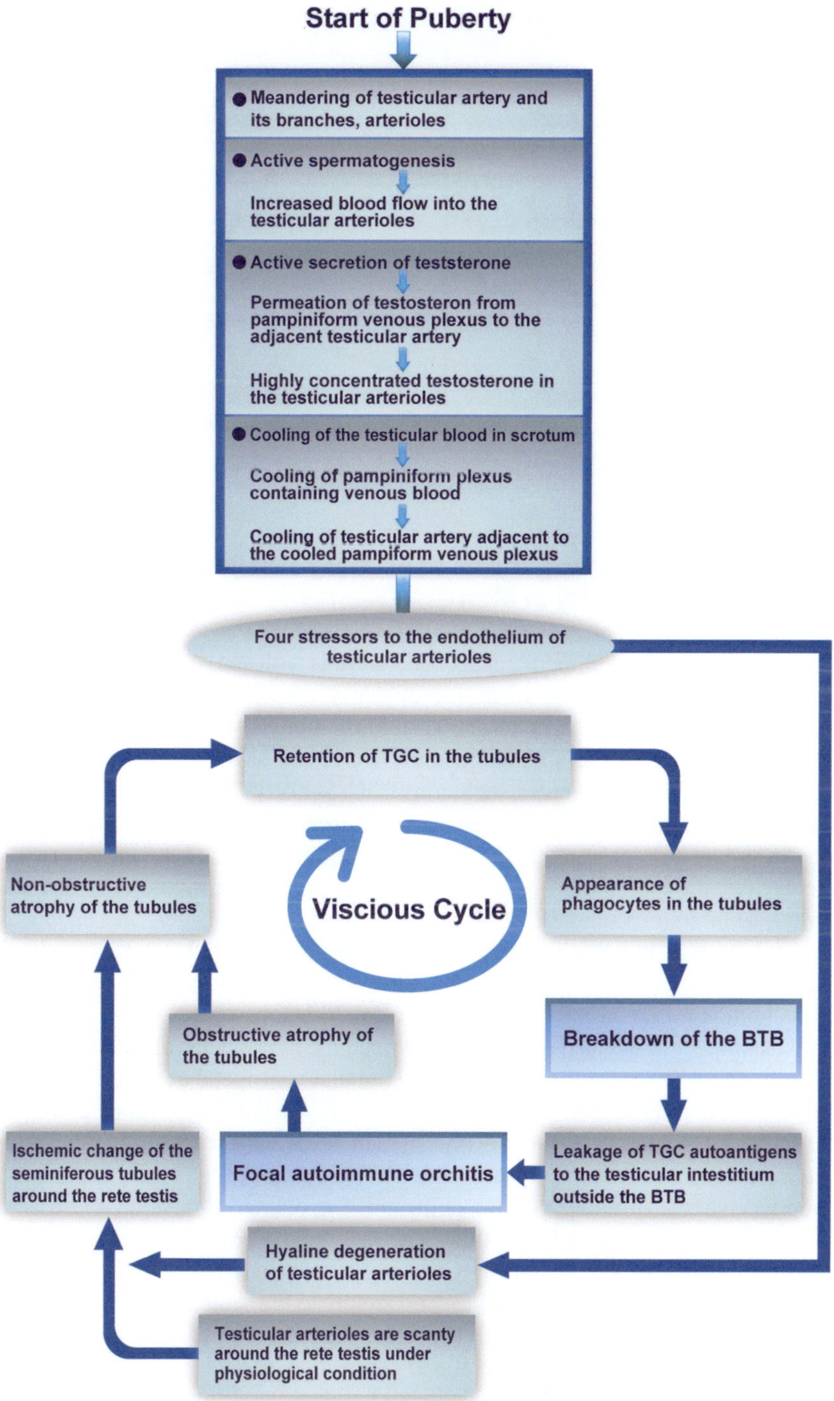

Fig. 3.5 A hypothesis for autoimmune orchitis composed of four stressors to the testicular arterioles and the following vicious cycle resulting in the spermatogenic disturbance after puberty in men (Hatakeyama 1984). *BTB* blood-testis barrier, *TGC* testicular germ cells

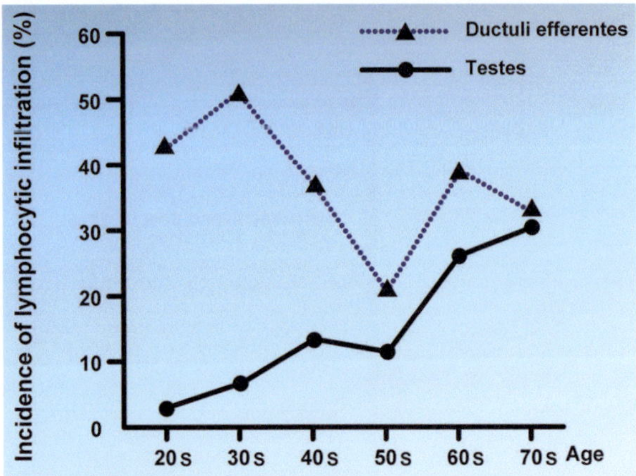

Fig. 3.6 Lymphocytic infiltration in the testis and the ductuli efferentes in men

3.8 Possible Pathogenesis of Primary Testicular Autoimmunity in Men

Primary testicular autoimmunity is isolated orchitis with autoantibodies against testicular antigens but without identified evidence of local or systemic disease or injury. It means that primary testicular autoimmunity is really idiopathic. Many studies pertaining to the spermatogenic disturbance have targeted the elements within the seminiferous tubules, including TGC, Sertoli cells, and their interactions. However, the involvement of tissue microenvironment outside the seminiferous tubules should be considered in the testicular autoimmunity. When viewed in a wide perspective, the spermatogenesis is supported by peritubular myoid cells surrounding the seminiferous tubules, Leydig cells, resident macrophages, and endothelial cells of blood and lymphatic capillaries (Fig. 3.6). Takizawa and Hatakeyama (1978) focused mostly on testis-specific vasculature. Age-associated architectural changes of the human testicular microvasculature from 70 autopsy cases were stereoscopically examined. In the testis of a young subject, the interlobular main arterioles run straight. The coiling phenomena of the interlobular centripetal or centrifugal arterioles are commonly seen in adult testis. It was confirmed that the coiling changes in the interlobular main arterioles of the human testis appear as an age-dependent alteration of the vasculature closely related to the volume of the testis. The practical importance of the spiraling, coiling, or meandering of arterioles is that it results in a considerable reduction of blood flow. The age-related coiling of the interlobular arterioles is virtually accompanied by varying degrees of collapse of the peritubular capillary networks. The reduction of blood supply to the seminiferous tubules plays an active role in promoting aging of the testis. The characteristics of age-associated coiling phenomena in the centripetal and centrifugal arterioles are summarized as follows: (1) coexistence of varying degrees of collapse or disappearance of the peritubular capillary networks, (2) irregular-pitched coiling of the arteriole occasionally with focal conglomeration, and (3) disorganized meandering of the main interlobular arterioles.

The testicular artery and its branches in rats and mice are particularly tortuous and run meanderingly, and fluid dynamic stress on the vascular endothelium is believed to be greater than that found in blood vessels in other organs (Terayama et al. 2005; Hirai and Itoh 2012). In addition, spermatogenesis beginning at puberty is accompanied by a rapid increase in intra-testicular blood flow, and testosterone secreted from Leydig cells passes from the pampiniform venous plexus to the adjacent testicular artery, causing an increase in the intra-arterial testosterone concentration. The venous blood, which is cooled down in the scrotum, lowers the temperature of the testicular artery running among the pampiniform venous plexus (Fig. 3.5). All these facts are believed to act as stressors on the endothelium of the testicular arterioles. Hyalinotic lesions of the testicular arterioles appeared in the beginning of puberty and reached the maximum at the third decade in severity and frequency. Hyaline impregnation begins in the subendothelial layer, most probably as a result of the enhanced transcellular permeability of the endothelium, i.e., cytopempsis or pinocytosis. Hyaline deposits are mainly composed of granular glycolipoprotein that originated from the imported plasmatic fluids and from the secondarily disintegrated basement membrane and elastic lamellae (Hatakeyama 1965; Hatakeyama et al. 1966). These changes terminate in scarring, and the scarred foci increase in number with aging. In addition, the hernia-like protrusion of seminiferous tubules, suggestive of a certain regenerative feature, probably plays more or less a certain role in distortion of delicate ringlike pattern of peritubular capillary networks. In Fig. 3.5, Hatakeyama's concept is represented schematically (Hirai and Itoh 2012). This indicates that physiological stressors to testicular blood vasculature in young adults result in focal ischemia, which damages the BTB, and the resultant leakage of TGC from the damaged BTB to the testicular interstitium evokes local autoimmune responses (focal autoimmune orchitis), which affect the adjacent BTB and injure it accompanied by further leakage of TGC. If this vicious cycle chronically continues, autoimmune orchitis may be developed in the whole testis, leading to male infertility later. Indeed, Nistal et al. (1997) reported granulomatous epididymal lesions of possible ischemic origin. To examine this hypothesis, more information on clinical studies and physiological studies in men should be accumulated.

Spermatogenic disturbance can be induced by various factors (Fig. 3.7). To resolve the pathophysiology, observation of the seminiferous tubules and the surrounding testicular interstitium together is needed in both clinical and experimental examination. In particular, in animal experiments, it is important to observe the whole testis in the following direction: seminiferous tubules→tubuli recti→rete testis→ductuli efferentes→epididymal ducts. Although only a limited area can be histologically examined in human testicular biopsies, we can observe histological changes in whole testis in experimental animals. Furthermore, investigation of spermatogenesis from viewpoints of the circulation of the blood and lymph, the systemic immunity, and the hypothalamic-pituitary-gonadal axis and their combination may be important (Fig. 3.8). Accumulation of these findings should make the pathogenesis in human male infertility of autoimmune origin more clear in the future.

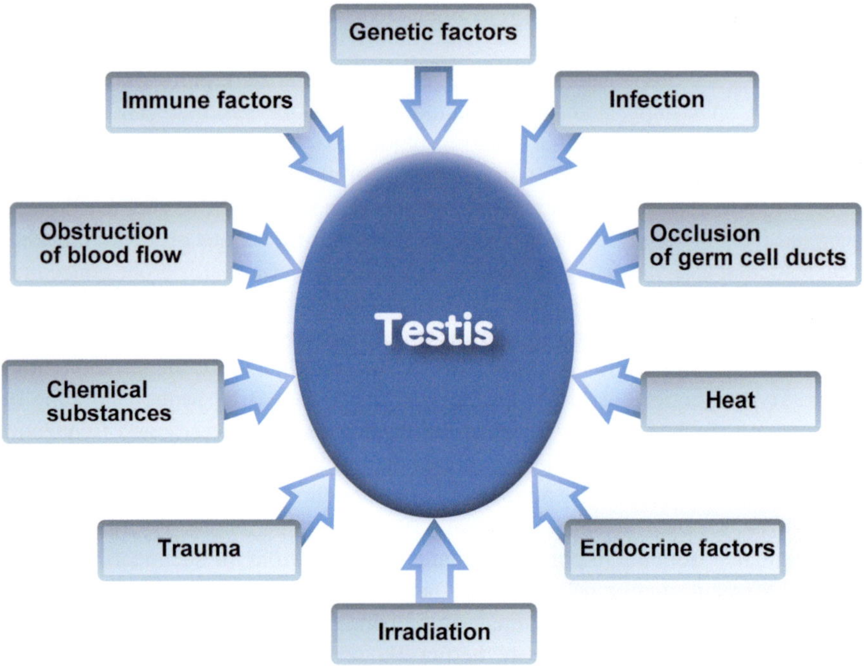

Fig. 3.7 Risk factors in the spermatogenesis

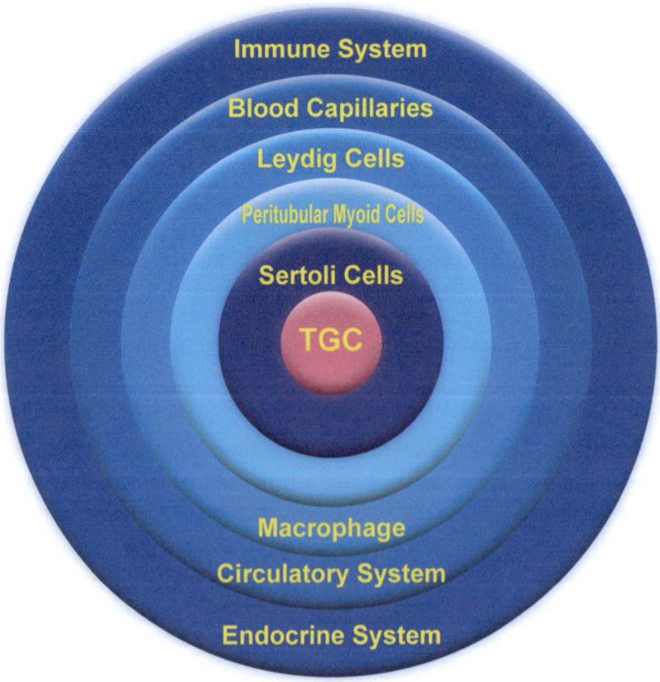

Fig. 3.8 Somatic cell system that surrounds testicular germ cells (TGC) in the testis

3.9 Human Autoimmune Orchitis and the Disease Model in Experimental Animals

Clinical studies that examined the relationship between autoimmune orchitis and male infertility in men have been still poor and limited. Generally, trial of a biopsy of the tubuli recti, the rete testis, and the ductuli efferentes is impossible because of potential obstruction of the passage of spermatozoa from the testes into the epididymis by the biopsy procedure. Therefore, from infertile patients, it is quite difficult to have biopsy data of these sites where the testicular inflammation may preferentially occur (Itoh et al. 2005; Hirai and Itoh 2012). Moreover, there is a possibility that testicular biopsy itself may cause damage to the BTB followed by induction of testicular autoimmunity. This iatrogenic obstruction of the tubular system results in anti-sperm antibody production (Linnet and Hjort 1977; Hjort et al. 1974; Hjort et al. 1982). Mechanical trauma due to the surgical removal of a biopsy specimen has been observed to cause damage to testicular tissue and produce a picture resembling autoimmune orchitis (Sjogren and Ploen 1988; Hendry et al. 1990).

In contrast to clinical data on the relationship between autoimmune orchitis and male infertility that are still lacking, research on experimental autoimmune orchitis (EAO) has been widely conducted in mice, rats, guinea pigs, and other animals as a model of acquired idiopathic spermatogenetic failure. Typical EAO is histologically characterized by lymphocytic inflammation accompanied by spermatogenic disturbance. However, we are aware of the fact that biopsies of human testes rarely show lymphocyte infiltration from reports on male infertility. Therefore, humans and mice may considerably differ in terms of sensitivity to autoimmune orchitis. However, as mentioned earlier, biopsy of the human testis allows for observation of only a very limited area, making identification of the cause of inflammation difficult. In general, patients will receive testicular biopsy after they have been diagnosed with male infertility. Therefore, even in cases of male infertility due to autoimmune orchitis, most patients do not receive testicular biopsy at the initial stage of inflammatory cell infiltration when they are not yet clinically diagnosed. This may result in that testicular biopsy is usually performed when the pathologic condition has reached an advanced stage, in which the inflammatory cell responses have subsided and only the spermatogenic disturbance remains (Fig. 3.3). The differences between the findings reported in autopsy cases and those confirmed in various clinical studies may be explained by the fact that Hatakeyama and his colleagues were able to observe the entire testis instead of only a portion of it and to examine testicular tissue in humans in whom male infertility had not yet developed (Hatakeyama 1984; Oshima et al. 1984). The focal orchitis observed in autopsy cases may have reflected the repair process subsequent to the destruction of the seminiferous tubules and the ductuli efferentes of the testis by focal ischemia, and it may also have involved an autoimmune reaction to the antigens of leaked TGC. Focal orchitis is presumably a chronic inflammation because it mainly involves an infiltration of lymphocytes but not polymorphonuclear leukocytes. In addition, significant deposits of complement, anti-TGC autoantibodies, and irrelevant immunoglobulins in the testes have been found in male infertility patients (Hatakeyama 1984; Oshima et al. 1984). Therefore, a relationship between focal orchitis in men and testicular autoimmunity is supposed to be highly significant (Fig. 3.5).

Conventionally, EAO had been easily induced in guinea pigs by subcutaneous injection of a testicular antigen mixed with complete Freund's adjuvant (CFA) containing killed *Mycobacterium tuberculosis*. For that reason, the use of guinea pigs had been common in the study of EAO; however, in the era of mouse immunology, the development of mouse models of experimental EAO has been desirable and produced by subcutaneously injecting testicular antigen and CFA, followed by intravenous injection of killed *Bordetella pertussis* (BP) antigens (Bernard et al. 1978; Sato et al. 1981; Kohno et al. 1983). Later, Itoh et al. (1991a, b, c) reported that EAO could be easily and simply induced using only subcutaneous injection of TGC freshly collected from syngeneic donor mice and that no adjuvant was necessary for the EAO induction. In animals with unilateral testicular trauma, Naito et al. (2009a) also succeeded in inducing experimental EAO in the testis on the opposite side (=sympathetic EAO) with no immunopotentiating drugs. In various organs other than the testis, experimental induction of autoimmune inflammation is hardly possible by only inflicting traumatic injury to target organs or active immunization with target antigens with no CFA and BP use. This suggests that TGC antigens contain very strong autoimmunogenicity not found in any other cells. In other words, the testicular tissue is most vulnerable for autoimmunity among the various tissues. Therefore, although the testis is regarded as an immune-privileged organ and resistant to inflammation, it is also highly susceptible to autoimmune inflammation (Fig. 3.9).

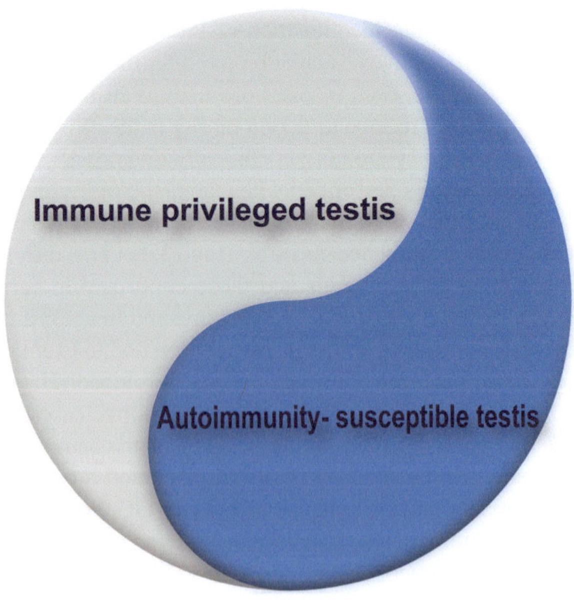

Fig. 3.9 Immunological dual nature of the testis

Since EAO can be induced by only exposing TGC to the immune system outside the BTB with no artificial immune enhancement (Itoh et al. 1991a), it can be said that this disease model is closer to the clinical cases, in which focal ischemia or traumatic injury in the testis damages the seminiferous tubules, followed by leakage of the TGC to the outside of the tubules. In this EAO model, rampant lymphocytic infiltration occurs during the active phase, whereas during the late stages of EAO, lymphocytic infiltration subsides, leaving only irreversible spermatogenetic disturbance (Naito and Itoh 2008; Naito et al. 2009b). At this point, this EAO at late stages closely resembles maturation arrest and Sertoli cell-only syndrome in humans (Fig. 3.3). In addition, as with clinical findings of infertile male patients, both the deposition of complement and immunoglobulins and the resulting thickening of the basal membrane of the seminiferous tubules were also found in the late stages of EAO (Naito et al. 2012a, b). Furthermore, the area of predilection of lymphocytic infiltration in the human testis and the pathological feature in the mouse EAO model are very similar. In both cases, inflammation preferentially developed in and near the mediastinum testis (interstitial tissue adjacent to the tubuli recti and the rete testis) (Naito and Itoh 2008; Naito et al. 2009a). Even under normal circumstances, the distribution of arterioles is poor at the mediastinum testis, making ischemia likely to occur (Hatakeyama 1984). In addition, macrophages are dense in the mediastinum testis, and a few lymphocytes and macrophages also invade the tubuli recti and rete testis (Osman 1979; Tung et al. 1987; Itoh et al. 1995, 1999; Naito et al. 2008; Tainosho et al. 2011). The tissue environment in the tunica albuginea adjacent to the mediastinum testis is also very specific, including components such as highly developed lymphatic capillaries (Hamasaki and Kumabe 1994; Itoh et al. 1998; Hirai et al. 2010, 2012, 2013). Clinically, biopsy at the mediastinum testis is associated with a risk of obstruction of the efferent duct system for germ cells. Thus, biopsy at the mediastinum testis is unsuitable for clinical laboratory tests. Therefore, even if no inflammatory lesion is found on biopsy at some peripheral sites in the testes of male infertility patients, the potential for inflammation at the mediastinum testis remains.

References

Agarwal S, Choudhury M, Banerjee A. Mast cells and idiopathic male infertility. Int J Fertil. 1987;32:283–6.

Agarwal V, Li JKH, Bard R. Lymphocytic orchitis: a case report. Hum Pathol. 1990;21:1080–2.

Aiman J, Brenner PF, MacDonald PC. Androgen and estrogen production in elderly men with gynecomastia and testicular atrophy after mumps orchitis. J Clin Endocrinol Metab. 1980;50:380–6.

Aitchison K, Mufti GR, Farrell J, Paterson PJ, Scott R. Granulomatous orchitis. Review of 15 cases. Br J Urol. 1990;66:312–4.

Alba MA, Moreno-Palacios J, Beca S, Cid MC. Urologic and male genital manifestations of granulomatosis with polyangitis. Autoimmun Rev. 2015;14:897–902.

Anderson DJ, Hill JA. Cell-mediated immunity in infertility. Am J Reprod Immunol Microbiol. 1998;17:22–30.

Apa DD, Cayan S, Polat A, Akbay E. Mast cells and fibrosis on testicular biopsies in male infertility. Arch Androl. 2002;48:337–44.

Aslani F, Schuppe HC, Guazzone VA, Bhushan S, Wahle E, Lochnit G, Lustig L, Meinhardt A, Fijak M. Targeting high mobility group box protein 1 ameliorates testicular inflammation in experimental autoimmune orchitis. Hum Reprod. 2014.; pii:deu320

Bernard CCA, Mitchell GF, Leydon J, Bargerbos A. Experimental autoimmune orchitis in T-cell-deficient mice. Int Arch Allergy Appl Immunol. 1978;56:256–63.

Bosilkovski M, Kamiloski V, Miskova S, Balalovski D, Kotevska V, Petrovski M. 2016. Testicular infection in brucellosis: report of 34 cases. J Microbiol Imunol Infect. pii: S1684–1182(16)30004–4.

Bouloux PMG, Wass JAH, Parslow JM, Hendry WF, Besser GM. Effect of cyclosporine A in male autoimmune infertility. Fertil Steril. 1986;46:81–5.

Bozhedomov VA, Lipatova NA, Rokhlikov IM, Alexeev RA, Ushakova IV, Sukhikh GT. Male fertility and varicocele: role of immune factors. Andrology. 2014;2:51–8.

Chabon AB, Stenger RJ, Grabstald H. Histopathology of testis in acquired immune deficiency syndrome. Urology. 1987;29:658–63.

Chandrashekar P, Sathiasekar AC, Namaratha K, Singarayan JL, Gnanam AP. A rare case of mumps orchitis. J Parm Bioallied Sci. 2015;7:S773–5.

Dahl EV, Baggenstoss AH, De Weerd JH. Testicular lesions of periarteritis nodosa, with special reference to diagnosis. Am J Med. 1960;28:222–8.

D'Cruz OJ, Haas GG, de La Rocha R, Lambert H. Occurrence of serum antisperm antibodies in patients with cystic fibrosis. Fertil Steril. 1991;56:519–27.

De Buy Wenniger LM, Scheltema JM, Verheij J, Beuers U. Testicular inflammation as a new manifestation of IgG4-associated disease. Urology. 2013;82:15–6.

De Kretser DM, Kerr JB, Paulsen CA. The peritubular tissue in the normal and pathological human testis. An ultrastructural study. Biol Reprod. 1975;12:317–24.

De Paepe ME, Waxman M. Testicular atrophy in AIDS: a study of 57 autopsy cases. Hum Pathol. 1989;20:210–4.

Diekman AB, Norton EJ, Westbrook A, Klotz KL, Naaby-Hansen S, Herr JC. Anti-sperm antibodies from infertile patients and their cognate sperm antigens: A Review. Identity between SAGA-1, the H6-3C4 antigen, and CD52. Am J Reprod Immunol. 2000;43:134–43.

Duan TG, CF Y, Novak N, Bieber T, Zhu CH, Schuppe HC, Haidl G, Allam JP. Immunodeviaiton towards a Th17 immune response associated with testicular damage in azoospermic men. Int J Androl. 2011;34:536–45.

Eid N, Shibata M, Ito Y, Kusakabe K, Hammad H, Otsuki Y. Involvement of Fas system and active caspases in apoptotic signaling in testicular germ cells of ethanol-treated rats. Int J Androl. 2002;25:159–67.

El-Demiry MI, Hargreave TB, Busuttil A, James K, Ritchie AWS, Chisholm GD. Lymphocyte subpopulation in the male genital tract. Br J Urol. 1985;57:769–74.

El-Demiry MI, Elton R, Hargreave TB, James K, Busuttil A, Chisholm GD. Immunocompetent cells in human testis in health and disease. Fertil Steril. 1987;48:470–9.

Eyselbergs M, D'Hauwe R, De Cuyper K, Camerlinck M, Van Aken B, Oyen R, Vanhoenacker FM. Testicular sarcoidosis. JBR-BTR. 2011;94:199–201.

Francavilla F, Romano R, Santucci R, La Verghetta G, D'Abrizio P, Francavilla S. Naturally-occurring antisperm antibodies in men: interference with fertility and implications for treatment. Front. Bioscience. 1999;4:e9–e25.

Francavilla F, Santucci R, Barbonetti A, Francavilla S. Naturally-occurring antisperm antibodies in men: Interference with fertility and clinical implications. An update. Front Biosci. 2007;12:2890–911.

Frick J, Kunit G, Joos H, Rovan E, Talwar GP. Effect of intratesticular administration of BCG on testicular function. Int Urol Nephrol. 1983;15:71–81.

Frungieri M, Calandra RS, Lustig L, Meineke V, Kohn FM, Vogt HJ, Mayerhofer A. Number, distribution pattern, and identification of macrophages in testes of infertile men. Fertil Steril. 2002;78:298–306.

Haidl G, Duan YG, Chen SJ, Kohn FM, Schuppe HC, Allam JP. The role of mast cells in male infertility. Expert Rev Clin Immunol. 2011;7:627–34.

Hall JL, Engel D, Naz RK. Significance of antibodies against human sperm FA-1 antigen in immunoinfertility. Arch Androl. 1994;32:25–30.
Hamasaki M, Kumabe T. Three-dimensional structure of two different lymphatic spaces in rat testis, and the route of flow fluxes of their lymphatic fluids. Kaibogaku Zassi. 1994;69:669–83.
Handelsman DJ, Conway AJ, Radonic I, Turtle JR. Prevalence, testicular function and seminal parameters in men with sperm antibodies. Clin Reprod Fertil. 1983;2:39–45.
Hassanin AM, Ayad E. The impact of chronic testicular inflammatory infiltration on spermatogenesis in azoospermic men, evidence-based pilot study. Middle East Fertility Society Journal 21 2016;(1):31–35.
Hatakeyama S. A study on the interstitial cells of the human testis, especially on their fine-structural pathology. Acta Pathol Jpn. 1965;15:155–96.
Hatakeyama S, Sengoku R, Takayama S. Histological and submicroscopic studies on arteriolar hyalinosis of the human testis. Bull Tokyo Med Dent Univ. 1966;13:511–30.
Hatakeyama S. Pathology of human testicular atrophy. J Jpn Soc Pathol. 1984;73:3–29.
Hedger MP. Immunophysiology and pathology of inflammation in the testis and epididymis. J Androl. 2011;32:625–40.
Hendry WF, Stedronska J, Hughes L, Cameron KM, Pugh RC. Steroid treatment of male subfertility caused by antisperm antibodies. Lancet. 1979;2(8141):498–501.
Hendry WF, Parslow JM, Parkinson C. Immune orchitis: A rare but treatable cause of azospermia in man. J Androl. 1985;6:54–9.
Hendry WF, Levison DA, Parkinson MC, Parslow JM, Royle MG. Testicular obstruction: clinicopathological studies. Ann R Coll Surg Engl. 1990;72:396–407.
Hernandez-Rodriguez J, Tan CD, Koening CL, Khasnis A, Rodriguez ER, Hoffman GS. Testicular vasculitis: findings differentiating isolated disease from systemic disease in 72 patients. Medicine. 2012;91:75–85.
Hirai S, Naito M, Terayama H, Qu N, Miura M, Shirakami G, Itoh M. Differences in abundance of blood and lymphatic capillaries in the murine epididymis. Med Mol Morphol. 2010;43:37–42.
Hirai S, Naito M, Terayama H, Qu N, Kuerban M, Musha M, Ikeda A, Miura M, Itoh M. The origin of lymphatic capillaries in murine testes. J Androl. 2012;33:745–51.
Hirai S, Itoh M. Testicular autoimmunity in men. Its suggestion that a Japanese pathologist left. Reprod Immunol Biol. 2012;27:7–13.
Hirai S, Naito M, Terayama H, Qu N, Kuerban M, Musha M, Itoh M. Lymphangiogenesis in chronic inflammation in the testis. Andrology. 2013;1:147–54.
Hjort T, Husted S, Linnet-Jepsen P. The effect of testis biopsy on autosensitization against spermatozoal antigens. Clin Exp Immunol. 1974;18:201–12.
Hjort T, Linnet L, Skakkebeak NE. Testicular biopsy: indications and complications. Eur J Periatr. 1982;138:23–5.
Hussein MR, Abou-Deif ES, Bedaiwy MA, Said TM, Mustafa MG, Nada E, Ezat A, Agarwal A. Phenotypic characterization of the immune and mast cell infiltrates in the human testis shows normal and abnormal spermatogenesis. Fertil Steril. 2005;83:1447–53.
Ike A, Tokuhiro K, Hirose M, Nozaki M, Nishimune Y, Tanaka H. Comprehensive analysis of gene expression in testes producing haploid germ cells using DNA microarray analysis. Int J Androl. 2007;30:462–75.
Irani AMA, Schwartz LB. Mast cell heterogeneity. Clin Exp Allergy. 1989;19:143–55.
Ishidori A, Dondero F, Lenzi A. Immunobiology of male infertility. Hum Reprod. 1988;3:75–7.
Itoh M, Hiramine C, Hojo K. A new murine model of autoimmune orchitis induced by immunization with viable syngeneic testicular germ cells alone. I. Immunological and histological studies. Clin Exp Immunol. 1991a;83:137–42.
Itoh M, Hiramine C, Tokunaga Y, Mukasa A, Hojo K. A new murine model of autoimmune orchitis induced by immunization with viable syngeneic testicular germ cells alone. II. Immunohistochemical findings of fully-developed lesion. Autoimmunity. 1991b;10:89–97.
Itoh M, Mukasa A, Tokunaga Y, Hiramine C, Hojo K. New experimental model for adoptive transfer of murine autoimmune orchitis. Andrologia. 1991c;23:415–20.
Itoh M, de-Rooij DG, Jansen A, Drexhage HA. Phenotypical heterogeneity of testicular macrophages/dendritic cells in normal adult mice: an immunohistochemical study. J Reprod Immunol. 1995;28:217–32.

Itoh M, Li XQ, Yano A, Xiw Q, Takeuchi Y. Patterns of efferent lymphatics of the mouse testis. Int J Androl. 1998;19:466–72.
Itoh M, Xie Q, Miyamoto K, Takeuchi Y. F4/80-positive cells rapidly accumulate around tubuli recti and rete testis between 3 and 4 weeks of age in the mouse: an immunohistochemical study. Am J Reprod Immunol. 1999;42:321–6.
Itoh M, Terayama H, Naito M, Ogawa Y, Tainosho S. Tissue microcircumstances for leukocytic infiltration into the testis and epididymis in mice. J Reprod Immunol. 2005;67:57–67.
Jahnukainen K, Jorgensen N, Pollanen P, Giwercman A, Skakebaek NE. Incidence of testicular mononuclear cell infiltrates in normal human males and in patients with germ cell neoplasia. Int J Androl. 1995;18:313–20.
Jala H, Bahadur G, Knowles W, Jin L, Brink N. Mumps epididymo-orchitis with prolonged detection of virus in semen and the development of anti-sperm antibodies. J Med Viol. 2004;73:147–50.
Jerne N. Toward a network theory of the immune system. Ann Immunol (Paris). 1974;125C:373–89.
Jezek D, Banek L, Hittmair A, Pezerovic-Panijan R, Goluza T, Schulze W. Mast cell in testicular biopsies of infertile men with 'mixed atrophy' of seminiferous tubules. Andrologia. 1999;31:203–10.
Jodot-van de Casseye M, De Bled G, Gepts W, Schoysman R. An immunohistochemical study for testicular biopsies in cases of male infertility. Andrologia. 1980;12:122–9.
Kahn RI, Mcaninch JW. Granulomatous disease of the testis. J Urol. 1980;123:868–71.
Karram S, Kao CS, Osunkoya AO, Ulbright TM, Epstein JI. Idiopathic granulomatous orchitis: morphology and evaluation of its relationship to IgG4 related disease. Hum Pathol. 2014;45:844–50.
Kekalainen E, Tuovinen H, Joensuu J, Gylling M, Franssila R, Pontynen N, Talvensaari K, Perheentupa J, Miettinen A, Arstila TP. A defect of regulatory T cells in patients with autoimmune polyendocrinopathy-candidiasis-ectodermal dystrophy. J Immunol. 2007;178:1208–15.
Kim SK, Yoon YD, Park TS, Seo JT, Kim JH. Involvement of the Fas-Fas ligand system and active caspase-3 in abnormal apoptosis in human testes with maturation arrest and Sertoli cell-only syndrome. Fertil Steril. 2007;87:547–53.
Klein FA, Vick CW, Schneider V. Bilateral granulomatous orchitis: manifestation of idiopathic systemic granulomatosis. J Urol. 1985;134:762–4.
Kleinman SZ, Robinson ND, Simon SA. Malakoplakia of testis. Urology. 1983;22:194–7.
Klune JR, Dhupar R, Cardinal J, Billiar TR, Tsung A. HMGB1: endogenous danger signaling. Mol Med. 2008;14:476–84.
Kohno S, Munoz JA, Williams TM, Teuscher C, Bernard CC, Tung KS. Immunopathology of murine experimental allergic orchitis. J Immunol. 1983;130:2675–82.
Kriegel MA, Lohmann T, Gabler C, Blank N, Kalden JR, Lorenz HM. Defective suppressor function of human $CD4^+CD25^+$ regulatory T cells in autoimmune polyglandular syndrome type II. J Exp Med. 2004;199:1285–91.
Kumar B, Raina A, Kaur S, Dash RJ, Samuel DE, Datta BN. Clinico-pathological study of testicular involvement in leprosy. Lepr India. 1982;54:48–55.
Lee R, Goldstein M, Ullery BW, Ehrlich J, Soares M, Razzano RA, Herman MP, Callahan MA, Li PS, Schlegel PN, Witkin SS. Value of serum antisperm antibodies in diagnosing obstructive azoospermia. J Urol. 2009;181:264–9.
Lehmann D, Temminck B, Litmanen K, Leibundgut B, Hadziselimovic F, Muller HJ. Autoimmune phenomena and cytogenetic findings in a patient with carcinoma (seminoma) in situ. Cancer. 1986;58:2013–7.
Lehmann D, Muller H. Analysis of the autoimmune response in an 'in situ' carcinoma of the testis. Int J Androl. 1987;10:163–8.
Lehmann D, Temminch D, Da-Rugna D, Leibundgut B, Sulmoni A, Muller HJ. Role of immunological factors in male infertility: immunohistochemical and serological evidence. Lab Investig. 1987;57:21–8.
Lehmann D, Emmons LR. Immunological phenomena observed in the testis and their possible role in infertility. Am J Reprod Immunol. 1989;19:43–52.

Lie JT. Isolated polyarteritis of testis in hairy-cell leukemia. Arch Pathol Lab Med. 1988;112:646–7.
Lin W, Lu S, Chen H, Wu Q, Fei Y, Li M, Zhang X, Tian X, Zeng W, Leng X, Xu D, Wang Q, Shen M, Wang L, Li J, Wu D, Zhao L, Wu C, Yang Y, Peng ZJ, Wang Y, Sha Y, Huang X, Jiao Y, Zeng X, Shi Q, Li P, Zhang S, Hu C, Deng C, Li Y, Zhang S, Liu J, Su J, Hou Y, Jiang Y, You X, Zhang H, Yan L, Zhang W, Zhao Y, Zeng X, Zhang F, Lipsky PE. Clinical characteristics of immunoglobulin G4-related disease: a prospective study of 118 Chinese patients. Rheumatology. 2015;54:1982–90.
Linnet L, Hjort T. Sperm agglutinins in seminal plasma and serum after vasectomy: correlation between immunological and clinical findings. Clin Exp Immunol. 1977;30:413–20.
Lustig L, Tung KS. Orchitis and male infertility. The autoimmune diseases. 4th ed. Amsterdam: Elsevier Academic Press; 2006. p. 841–7.
Maclaren N, Chen QY, Kukreja A, Marker J, Zhang CH, Sun ZS. Autoimmune hypogonadism as part of an autoimmune polyglandular syndrome. J Soc Gynecol Investig. 2001;8:52–4.
Maseki T, Miyake K, Mitsuya H, Kitamura H, Yamada K. Mastocytosis occurring in the testes from patients with idiopathic male infertility. Fertil Steril. 1981;36:814–7.
Mathur S, Williamson HO, Baker ER, Fudenberg HH. Immunoglobulin E levels and antisperm antibody titiers in infertile couples. Am J Obstet Gynecol. 1981;140:923–30.
Matsuki S, Sasagawa I, Suzuki Y, Yazawa H, Tateno T, Hashimoto T, Nakada T, Saito H, Hiroi M. The use of ebastine, a mast cell blocker, for treatment of oligozoospermia. Arch Androl. 2000;44:129–32.
Matsumura M, Taketani T, Horie A, Mizota Y, Nakata S, Kumori K, Nagase M, Harada Y, Tanaka Y, Yamaguchi S. Pediatric granulomatous orchitis: Case report and review of the literature. Padiat Int. 2016;58:155–8.
Melaine N, Ruffault A, Dejucq-Rainsford N, Jegou B. Experimental inoculation of the adult rat testis with Sendai virus: effect on testicular morphology and leukocyte population. Hum Reprod. 2003;18:1574–9.
Menge AC, Christman GM, Ohl DA, Naz RK. 1999. Fertilization antigen-1 removes antisperm autoantibodies from spermatozoa of infertile men and results in increased rates of acrosome reaction. 71, 256–260.
Migita K, Miyashita T, Mizuno A, Jiuchi Y, Ito M, Matsuo M, Izumi Y, Takeoka A, Nishino A, Hayashi M. IgG4-related epididymo-orchitis associated with bladder cancer: possible involvement of BAFF/BAFF-R interaction in IgG4-related urogenital disease. Mod Rheumatol. 2014;24:188–94.
Morgan AD. Inflammation and infestation of the testis and paratesticular structures. In: Pugh, RCB, pathology of the testis. Oxford: Blackwell; 1976. p. 79–138.
Nagai T, Takaba H, Miyake K, Hirabayashi Y, Yamada K. Testicular mast cell heterogeneity in idiopathic male infertility. Fertil Steril. 1992;57:1331–6.
Nagarkatti PS, Shanta RS. Cell-mediated immunity to homologous spermatozoa following vasectomy in the human male. Clin Exp Immunol. 1976;26:239–42.
Naito M, Terayama H, Hirai S, Qu N, Moriyama H, Itoh M. The presence of intra-tubular lymphocytes in normal testis of the mouse. Okajimas Folia Anat Jpn. 2008;85:91–6.
Naito M, Itoh M. Patterns of infiltration of lymphocytes into the testis under normal and pathological conditions in mice. Am J Reprod Immunol. 2008;59:55–61.
Naito M, Sakamoto Y, Terayama H, Hirai S, Qu N, Aota Y, Itoh M. Effect of unilateral testicular rupture on histopathology and germ cell delayed-type hypersensitivity in C3H/He and A/J mice. J Reprod Immunol. 2009a;81:55–61.
Naito M, Terayama H, Hirai S, Qu N, Kawata S, Itoh M. Histopathology of the tubuli recti at the start of experimental autoimmune orchitis in mice. Med Mo Morphol. 2009b;42:230–5.
Naito M, Hirai S, Terayama H, Qu N, Kuerban M, Musha M, Kitaoka M, Ogawa Y, Itoh M. Post-inflammation stage of autoimmune orchitis induced by immunization with syngeneic testicular germ cells alone in mice. Med Mol Morphol. 2012a;45:35–44.
Naito M, Terayama H, Hirai S, Qu N, Lustig L, Itoh M. Experimental autoimmune orchitis as a model of immunological male infertility. Med Mol Morphol. 2012b;45:185–9.
Naz RK. Human synthetic peptide vaccine for contraception targeting sperm. Arch Androl. 2004;50:113–9.

Nistal M, Santamaria L, Paniagua R. Mast cells in the human testis and epididymis from birth to adulthood. Acta Anat. 1984;119:155–60.
Nistal M, Mate A, Paniagua R. Granulomatous epididymal lesion of possible ischemic origin. Am J Surg Pathol. 1997;21:951–6.
Nistal M, Riestra ML, Paniagua R. Focal orchitis in undescended testes. Arch Pathol Lab Med. 2002;126:64–9.
Oshima S, Okayasu I, Uchima H, Hatakeyama S. Histopathological and morphometrical study of the human epididymis and testis. Acta Pathol Jpn. 1984;34:1327–42.
Osman DI. A comparative ultrastructural study on typical and modified Sertoli cells before and after ligation of the efferent ductules in the rabbit. Zbl Vet Med C Anat Histo Embryo. 1979;8:114–23.
Pannek J, Haupt G. Orchitis due to vasculitis in autoimmune diseases. Scand J Rheumatol. 1997;26:151–4.
Perimenis P, Athanasopoulos A, Venetsanou-Petrochilou C, Barbalias G. Idiopathic granulomatous orchitis. Eur Urol. 1991;19:118–20.
Piton N, Roquet ML, Sibert L, Sabourin JC. Focal non-granulomatous orchitis in a patient with Crohn's disease. Diagn Pathol. 2015;10:39. doi:10.1186/s13000-015-0273-5.
Polidori R, Ambrogi F, Izzo PL, Mariani M, Grassi B, Menchini Fabris GF. Cell-mediated immunity in male fertility. Immunological infertility in man. Andrologia. 1980;12:141–5.
Pudney J, Anderson D. Orchitis and human immunodeficiency virus type I infected cells in reproductive tissues from men with the acquired immune deficiency syndrome. Am J Pathol. 1991;139:149–60.
Ramonda R, Foresta C, Ortolan A, Bertoldo A, Oliviero F, Lorenzin M, Pizzol D, Punzi L, Garolla A. Influence of tumor necrosis factor alpha inhibitors on testicular function and semen in spondyloarthritis patients. Fertil Steril. 2014;101:359–65.
Reimand K, Perheentupa J, Link M, Krohn K, Peterson P, Uibo R. Testis-expressed protein TSGA10 an auto-antigen in autoimmune polyendocrine syndrome type I. Int Immunol. 2008;20:39–44.
Rogers C, Klatt EC. Pathology of the testis in acquired immunodeficiency syndrome. Histopathology. 1988;12:659–65.
Rosi P, Carini M, Gambacorta G, Mottola A, Selli C. Granulomatous orchitis: clinical and pathologic aspects. Eur Urol. 1984;10:130–2.
Roy S, Hosoda S, Parwani AV. Idiopathic granulomatous orchitis. Pathol Res Pract. 2011;207:275–8.
Salomon F, Hedinger CE. Abnormal basement membrane structures of seminiferous tubules in infertile men. Lab Investig. 1982;47:543–54.
Salomon F, Saremaslani P, Jakob M, Hedinger CF. Immune complex orchitis in infertile men. Immunoelectron microscopy of abnormal basement membrane structures. Lab Investig. 1982;47:555–67.
Sato K, Hirokawa K, Hatakeyama S. Experimental allergic orchitis in mice. Histopathological and immunological studies. Virchows Arch A Pathol Anat Histol. 1981;392:147–58.
Schwartz LB, Austen KF. Structure and function of the chemical mediators of mast cells. Prog Allergy. 1984;34:271–321.
Shibahara H, Shiraishi Y, Suzuki M. Diagnosis and treatment of immunologically infertile males with antisperm antibodies. Reprod Med Biol. 2005;4:133–41.
Shiraishi Y, Shibahara H, Koriyama J, Hirano Y, Okazaki H, Minota S, Suzuki M. Incidence of antisperm antibodies in males with systemic autoimmune diseases. Am J Reprod Immunol. 2009;61:183–9. doi:10.1111/j1600-0897.
Shurbaji MS, Epstein JI. Testicular vasculitis. Hum Pathol. 1988;19:186–9.
Silva CA, Cocuzza M, Borba EF, Bonfa E. Cutting-edge issues in autoimmune orchitis. Clinic Rev Allerg Immunol. 2012;42:256–63.
Silva CA, Cocuzza M, Carvalho JF, Bonfa E. Diagnosis and classification of autoimmune orchitis. Autoimmun Rev. 2014;13:431–4.
Sjogren I, Ploen L. Restricted lesions after testicular biopsies in young and adult rats. Int J Androl. 1988;11:525–31.

Smith CJ, Oscarson M, Ronnblom L, Alimohammadi M, Perheentupa J, Husebye ES, Gustafsson J, Nordmark G, Meloni A, Crock PA, Kampe O, Bensing S. TSGA10 – A target for autoantibodies in autoimmune polyendocrine syndrome type 1 and systemic lupus erythematosus. Scand J Immunol. 2011;73:147–53.

Sporer A, Seebode JJ. Granulomatous orchitis. Urology. 1982;19:319–21.

Suominen J, Soderstrom KO. Lymphocytic infiltration in human testicular biopsies. Int J Androl. 1982;5:461–6.

Suominen J. Sympathetic auto-immune orchitis. Andrologia. 1995;27:213–6.

Tainosho S, Naito M, Hirai S, Terayama H, Qu N, Itoh M. Multilayered structure of the basal lamina of tubuli recti in normal mice. Med Mol Morphol. 2011;44:34–8.

Takizawa T, Hatakeyama S. Age-associated changes in microvasculature of human adult testis. Acta Pathol Jpn. 1978;28:541–54.

Tarabuta-Cordun G. "Nonspecific" granulomatous orchitis. Morphol Embryol. 1983;29:103–8.

Taylor TA, Scott DG, Anderson CK, Jones N, Stewart PAH. Immunological studies of testicular tissue in oligozoospermic and azoospermic patients. J Urol. 1978;50:419–22.

Tchiokadze SH, Galdava G. Clinical and anamnestic characteristics of development of antisperm immunity in infertile men. Georgian Med News. 2015;246:18–22.

Terada T, Hatakeyama S. Morphological evidence for two types of idiopathic 'Sertoli-cell-only' syndrome. Int J Androl. 1991;14:117–26.

Terayama H, Naito M, Nakamura Y, Iimura A, Itoh M, Tamatsu Y, Shimada K. Corrosion casts of convoluted testicular arteries in mice and rats. Arch Androl. 2005;51:471–80.

Tsatsoulis A, Shalet SM. Antisperm antibodies in the polyglandular autoimmune (PGA) syndrome type I: response to cyclical steroid therapy. Clin Endocrinol. 1991;35:299–303.

Tung KS, Cooke WD, McCarty TA, Robitaille P. Human sperm antigens and antisperm antibodies. II. Age-related incidence of antisperm antibodies. Clin Exp Immunol. 1976;25:73–9.

Tung KS, Yule TD, Mahi-Brown CA, Listrom MB. Distribution of histopathology and Ia positive cells in actively induced and passively transferred experimental autoimmune orchitis. J Immunol. 1987;138:752–9.

Tung KS. Autoimmune disease of the testis and the ovary. The autoimmune diseases. 3rd ed. California: Academic Press; 1998. p. 687–704.

Ulcova-Gallova Z, Gruberova J, Bibkova K, Micanova Z, Novotny Z, Rokyta Z. Antibodies against laminin-1 and sperm, intraacrosomal proteins in semen from infertile couples. Syst Biol Reprod Med. 2008;54:211–6.

Villiger PM, Caliezi G, Cottin V, Forger F, Senn A, Ostensen M. Effects of TNF antagonists on sperm characteristics in patients with spondyloarthritis. Ann Rheum Dis. 2010;69:1842–4.

Vu Van H, Grimaud JA, Cognat M. Immunoglobulin deposits and testis tubular membrane pathology in human sterility. Arch Androl. 1978;1:351–3.

Wall JR, Stedronska J, Lessof MH. Antibodies against Sertoli cells in human infertility. Clin Endocrinol. 1974;3:187–94.

Wang W, Zhu Y, Wu H, Jiao Y, Van Halm-Lutterodt N, Li W. IL-6 and IFN-gamma are elevated in severe mumps cases: a study of 960 mumps patients in China. J Infect Dev Ctries. 2014;8:208–14.

Wegner HEH, Loy V, Diekmann KP. Granulomatous orchitis – an analysis of clinical presentation, pathological anatomic features and possible etiologic factors. Eur Urol. 1994;26:56–60.

Welter H, Kohn FM, Mayerhofer A. Mast cells in human testicular biopsies from patients with mixed atrophy: increased numbers, heterogeneity, and expression of cyclooxygenase 2 and prostaglandin D2 synthase. Fertil Steril. 2011;96:309–13. doi:10.1016/j.fertnstert.2011.05.035.

Witkin SS, Zelikovsky G, Bongiovanni AN, Geller N, Good RA, Day NK. Sperm-related antigens, antibodies, and circulating immune complexes in sera of recently vasectomized men. J Clin Invest. 1982;70:33–40.

Wu H, Shi L, Wang Q, Cheng L, Zhao X, Chen Q, Jiang Q, Feng M, Li Q, Han D. Mumps virus-induced innate immune responses in mouse Sertoli and Leydig cells. Sci Rep. 2016;6:19507. doi:10.1038/srep19507.

Yamamoto M, Hibi H, Miyake K. New treatment of idiopathic severe oligoospermia with mast cells blocker: results of a single-blind study. Fertil Steril. 1995;64:1221–3.

Yoshikawa Y, Truong LD, Fraire AE, Kim HS. The spectrum of histopathology of the testis in acquired immunodeficiency syndrome. Mol Pathol. 1989;2:233–8.

Zanchetta R, Mastrogiacomo I, Graziotti P, Foresta C, Betterle C. Autoantibodies against Leydig cells in patients after spermatic cord torsion. Clin Exp Immunol. 1984;55:49–57.

Testicular Autoimmunity by Immunization with Testicular Antigens Alone in Experimental Animals

4

4.1 Introduction of Autoimmune Orchitis in Experimental Animals

Testicular autoimmunity in experimental animals can be divided into "spontaneous" and "experimental" autoimmune orchitis (EAO).

Spontaneous autoimmune orchitis was reported in the dog (Fritz et al. 1976; Davidson et al. 2015), the mink (Tung et al. 1981, 1984; Pelletier et al. 2009), the rat (Furbeth et al. 1989), and the mouse (Robinson et al. 1994). The pathology of the spontaneous orchitis involves lymphocytic infiltration, spermatogenic disturbance, and deposits of immune complexes in the basal lamina of seminiferous tubules with appearance of serum anti-TGC autoantibodies; however, its pathophysiology remains unclear. In the mink, there are two pathological patterns: one has massive granulomatous inflammatory lesion, and another has extensive TGC loss with little inflammation (Lustig et al. 2014). It is noted in the mink that there is an association of spontaneous autoimmune orchitis with abnormal hypothalamic-pituitary-testicular axis since correction of the hormonal defect prevented the orchitis (Tung et al. 1984). Pelletier et al. (2009) identified aberrations leading to spontaneous autoimmune orchitis, in which a malfunction of the clearance mechanisms for apoptotic cell debris arising from imbalance in phagocyte receptors or cytokines acting on Sertoli cells was observed with increased serum levels of TNF-alpha and IL-6 in the mink. Western blot analyses revealed that serum from minks with the orchitis reacted specifically to 23 and 50 kDa proteins of TGC. With the advance of the spontaneous autoimmune orchitis, expression of connexin 43, a gap junction protein, decreased (Pelletier et al. 2011).

On the other hand, EAO are experimentally induced by various protocols for immunization with testicular autoantigens or for alteration of the immune system without injecting testicular autoantigens. The first model of EAO was developed by Freund et al. (1953). The EAO lesions contained immunopathological evidence of

The original version of this chapter was revised. An erratum to this chapter can be found at DOI 10.1007/978-4-431-54460-9_9

M. Itoh, *Testicular Autoimmunity*, DOI 10.1007/978-4-431-54460-9_4

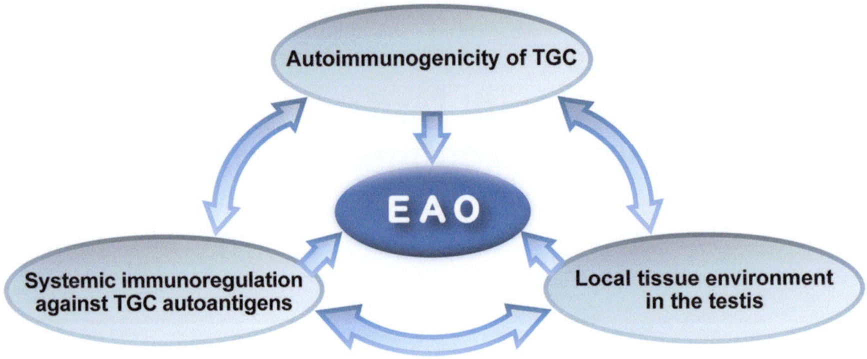

Fig. 4.1 Three main factors for induction or suppression of experimental autoimmune orchitis (EAO)

granulomatous or non-granulomatous orchitis, testicular immune complexes, and epididymal granuloma of noninfectious origin. Similar changes have been often found in testicular biopsies from infertile men. In general, EAO is $CD4^+$ T cell dependent and characterized by lymphocytic inflammation with damage to the seminiferous epithelium, that is, the shedding and apoptosis of TGC. The complete histopathological lesion is produced by both cellular and humoral immune responses. EAO has been investigated in guinea pigs, rats, mice, and other animals for more than 60 years, and, at present, the mouse has the distinct advantage of the availability of a wide range of immunological markers and a well-defined genetic background.

Chapters 4–7 review research on various EAO models. Its aim is to review and attempt to understand the regulatory mechanisms that normally prevent EAO from occurring, the events that overcome these control mechanisms, and, once initiated, the mechanisms that amplify the disease process (Fig. 4.1).

4.2 Various EAO Models by Immunization with Testicular Antigens Alone

4.2.1 EAO Induced by Immunizations with Syngeneic TGC Alone

4.2.1.1 Induction of Active EAO

Active EAO is produced in both C3H/He and A/J mice with as high as 100% incidence by two subcutaneous injections of 1×10^7 viable syngeneic TGC on days 0 and 14 without resorting to any adjuvants or other artificial immuno-potentiation (Fig. 4.2a) (Itoh et al. 1991a). Prepared TGC contained all kinds of spermatogenic cells including spermatogonia, spermatocytes, spermatids, and spermatozoa. This EAO develops fully within 40 days through three different phases: a preclinical phase (until day 20), the disease onset phase (from day 20 to day 25), and the disease developing phase (from day 25 to day 40) (Itoh et al. 1995a; Naito and Itoh 2008; Naito et al. 2012a, b). The autoimmune nature of this model may be evidenced by a steady occurrence of both antibody and DTH responses against syngeneic TGC (Hirai et al. 2013a; Qu et al. 2014). In particular, the level of DTH

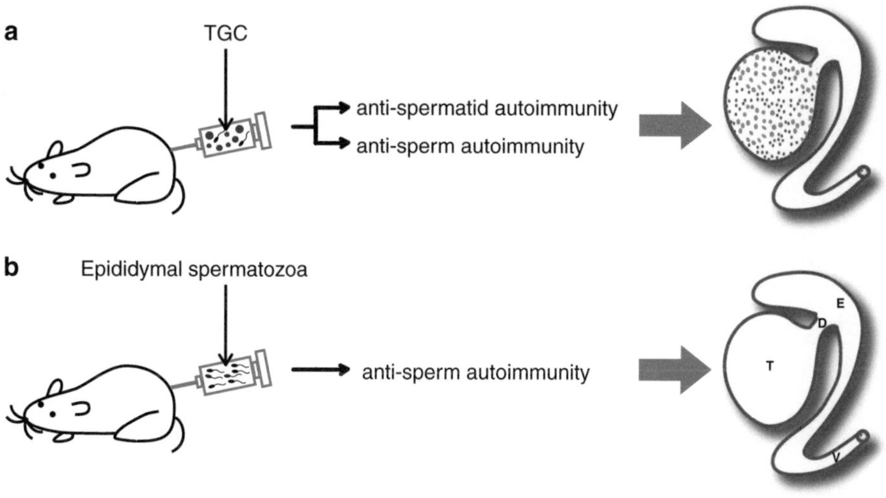

Fig. 4.2 Comparison of autoimmune inflammation between TGC- and epididymal spermatozoa-immunized mice. **a**, mice immunized with TGC. **b**, mice immunized with epididymal spermatozoa. *Dotted* area indicates the presence of the lymphocytic inflammation. D, ductuli efferentes. E, epididymis. T, testis. V, vas deferens

response to TGC protein was highly relevant to the pathology of EAO development. As this EAO model can be induced without the immune responses against adjuvants, it is simply autoimmune in nature. It is also noted that immunization with syngeneic epididymal spermatozoa failed to induce EAO (Fig. 4.2b).

4.2.1.2 Histopathology of Testicular Inflammation

In this EAO model, lymphocytes first appear around the tubuli recti, surround them, and then spread to the peripheral interstitium, resulting in induction of spermatogenic disturbance (Naito and Itoh 2008; Naito et al. 2009) (Fig. 4.3). Therefore, the pathologic lesions preferentially involve the tubuli recti where the BTB may be incomplete. A number of F4/80$^+$ and class II MHC antigen$^+$ cells were located in and around the tubuli recti of the TGC-immunized mice. This model is very unique in that epididymitis and vasitis are completely lacked (Itoh et al. 1991a, b) (Fig. 4.2). Therefore, the immune responses involved in this model may be mainly directed to testis-specific antigens on TGC but not to specific antigens on epididymal spermatozoa bearing late developing male antigens. The antigenic determinants of TGC, which diminish or disappear as the spermatogenic cells differentiate to mature sperm, may be chiefly responsible for the induction of this EAO model. Unexpectedly, subcutaneous injections of viable epididymal spermatozoa did not evoke any autoimmune inflammation in the epididymides (Fig. 4.2). Therefore, the testis rather than the epididymis may easily become an unprivileged organ as to autoimmunity in this experimental model. It may be that testicular but not epididymal haploid cells, spermatids but not spermatozoa, have critical autoantigens for this EAO.

Both cellular (CD4$^+$ T cells and CD8$^+$ T cells) and humoral (B cells and plasma cells) immunity participate in immunohistochemical manifestation of the EAO

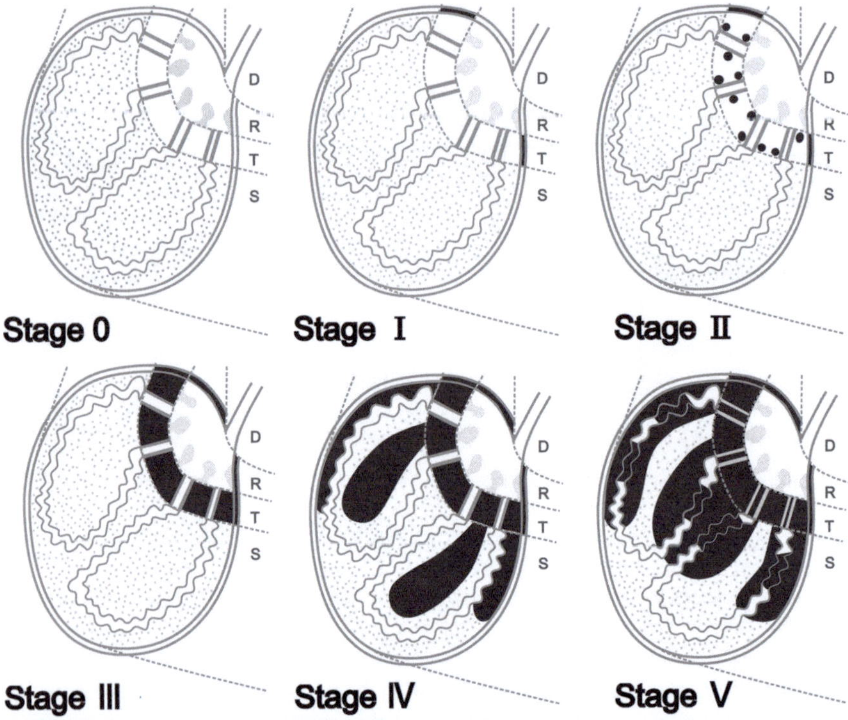

Stage 0	No inflammation
Stage I	Focal inflammation in the tunica albuginea
Stage II	Focal inflammation adjacent to the tubuli recti
Stage III	Inflammation surrounding the tubuli recti
Stage IV	Inflammation spreading around the seminiferous tubules
Stage V	Widespread inflammation involving the tubuli recti and seminiferous tubules

Fig. 4.3 Histopathological stages of EAO. D, ductuli efferentes. R, rete testis. S, seminiferous tubules. T, tubuli recti. *Dark-colored* area indicates the presence of the lymphocytic inflammation

lesion. T cells in the testes were as numerous as cytoplasmic Ig-bearing cells (approximately 30% of all inflammatory infiltrating cells). The T cells and cytoplasmic Ig-bearing cells were diffusely distributed through the interstitium, while B220$^+$ cells formed focal collections and were predominantly located in the subcapsular lesion. Major phenotype of T cells in the lesion was CD4$^+$ (approximately 85%) with the remainder (approximately 15%) being CD8$^+$. Deposits of immunoglobulins and complements were identified on the basement membrane of the seminiferous tubular wall, interstitium between the seminiferous tubules, blood capillary endothelium, and degenerated TGC. Inflammatory cells (including macrophages, B cells, and, probably, some activated T cells) in the lesion were class II MHC antigens⁺ (Itoh et al. 1991b). However, Leydig cells, Sertoli cells, and TGC did not exhibit class II MHC antigens at all. In addition, after the active inflammation stage of this model, the seminiferous epithelium is damaged irreversibly, resembling the histopathology of human male idiopathic spermatogenic disturbance (Naito et al. 2012a).

During EAO, lymphangiogenesis occurred along the undersurface of the tunica albuginea but not into the interstitium proper between the seminiferous tubules (Hirai et al. 2012, 2013b). It was noted that some F4/80$^+$ macrophages expressed lymphatic vessel endothelial hyaluronan receptor (LYVE)-1, a lymphatic endothelial cell marker, at the undersurface of the tunica albuginea and also in the testicular interstitium proper between the seminiferous tubules, indicating that activated macrophages play an important role in the process of testicular lymphangiogenesis. All LYVE-1$^+$ cells between the seminiferous tubules are positive for F4/80 and negative for CD31, an endothelial marker. There is no LYVE-1$^+$ cell in normal testicular interstitium proper between the seminiferous tubules (Hirai et al. 2010, 2012). These data suggested that LYVE-1$^+$ cells in the testicular interstitium proper in testicular inflammation are mature macrophages but not endothelia of lymphatic capillary. LYVE-1$^+$ cells in EAO were frequently detected around blood capillaries but did not form capillary structure in the testicular interstitium proper. However, the interstitium under the tunica albuginea, the lymphatic capillary structure, was identified, and some LYVE-1$^+$ macrophages were incorporated into the wall of lymphatic capillaries. This suggests that some F4/80$^+$ mature macrophages expressing LYVE-1 migrate and are incorporated into the lymphatic capillaries for lymphangiogenesis during inflammatory testis. Real-time RT-PCR analysis revealed that the expression of vascular endothelial growth factor (VEGF)-A, VEGF-D, and TNF-alpha were significantly increased but that of VEGF-C remained unchanged in the inflammatory testes. The interstitial area in EAO was expanded on active inflammatory condition and then reduced with resolution of lymphocytic inflammation under post-inflammatory condition (Naito et al. 2012a). In EAO, lymphatic capillaries extend along the undersurface of the tunica albuginea, indicating that increased lymphatic capillaries preferentially surround inflammatory lesions and play important roles in draining both the increased interstitial fluid including the infiltrating lymphocytes effectively (Hirai et al. 2012, 2013b).

4.2.1.3 Histopathology of the Spermatogenic Disturbance

A significant spermatogenic disturbance was consistently induced after the appearance of inflammatory cell responses around the tubuli recti (Itoh et al. 1995a, b). The histopathology of the seminiferous tubules in the early phase ranged from partial degeneration and depletion of all kinds of TGC to complete loss of spermatocytes, spermatids, and spermatozoa, with some remaining spermatogonia, while both Sertoli cells and the basal lamina of the tubules appeared relatively intact. The disturbance of spermatogenesis which had started near the tubuli recti region spread to the peripheral area in spite of the fact that the inflammatory cell infiltration was still limited to the tubuli recti region. Thus, the damage to seminiferous epithelium was not dependent on a direct contact of the inflammatory cells with the epithelium. In the late phase, loss of contact between TGC, appearance of some round-shaped degenerating ones, depletion of some Sertoli cells with detachment of the cells from the basal membrane, distortion and dissociation of the tubular wall layers, appearance of malformed spermatids with signet ring nuclei, depletion of immature TGC with remaining elongated spermatids, or complete loss of the seminiferous epithelium were observed in addition to the early histopathological features. Some Sertoli cells and a few spermatogonia were sometimes remained even when the tubules were infiltrated by inflammatory cells, showing that they, especially Sertoli cells, are relatively resistant to this autoimmunity. In the most severely damaged tubules, the whole tubular architecture was destroyed by the invading inflammatory cells and replaced by granulomatous tissue. Considering that this EAO model is induced by spermatid-specific autoimmunity, the histological feature of the seminiferous tubules in the lesions apparently shows depletion of elements of the seminiferous epithelium in an antigen-nonspecific fashion. These features support the theory that a disturbance of TGC development rather than a specifically immunological depletion of TGC may be critical for producing such lesions (Fig. 4.4).

Previously, the pathogenesis for TGC depletion in EAO-affected seminiferous tubules was often attributed to an influx of specific autoantibodies into the germ cell ducts with a leaky BTB. However, this theory is not suitable for the antigen-nonspecific TGC depletion in EAO. At least three causes can be considered for the disturbance of

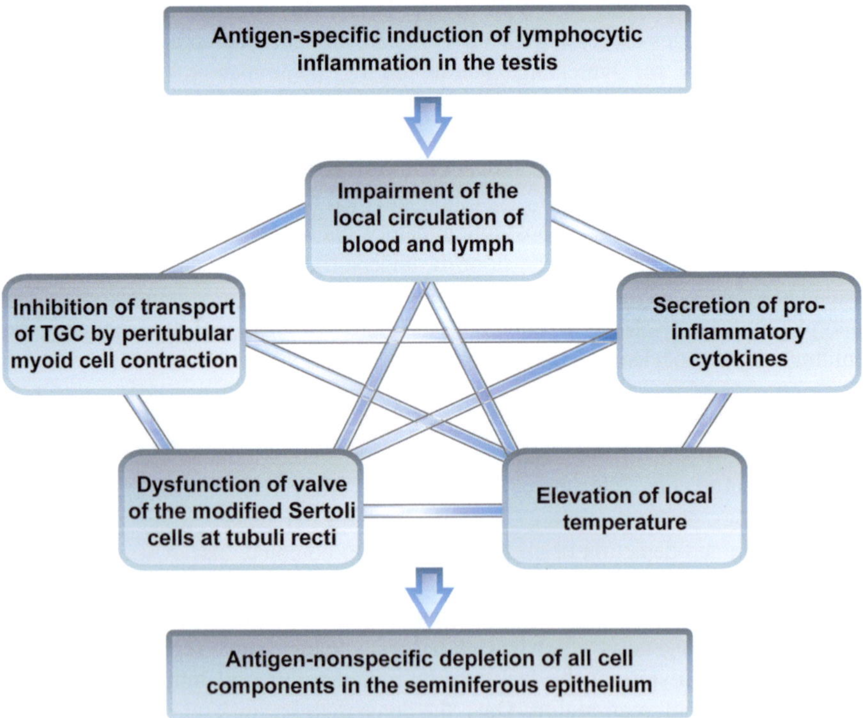

Fig. 4.4 Modes of lymphocytic inflammation and the following spermatogenic disturbance during EAO

spermatogenesis. The first is that the presence of the testicular inflammation induces an impairment of the local circulation of blood and lymph in the testis, leading to an inhibition of TGC development. The circulatory impairment in the testis is evidenced by the presence of congestion and widened lymphatic space in the lesion. The circulatory impairment may also inhibit transport of TGC by peritubular myoid cell contraction. The local congestion may also elevate intratesticular temperature, with the resultant physical damage to the seminiferous epithelium. The second is that intense inflammation surrounding the tubuli recti may cause dysfunction of the valve of the modified Sertoli cells at tubuli recti for regulation of intra-seminiferous tubular pressure. The valve dysfunction may evoke increase in the intratubular pressure, resulting in damage to the seminiferous epithelium. The third is that the inflammatory cells in EAO lesion locally secrete various cytokines (such as IL-1, IL-2, IFN-gamma, and TNF-alpha), which may be harmful to the TGC development (Fig. 4.4).

It has been demonstrated that Fas/Fas ligand- and Bax/Bcl-2-mediated apoptoses are two of the main causes of TGC death under various conditions, including cryptorchidism, vasectomized testis, and testicular torsion (Koji 2001; Koji et al. 2001; Kuerban et al. 2012). In TGC-induced EAO, some TGC still exist in the seminiferous tubules when lymphocytic infiltration has finally resolved (Naito et al. 2012a, b). It was also found that both the proliferation and death of TGC occurred simultaneously in the seminiferous tubules during the post-active inflammation stage of TGC-induced EAO. To get more detailed pathogenic information on TGC death during EAO, involvements of Fas/Fas ligand and Bax/Bcl-2 systems in TGC death following immunization with TGC were studied (Kuerban et al. 2012). Many TUNEL-stained TGC were present in the seminiferous tubules during the active inflammation stage, and these cells were persistently observed in the seminiferous epithelium until the post-active inflammation stage. Intra-testicular mRNA expression levels of both Fas and Bax were increased during the active inflammation stage and were dramatically decreased during the post-active inflammation stage. In contrast, the intra-testicular mRNA expression levels of both Fas ligand and Bcl-2 did not show significant changes during the active inflammation stage. Immunohistochemically, some Fas- and Bax-positive germ cells were detected during the active inflammation stage, but these were hardly found during the post-active inflammation stage. In contrast, some Fas ligand- and Bcl-2-positive TGC were immunohistochemically found during the active inflammation stage, and many of these were also observed during the post-active inflammation stage. These results indicate that TGC death during TGC-induced EAO is mediated by the Fas/Fas ligand and Bax/Bcl-2 systems during the active inflammation stage but not the post-active inflammation stage. Therefore, TGC death during the post-active inflammation stage should occur through mechanisms other than the Fas/Fas ligand or Bax/Bcl-2 system in TGC-induced EAO. The intra-testicular mRNA expression levels of caspase 3 and caspase 8 increased during the active inflammation stage; however, the expression level of caspase 9 decreased during this stage. This implies that TGC apoptosis during the active inflammation stage is primarily mediated by the Fas/Fas ligand system rather than the Bax/Bcl-2 system. During the post-active inflammation stage, the intra-testicular mRNA expression levels of caspase 3 and caspase 8 did not change significantly, whereas the expression level of caspase 9 decreased. Considering that TUNEL-positive TGC were detected at higher levels than those of normal mice during the post-active inflammation stage, most TGC deaths are probably non-apoptotic during the post-active inflammation stage. In general, cells that show increased resistance to stress require higher stimulus levels to induce cell death. The ability to evade apoptosis is induced by a range of different alterations, inducing physiological changes such as the activation/upregulation of mitogenic signaling pathways, inactivation/downregulation of certain apoptotic molecules, and upregulation of a number of anti-apoptotic genes. In normal condition, Fas- and/or Bax-positive TGC and Fas- and Bax-negative TGC exist simultaneously; however, Fas- and/or Bax-positive TGC were increased during the active inflammation stage, but Fas- and Bax-negative TGC remained alive during the post-active inflammation stage. There is a possibility that the upregulation of Fas ligand and Bcl-2 during the post-active inflammation stage is a reaction against the inactivation of Fas- and the Bax-mediated TGC death, respectively (Kuerban et al. 2012).

4.2.1.4 Passive EAO by Adoptive Transfer of Lymphocytes

For analysis of immunological events at the beginning and the course of this autoimmune reaction, the adoptive transfer system offers an important approach. In a simple protocol for adoptive transfer of EAO, cell donors were mice that received subcutaneous injections twice with TGC alone (Itoh et al. 1991c). Spleen cells from the donor mice were stimulated in vitro with TGC, propagated in IL-2-containing medium, and then injected intraperitoneally or intravenously to naive recipient mice. This procedure induced severe orchitis and spermatogenic disturbance in the recipients at high incidence, with often involvement of inflammation in the epididymis and the vas deferens. Elimination of all T cells or $CD4^+$ T cells before the transfer produced no histopathological signs in the recipients, whereas that of the $CD8^+$ T cells or B cells had no inhibitory effects on the disease transfer, indicating that the effector cells are $CD4^+$ T cells (Itoh et al. 1991c). Therefore, the $CD4^+$ T cells are critical cells for EAO induction and the $CD8^+$ cells (approximately 15% of infiltrating leukocytes in EAO lesion), B cells, and plasma cells (approximately 50% of infiltrating leukocytes) may be involved in further development of EAO lesion (Itoh et al. 1991b). It is known that $CD4^+$ T cells recognize peptides in association with class II MHC molecules, although MHC class II-positive cells in normal mouse testis are quite sparse.

In the experimental system using mice immunized with TGC alone, it is also noted that mode of inflammatory cell infiltration in adoptively transferred EAO to recipients (passive EAO) differs from that in EAO induced by subcutaneous injections with TGC (active EAO). Although the orchitis affecting the tubuli recti and seminiferous tubules at various sites was common between passive and active EAO, epididymitis and vasitis were accompanied only in the passive EAO (Itoh et al. 1991a, b, c). The reason for producing the different histopathology is unknown. Differences in migration property of lymphocytes to the target organ may exist between the transferred lymphocytes stimulated in vitro in passive EAO and lymphocytes stimulated in vivo in active EAO. At present, the precise mechanism of migration of the transferred TGC-specific lymphocytes into the male reproductive tissues is still unanswerable. The donor lymphocytes introduced into naive recipients were able to home to the testis and induce EAO without depending on artificial perturbation of the BTB. This indicates that a part of TGC autoantigens are not immunologically sequestered by the BTB and accessible by exogenously administered TGC-specific CD4$^+$ T cells in normal recipient mice.

Subsequently, a CD4$^+$ T cell line was derived from mice immunized with TGC alone by subsequent repeated selection of the lymphocytes in vitro with soluble testicular antigens (Itoh et al. 1992a). Intraperitoneal or intravenous inoculation of as few as 1×10^5 lined cells that had been stimulated in vitro with testicular antigens before inoculation was capable of transferring EAO to naive recipients. The transferred lesion was characterized by infiltration of inflammatory cells into the epididymis and rete testis (epididymo-orchitis) and the following widespread spermatogenic disturbance in the testis. Therefore, this passive EAO by CD4$^+$T cell line is quite different from active EAO (orchitis without epididymitis) in regard to mode of inflammatory cell infiltration. In the T cell line-induced EAO, lymphocytic infiltration consistently started in the epididymis before spreading to the rete testis (Fig. 4.5). In vitro characterization of the biological activity of the lined cells revealed that the cells had no cytolytic or cytotoxic activity against TGC, but the culture supernatant had macrophage migration inhibitory activity involved in the DTH response (Itoh et al. 1993). Therefore, the DTH responsiveness transferred by the T cell line was found to correlate with their EAO-inducing capacity. It is also important to stress that the transferred T cell line must be stimulated with testicular antigens before the cell

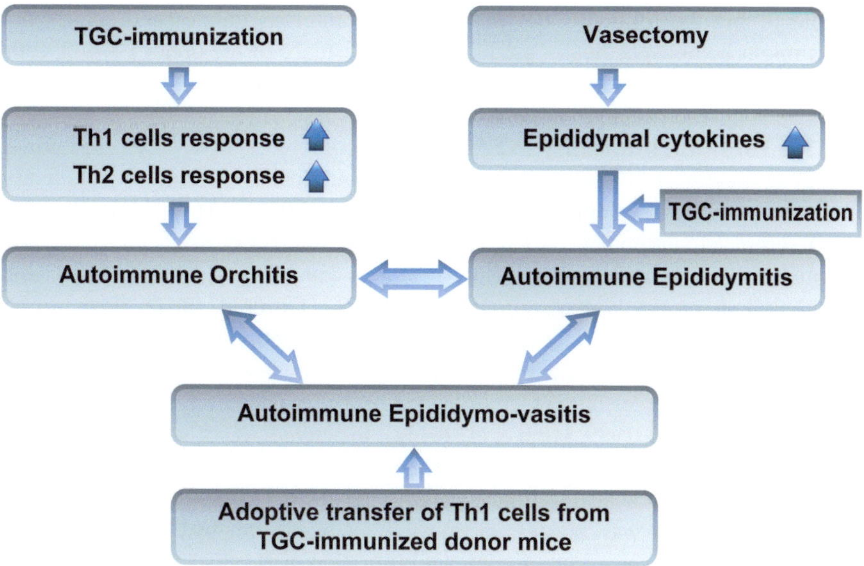

Fig. 4.5 Autoimmune orchitis, epididymitis, and vasitis by TGC-specific lymphocytes

transfer for the successful induction of EAO. The lined T cells cultured in the absence of stimulation with testicular antigen revert to the resting state and lose their EAO-inducing capacity. Although it is supposed that the activated cells may home in on the testis and epididymis more efficiently than the resting cells, it is not yet clear what differences exist at the molecular level between the activated and resting lined cells in this EAO transfer model. In the relevant experiments, when the lined orchitogenic CD4⁺ T cells were seeded onto cultured monolayers of syngeneic Sertoli cells and dermal fibroblasts, they immediately induced detachment of the both monolayers in an antigen-nonspecific manner (Itoh et al. 1993). The disease transfer was antigen specific, because no inflammatory lesion was found in any organs other than epididymis and testis by intraperitoneal transfer of the T cell line. Therefore, activated T cell line might specifically home in on the epididymal and testicular vasculatures, migrate into their interstitium, and then break the integrity of the blood-epididymal barrier and the BTB, in an antigen-nonspecific fashion through the secretion of some cytokines or direct cell contact. Furthermore, with loss of the blood-epididymal barrier and the BTB, more germ cell autoantigens might leak from the epididymal ducts and the seminiferous tubules, and a continuous source of the autoantigens for immune stimulation might be provided. Indeed, the culture supernatant of the T cell line induced nonspecific local inflammation when injected into subdermal tissue of normal syngeneic mice. Therefore, the lined T cells were shown to devastate a tissue integrity and cause attraction and activation of inflammatory cells of the recipient origin in a local environment. The injection of culture supernatant from the lined T cells with irradiated spleen cells caused more intense subdermal inflammation compared to that of the culture supernatant alone. These results suggest that the transferred lined CD4⁺ T cells will specifically home in to the testis and epididymis of recipients, but the following devastation of seminiferous tubules and epididymal ducts might be nonspecifically produced by coexistence of the donor CD4⁺ T cells and other inflammatory cells of recipient origin in the lesion.

4.2.1.5 Humoral Immunity in EAO

Serum autoantibody titers against TGC and epididymal spermatozoa gradually increased with the development of EAO (Hirai et al. 2013a). At the initial stage of EAO, serum autoantibodies reacted with only a few antigens of TGC and epididymal spermatozoa, while in the later stage, the reactions with various antigens of TGC and epididymal spermatozoa occurred (Itoh et al. 1994; Qu et al. 2010; Musha et al. 2013). However, the autoantibodies were specific to the testis and epididymis but not to other organs (seminal vesicle, brain, heart, lung, thymus, salivary gland, small intestine, liver, pancreas, kidney, muscle, and ovary) in enzyme-linked immunosorbent assay (Itoh et al. 1989; Hirai et al. 2013a). In active EAO of which induction is CD4⁺ T cell-dependent, B cell lineage (B cells and plasma cells) was found to be approximately 50% of all infiltrating cells in the testis lesion (Itoh et al. 1991b). Although the disease was transferrable to naive recipients only by CD4⁺ T cells from TGC-immunized donor mice, a significant infiltration of B cells and plasma cells in EAO lesion suggests that the local humoral immunity also might affect the integrity of seminiferous epithelium and the supporting tissue in the testis. Many plasma cells preferentially infiltrated around the tubuli recti already from the early stage of EAO (Naito et al. 2009, 2012b). A number of these cytoplasmic Ig-bearing cells contained IgG or IgA. It is noted that there was a good correlation between the serum level of anti-TGC antibodies of IgG class and the intensity of IgG deposition in the testis lesion, but serum IgA autoantibodies were not detected in spite of evidence of IgA deposition on degenerated cells inside the epididymal ducts. There were no cytoplasmic IgA-bearing cells in any portion of the epididymal interstitium in TGC-induced active EAO. It appears most likely that the IgA deposits on degenerated cells inside the epididymal ducts were derived from TGC reacted with intra-seminiferous tubular-specific IgA antibodies secreted by a number of IgA-producing cells residing in the testis lesion. There is another possibility that degenerated IgA-producing plasma cells themselves which had infiltrated into the seminiferous tubules were finally flowed to the epididymal ducts. The circulating antibodies of IgG class reacted strongly with the acrosomal portion of round and elongating spermatids but only weakly with that of mature spermatozoa (Itoh et al. 1991b, 1994). Although the IgM antibodies reactive with the acrosomal area of immature TGC were also identified, the same class of antibodies reactive with the acrosome of mature spermatozoa was undetectable (Itoh et al. 1991b). It seems therefore that this testicular autoimmunity may be primarily directed to immature acrosomal proteins of developing haploid cells which diminish as the spermatids differentiate to mature sperm, with the resultant orchitis but not epididymo-vasitis (Fig. 4.2). Anti-TGC antisera primarily reacted with the acrosomal and proacrosomal portion of spermatids of mice as early as 3 weeks (Soramoto et al. 1993; Itoh et al. 1994). As shown in enzyme-linked immunosorbent assay, immunohistochemical stainings obtained by reaction of the immune sera with liver, kidney, and ovary sections were also negative. Therefore, the results indicate that the circulating antibodies are quite organ specific (Itoh et al. 1994; Hirai et al. 2013a). However, it cannot be excluded that circulating autoantibodies against spermatogonia, spermatocytes, Sertoli cells, the basal lamina of the seminiferous tubules, and the Leydig cells are also produced in TGC-immunized mice but deposited in the testicular tissue of the host, resulting in absorption of the autoantibodies against testicular cells other than the spermatids and spermatozoa from the blood circulation, because the testicular tissues outside the BTB formed by inter-Sertoli cell junction apparently has free access to the products delivered from the blood circulatory system. In fact, the immune deposits had been detected on outside the BTB in the lesion of this EAO (Itoh et al. 1991b; Naito et al. 2012a, b). In this way the autoantibodies would easily react with the testicular tissue of the host and disappear from the serum samples. To test this possibility, an immunohistochemical examination was performed by using the immune sera from mice that were castrated before receiving the first TGC injection 7 days later. However, even in this case, the serum autoantibodies were against round, oval, and elongated-shaped spermatids but never on less mature TGC resting on the basal lamina, Sertoli cells, basal lamina, or testicular interstitial cells. Therefore, intra-testicular plasma cells may secrete autoantibodies against spermatids and spermatozoa. Furthermore, the preferential involvement of the tubuli recti might be due to that infiltrating class II MHC-positive B cells around the tubuli recti function as antigen-presenting cells and attract more lymphocytes (Naito et al. 2009). Furthermore, antibodies secreted from plasma cells in situ may cause further damage to basal lamina of the tubuli recti and the seminiferous tubules.

4.2.1.6 Developmental Autoimmunogenicity of TGC

Trials to induce EAO by immunization with TGC obtained from various aged mice revealed that TGC from donor mice younger than 3 weeks of age did not exhibit the capability to induce the disease; however, TGC from donor mice older than 4 weeks of age showed the EAO-inducing capability (Soramoto et al. 1993). Developmental studies using various aged mice demonstrated that TGC from 6- rather than 5-week-old mice had more strong capability of inducing EAO (orchitogenicity) (Fig. 4.6). Both DTH-inducing and anti-TGC antibody-eliciting capabilities were observed in mice immunized with TGC from donor mice older than 4 weeks of age. Therefore, this implies that the testis becomes vulnerable to localized autoimmunity as early as 4 weeks of age when spermatids first start to differentiate in the seminiferous tubules. To assess the cytokine release from specific lymphocytes stimulated with syngeneic TGC derived from mice at various ages, levels of IL-2 and IFN-gamma in the supernatants obtained from co-culture of lymphocytes with each TGC were determined. The spleen cells did not secrete detectable levels of IL-2 and IFN-gamma in response to TGC from 3-week-old mice but did upon stimulation with TGC from 4 weeks or older (Soramoto et al. 1993).

In biochemical studies for detection of autoantigens of TGC, the fragility of TGC plasma membrane following exposure to chemical treatment must be kept in mind. By using SDS-polyacrylamide gel electrophoresis and immunoblotting in reaction of normal sera with normal murine testicular homogenates, two immunoreactive bands corresponding to approximately 45 and 100 kDa were detected (Qu et al. 2010; Musha et al. 2013). These two natural autoantibodies were more definitely detected in sera of TGC-induced EAO. Furthermore, the immune serum samples also reacted with three additional autoantigens of approximately 25, 40, and 250 kDa.

Later, Terayama et al. (2016) tried to identify TGC-specific autoantigens relevant to EAO. In that study, 11 TGC-specific autoantigens including (1) tubulin, beta 2cl; (2) ATPase, H^+ transporting, lysosomal V1 subunit A; (3) pyruvate dehydrogenase lipoamide beta; (4) heat shock protein 1-like; (5) fructose bisphosphatase 1; (6) leucine-rich repeat containing 34; (7) aspartyl aminopeptidase isoform b; (8) glyceraldehyde-3-phosphate dehydrogenase, spermatogenic; (9) pyruvate dehydrogenase E1 alpha 2; (10) DAZ-associated protein 1; and (11) unnamed protein product (fumarate hydratase-related protein) were specifically reacted with serum IgG from TGC-immunized mice by TGC liquid chromatography-tandem mass spectrometry analysis, followed by two-dimensional gel electrophoresis. Real-time RT-PCR analysis by the use of various organs such as the testis, epididymis, submandibular gland, spleen, heart, kidney, skeletal muscle, small intestine, liver, brain, lung, and pancreas showed that the mRNA expressions of 9 of identified 11 TGC-specific autoantigens except for (2) ATPase, H^+ transporting, lysosomal V1 subunit A, and (7) aspartyl aminopeptidase isoform b were extremely higher in the testis compared to in other organs. Moreover, mRNA expressions of (1) tubulin, beta 2 cl, (2) ATPase,

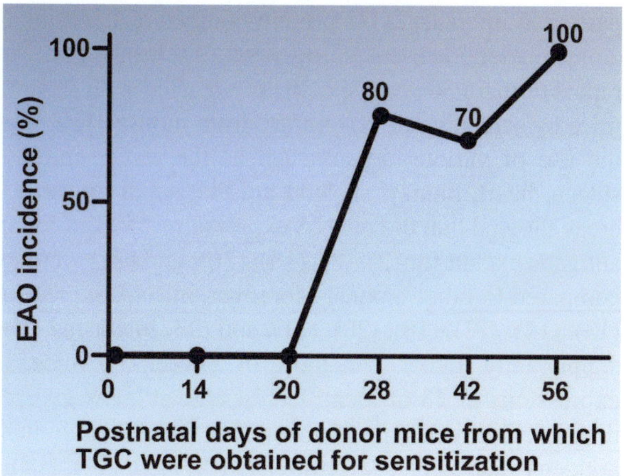

Fig. 4.6 Ontogeny of TGC autoimmunogenicity for EAO induction. Immunization with TGC obtained from donor mice older than 4 weeks of age has a sensitizing capability to induce EAO in the recipients

H+ transporting, lysosomal V1 subunit A, (4) heat shock protein 1-like, (5) fructose bisphosphatase 1, (6) leucine-rich repeat containing 34, (8) glyceraldehyde-3-phosphate dehydrogenase, spermatogenic, and (10) DAZ-associated protein 1 in normal testes of 8-week-old mice were significantly higher than those of 2-week-old mice. Exceptionally, only mRNA expression of (7) aspartyl aminopeptidase isoform b in normal testes of 8-week-old mice appeared lower than those of 2-week-old mice. It is also noted that mRNA expressions of 10 of identified 11 autoantigens except for (7) aspartyl aminopeptidase isoform b were more in TGC than in epididymal spermatozoa. Moreover, the identified each protein was produced by HEK293T cells that were transfected plasma vector with each candidate gene and then reacted with serum antibodies from EAO-induced mice by the Western blot analysis. The results showed that (2) ATPase, H^+ transporting, lysosomal V1 subunit A, (4) heat shock protein 1-like, (5) fructose bisphosphatase 1, (9) pyruvate dehydrogenase E1 alpha 2, and (10) DAZ-associated protein 1 specifically reacted with the immune sera, but not control ones. Therefore, three proteins composed of (4) heat shock protein 1-like, (5) fructose bisphosphatase 1, and (10) DAZ-associated protein 1 are important target autoantigens for EAO. In particular, in adult human testes, (4) Heat shock protein 1-like and (10) DAZ-associated protein 1 but not (5) fructose bisphosphatase 1 are specifically detected in round and elongated spermatids, indicating that these two proteins are critical for EAO induction (Uhlen et al. 2010, 2015).

By subtracted cDNA library screening, Nagahori et al. (2017) also tried identification of TGC-specific autoantigens related to EAO. In that study, 24 TGC-specific autoantigens including (1) 1700034O15, (2) diazepam binding inhibitor, (3) 1700093K21, (4) ADP-ribosylation factor-like 4A, (5) 2210012G02, (6) N-acetyltransferase 9, (7) 1700054F22, (8) interferon-stimulated protein, (9) zinc and ring finger 4, (10) Y box protein 2, (11) Y box protein 1, (12) abhydrolase domain containing 6, (13) syntaxin 18, (14) germ cell-specific gene 1, (15) peroxisomal biogenesis factor 3, (16) ubiquinol cytochrome c reductase core protein 2, (17) eukaryotic translation initiation factor 3, subunit E, (18) atlastin GTPase 3, (19) Zona pellucida 3 receptor, (20) LIM domain containing preferred translocation partner in lipoma, (21) G-protein-coupled receptor kinase-interactor 1, (22) nicotinamide nucleotide transhydrogenase, (23) heat shock protein 4-like, and (24) ankyrin repeat domain 36 were specifically reacted with serum IgM from TGC-immunized mice by screening cDNA library from mouse TGC. Real-time RT-PCR analysis by the use of various organs such as the testis, epididymis, submandibular gland, spleen, heart, kidney, skeletal muscle, small intestine, liver, brain, lung, and pancreas showed that the mRNA expressions of 19 of identified 24 TGC-specific autoantigens except for (2), (8), (16), (20), and (22) were extremely higher in the testis compared to other organs. Moreover, mRNA expressions of (1), (3), (6), (9), (10), (13), (14), (17), (18), (20), (21), and (23) in normal testes of 8-week-old mice were significantly higher than those of 2-week-old mice. It is also noted that mRNA expressions of 23 of identified 24 autoantigens except for (2) were more in TGC than in epididymal spermatozoa. Therefore, it is indicated that TGC-specific autoantigens such as (1), (3), (6), (9), (10), (13), (14), (17), (18), (21), and (23) are relevant target autoantigens for EAO. In adult human testis, (3), (14), and (21) are detected on various-staged TGC, and (6), (13), and (17) are detected on not only various-staged TGC abut also Leydig cells (Uhlen et al. 2010, 2015). In contrast, both (10) Y box protein 2 and (23) heat shock protein 4-like are detected definitely on round spermatids and faintly on other immature TGC, implying that these two antigens are critical for EAO induction.

4.2.1.7 Cytokines and Hormones in EAO

Both IFN-gamma and TNF-alpha were detected from cultured spleen cells and lymph node cells in EAO-induced mice in vitro (Tokunaga et al. 2007). A significant stimulation of IL-5 and IL-6 (Th2 cytokines) production by sensitized spleen cells was detectable when the TGC from 3-week or older mice were used as stimulants (Soramoto et al. 1993). IL-2 and IFN-gamma (Th1 cytokines) production was detected by immunization with TGC from 4-week or older mice. From this evidence, it is suggested that both Th1 and Th2 cells are involved in the immunization process of this EAO model. No IL-4 production by TGC-immunized spleen cells was detectable in C3H/He mice. The one reason for this result is that higher levels of IFN-gamma production may inhibit IL-4 production. For another reason, it is thought that levels of IL-4 production may be innately low in C3H/He compared with BALB/c mice. Actually, it has been shown that soon after *Leishmania* major infection, lymphocytes from a resistant strain C3H/He mice secrete higher levels of IFN-gamma and no IL-4, whereas lymphocytes from a susceptible strain BALB/c mice secrete IL-4 but little IFN-gamma (Scott 1991; Coffman et al. 1991). Splenic production of both Th1- and Th2-related cytokines increased after the second but not the first immunization with TGC, indicating that secondary immune responses are critical for the EAO induction (Tokunaga et al. 2007). Furthermore, the production of Th1-related cytokines became predominant at the clinical stage of EAO. In particular, IFN-gamma, a Th1-producing cytokine, significantly increased after the second immunization with TGC, decreased temporally at the preclinical phase of the EAO, but increased again at the clinical phase. Similar kinetics of cytokine secretion were observed for both IL-3 and granulocyte-macrophage colony-stimulating factor, which are produced by both Th1 and Th2 cells. The secretion of IL-2, another Th1-producing cytokines, gradually increased up to the clinical phase. IL-1, a DTH-related cytokine derived from macrophages, was also continuously produced after the second immunization. In contrast, IL-4, a Th2-producing cytokine, was not produced by the cultured spleen cells. Furthermore, the levels of other Th2-producing cytokines such as IL-5 and IL-10 were temporally increased after the second immunization with TGC but decreased later. However, IL-6, another Th2-producing cytokine, was continuously produced after the second immunization (Tokunaga et al. 2007).

Both IFN-gamma and TNF-alpha are representative cytokines of Th1 cells and exert local toxicity toward the seminiferous epithelium in vivo. For analyses of the tissue micro-circumstances of EAO, it is important to know about the cytokine expression in not only lymphoid organs but also the testes as target organs. Indeed, the intra-testicular mRNAs for both IFN-gamma and TNF-alpha significantly increased, while other cytokines such as IL-1-alpha, IL-1-beta, IL-6, and transforming growth factor-beta did not show significant changes in the TGC-immunized mice (Terayama et al. 2011a). These results suggest that secretion of significant amounts of IFN-gamma and TNF-alpha in situ contributes to the spermatogenic disturbance. In other studies, local injection of IFN-gamma and TNF-alpha into normal testes was shown to induce cytotoxicity to the seminiferous epithelium in vivo (Mealy et al. 1990; Natwar et al. 1995). This means that interference with spermatogenesis is inducible without specific cytotoxic T cells or specific autoantibodies (Fig. 4.4).

Real-time RT-PCR analyses revealed that Fas mRNA expression significantly increased in EAO-affected testes compared with the control testes. In contrast, Fas ligand expression did not show significant changes between EAO-affected and control testes (Kuerban et al. 2012).

Additionally, the serum follicle-stimulating hormone and inhibin B levels on days 60 and 120 were significantly high and low, respectively. In contrast, the serum luteinizing hormone level was not significantly changed. It was also noted that testosterone level was significantly increased on day 35 when EAO was in development, indicating no or little damage to Leydig cells in EAO lesion (Tokunaga et al. 2007).

4.2.1.8 Genetic Susceptibility of EAO

Various strains of inbred mice respond differentially to EAO induction, indicating that susceptibility is genetically controlled. Among various different inbred strains including C3H/He, A/J, C57BL/6, AKR, Balb/c, CBA, MRL/lpr, and DBA/2, both C3H/He (H-2^k) and A/J (H-2^a) strains are most susceptible to this EAO (Tokunaga et al. 1993a, b). AKR, CBA, and MRL/lpr mice, other H-2 k strains, are less susceptible to the disease induction than C3H/He (H-2^k) mice. This finding suggests that a genetic susceptibility associated with gens outside the H-2 haplotype may contribute to the development of this EAO (Itoh et al. 1991a). C57BL/6 (H-2^b), Balb/c (H-2^d), and DBA/2 (H-2^d) are also less susceptible. The highly susceptible C3H/He and A/J strains that received TGC immunization developed a significant increase in both levels of DTH and antibody responses against TGC. C57BL/6, Balb/c, and CBA strains were also positive for both DTH and antibody response. In contrast, AKR strain was negative for both DTH and antibody response, and DBA and MRL/MpJ strains showed negative DTH and positive antibody response (Tokunaga et al. 1993a). In general, susceptibility to experimental organ-specific autoimmune diseases has been considered to be due to genetic differences in response to autoantigens or to adjuvants. Thus, in this EAO model, it is not necessary to take genes controlling complete Freund's adjuvant (CFA) or *Bordetella pertussis* (BP)-induced inflammatory responses into consideration. In regard to the immunogenicity of TGC, it was found that TGC obtained from low susceptible and resistant mice both having H-2^k haplotype can also induce a high incidence of EAO in highly susceptible C3H/He mice (Tokunaga et al. 1993b). Therefore, it seems unlikely that TGC derived from the low susceptible or resistant strains are less immunogenic than those from the highly susceptible strain. In other words, immune susceptibility for TGC injection but not autoimmunogenicity of the injected TGC is critical for EAO induction.

The H-2 identical background disparate (highly susceptible × low susceptible)F1 hybrids, (C3H/He × C3H/HeJ)F1 and (C3H/HeJ × C3H/He) F1 mice, were highly susceptible to the induction of EAO, indicating that susceptibility equivalent to that of the highly susceptible parents was inherited as a dominant autosomal trait. However, the H-2 identical background disparate (highly susceptible x resistant)F1 hybrids, (C3H/He × C3H/HeBiKi)F1 and (C3H/HeBiKi × C3H/He) F1 mice, were low susceptible to the induction of EAO. In this case, the genes controlling the unresponsiveness of C3H/BiKi mice or complementation of gens may have an effect on the susceptibility to EAO in these F1 bidirectional hybrids. Both H-2 and background disparate (highly susceptible × resistant)F1 hybrids, the (C3H/He × DBA/2)F1 and (DBA/2 × C3H/He)F1 mice, were equally resistant to EAO induction. This indicates that the resistance of DBA/2 mice can be inherited as a dominant autosomal trait effectively negating the EAO susceptibility of C3H/He mice, which is an exception to the general rule: for most of genetically controlled antigens, high responsiveness to the antigen is dominantly inherited. In the susceptible hybrids, both DTH and antibody responses to TGC increased. On the other hand, in the resistant hybrids, the levels of anti-TGC antibodies were elevated; however, the DTH to TGC remains depressed. This suggests that the antibody production and induction of DTH may be under different genetic controls and that cellular rather than humoral immunity plays an important role in this EAO induction (Tokunaga et al. 1993a, b).

In order to search for the basis for low susceptible C3H/HeJ and resistant C3H/BiKi mice, these mice received EAO-inducible spleen cells from C3H/He mice. C3H/HeJ recipient mice became highly susceptible to passive EAO. In contrast, disease-resistant C3H/HeBiKi recipient mice failed to develop passive EAO. Furthermore, a study was examined whether or not Treg capable of preventing EAO induction were generated in low susceptible C3H/HeJ and resistant C3H/BiKi mice immunized with TGC (Tokunaga et al. 1993b). The results showed that transfer of spleen cells from TGC-immunized C3H/HeJ and C3/HeBiKi mice into C3H/He mice before the EAO challenge had no suppressive effect on subsequent disease induction. This means that Treg might be not involved in the low susceptibility of C3H/HeJ and C3H/HeBiKi mice. Some mechanisms other than Treg must be considered. It is known that C3H/HeJ mice are unresponsive to lipopolysaccharide and behave as low responders with respect to lipopolysaccharide-induced autoimmune reactivity (Bloembergen et al. 1988). In addition, C3H/HeJ mice display an ill-defined complement defect (Hoffmann 1978). Whether there exists a relation among the unresponsiveness to LPS, complement defect and resistance to EAO are unclear. There may be another possibility of unknown background (non-H-2) locus controlling resistance to EAO.

4.2.1.9 Regulation of EAO

TGC-induced EAO can be inhibited by intravenous administration with soluble testicular antigens (Mukasa et al. 1992). This suppression model was made by repeated intravenous injections with the tolerogenic form of testicular antigens before subcutaneous injections with TGC on days 0 and 14 for EAO induction. The testicular antigens were prepared by acid extraction and ammonium sulfate precipitation of defatted testes and epididymides. In the soluble testicular antigen-pretreated mice, the development of EAO and relevant DTH was suppressed in an antigen-specific fashion, but anti-TGC antibody formation was not affected after EAO challenge. This indicates that the soluble testicular antigen-induced suppression is exclusively directed against the cellular immunity but not against the humoral one. Also, the DTH reaction to sheep red blood cells, another antigen unrelated to testicular antigens, was unaffected by intravenous pretreatment of mice with the soluble testicular antigens, showing the suppression of cellular immunity in an antigen-specific manner. A single dose of cyclophosphamide at 2 days after the intravenous administration of the testicular antigens abrogated the unresponsiveness to EAO. $CD8^+$ T cells isolated from the spleen of mice that had been intravenously pretreated with the soluble testicular antigens could adoptively transfer suppression against EAO into naive recipients, whereas $CD4^+$ T cells failed to transfer the suppression.

Later, $CD8^+$ TCR alpha-beta + line of Treg was generated from the spleen cells of C3H/He mice which had received three intravenous injections of the soluble testicular antigens, followed by in vitro repeated selection of these spleen cells by stimulation with the soluble testicular antigens (Mukasa et al. 1994). Transfer of the lined $CD8^+$ Treg into naive animals 2 days before subcutaneous injections with TGC on days 0 and 14 for EAO induction resulted in an apparent reduction in both the incidence and severity of disease on day 40. In contrast, there was no downregulation of the disease when the lined Treg were transferred on the other days such as day 14 or day 21. These data suggest that the lined cells acted as regulatory cells on the inductive phase (afferent limb) of testicular autoimmune responses. The transferred lined $CD8^+$ Treg significantly inhibited the DTH to TGC in the recipients in an antigen-specific manner, but these cells had no inhibitory effect on the humoral immune response to TGC. This line could also inhibit in vitro TGC-driven proliferation of orchitogenic lymphocytes.

There is another model for the suppression of TGC-induced EAO by lined $CD4^+$ Treg (Itoh et al. 1992b). The lined $CD4^+$ Treg were derived from C3/He mice that were injected with 1×10^7 TGC subcutaneously ten times at 2-week intervals. When the lined cells were transferred immediately before the first injection of TGC on day 0, there was no suppression of EAO in recipient mice. However, the activated Treg,

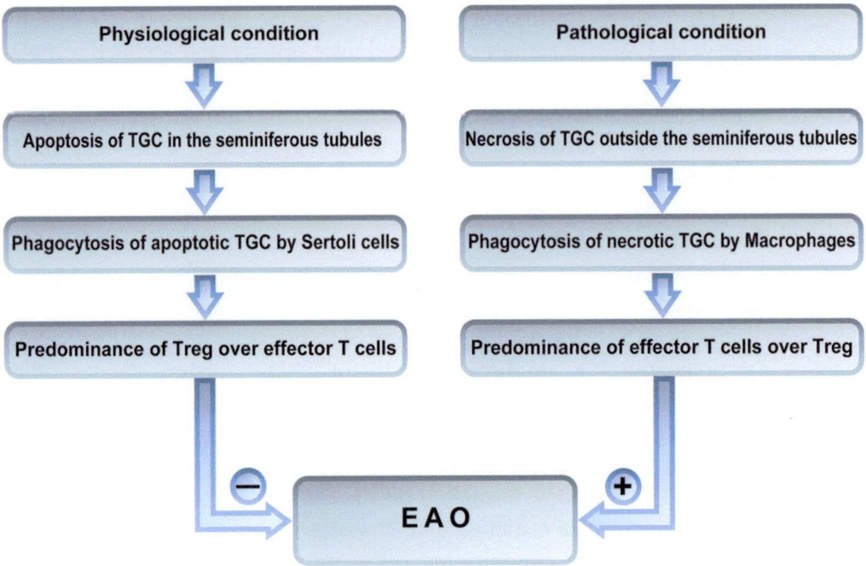

Fig. 4.7 Balance between effector and regulatory T cells in testicular autoimmunity

when transferred on day 21 (just before the onset of EAO), interfered with the ongoing anti-TGC immunity of both DTH and antibody responses and suppressed EAO induction, indicating that this cell line could downregulate the efferent limb of testicular autoimmune response. Antibody response against sheep red blood cells was not significantly affected by the transfer of lined $CD4^+$ Treg, suggesting the achievement of antigen-specific downregulation by the cell line. In contrast to the $CD8^+$ Treg described above, the $CD4^+$ Treg suppressed both the cellular and humoral responses to TGC in TGC-specific manner (Itoh et al. 1992b).

Taken together, both the $CD4^+$ Treg and the $CD8^+$ Treg may be important regulatory elements governing the suppression of EAO in mice (Fig. 4.1), and there must be different suppressive mechanisms between the $CD4^+$ Treg and the $CD8^+$ Treg. Under normal conditions, many TGC undergo cell death in the seminiferous tubules, followed by latent leakage of TGC autoantigens for a possible stimulation of antigen-specific Treg (Fig. 4.7). On the other hand, TGC injected outside the testis augment antigen-specific effector $CD4^+$ T cells (Th1 and Th2 cells) and may overwhelm the Treg (Fig. 4.7). It is yet unknown whether these Treg suppress the $CD4^+$ effector T cells directly or indirectly in association with a regulatory network or circuit. Moreover, it will be needed to determine whether the suppression of EAO is operated by contact-mediated suppression or suppression mediated by some diffusible factors.

4.2.1.10 Modulation of EAO by Vasectomy

Mice receiving sham-vasectomy and the following TGC immunization on days 0 and 14 had EAO with no epididymitis. In sharp contrast, no EAO was found in the testes of any mice receiving vasectomy and the following TGC immunization.

Instead, caput epididymitis involving infiltration of CD4⁺ T cells, CD8⁺ T cells, B cells, and macrophages was induced in them with striking elevation of the epididymal tissue levels of both IL-6 and IL-10 mRNA (Qu et al. 2008). Therefore, vasectomy suppressed EAO and alternatively induced caput epididymitis (Fig. 4.5). Furthermore, serum autoantibodies induced by sham-vasectomy and the following TGC immunization were reactive with both round (immature) and elongating (mature) spermatids; however, those induced by vasectomy and the following TGC immunization were more specific to elongating spermatids and spermatozoa. This indicates that vasectomy may induce the immune mode by which autoreactive lymphocytes gain access to TGC autoantigens in the epididymides, leading to autoimmune responses against the autoantigens of mature rather than immature spermatids (Qu et al. 2008).

Mice receiving vasectomy alone exhibited no significant inflammatory cell response in either the testis or epididymides. However, some studies revealed the induction of humoral and cell-mediated autoimmune responses directed against sperm antigens after vasectomy (Ansbacher 1973; Alexander and Tung 1977; Herr et al. 1987; Nashan et al. 1990; Flickinger et al. 1994, 1995, 1996). It has been reported that the ducts of caput epididymis are the sited of absorption of various materials leaving the testis (Hamilton 1980). Therefore, vasectomy may allow the epididymal ducts to absorb testis-secreting materials including autoantigens of mature spermatids more strongly with the resultant leakage or excretion of significant amounts of absorbed autoantigens to the outside of the ducts. Actually, Johnson and Howards (1975) reported the leakage of epididymal spermatozoa from the ducts of the caput epididymis after vasectomy in hamsters. It has been demonstrated that autoreactive lymphocytes could preferentially gain access to the tubuli recti and the rete testis where BTB is incomplete. (Dym and Fawcett 1970; Aoki and Fawcett 1975; Itoh et al. 1995c, 1998a). However, vasectomy may increase the hydrostatic pressure in the epididymal ducts rather than the tubuli recti and the rete testis, resulting in possible leakage of more germ cell autoantigens into the epididymal interstitium. There may be another possibility that blood flow or lymphatic drainage in the testis and epididymis is changed by vasectomy, because some blood and lymph capillaries leave testis from its inferior portion and then run along the vas deferens (Itoh et al. 1998b). It was also found that the levels of IFN-gamma, IL-6, and IL-10 in the epididymides strikingly increased with vasectomy alone (Qu et al. 2008).

Antisera obtained from mice with EAO lesions specifically defined testicular antigens with molecular weights of 15, 40, 75, and >200 kDa from 4 weeks of age, but the antisera obtained from vasectomized mice with autoimmune epididymitis strongly defined both testicular and epididymal antigens of 25 KDa from 5 to 8 weeks of ages, respectively. In mice with EAO, immune reactivity with at least nine bands of testicular autoantigens were detected by Western blotting, while only four bands of testicular autoantigens were clearly defined for autoimmune epididymitis in mice receiving vasectomy + TGC immunization. On the contrary, the epididymal autoantigens were similarly detected by antisera between mice with EAO and mice autoimmune epididymitis (Qu et al. 2008, 2010). Immunohistochemical analysis showed that the autoantigens relevant to EAO appeared from 3 weeks of age, while those relevant to autoimmune epididymitis appeared from 4 weeks of age. It suggests that vasectomy changes the target autoantigens in TGC-induced autoimmunity. In antisera of autoimmune epididymitis, it is noted that 25 kDa testicular antigens were definitely detected. Moreover, 25 kDa epididymal antigens were only detected in autoimmune epididymitis but not EAO. Therefore, the 25 kDa antigens in both the testes and epididymides may be a key autoantigen relevant to the pathophysiology of autoimmune epididymitis. The persistence of 25 kDa antigen-bearing germ cells in the epididymal ducts is prolonged after vasectomy, and some of the antigens may then leak outside of the ducts, resulting in autoimmune epididymitis rather than EAO. However, the localization of 25 kDa antigen has not yet been determined.

Although it remains unclear why testicular inflammation does not occur on TGC immunization after vasectomy, significant lymphocytic inflammation was induced in the initial segment of the epididymis instead of EAO, suggesting that the initial segment is an immunological fragile site, as is the tubuli recti. It may be that TGC autoantigens are mainly absorbed at the tubuli recti under physiological conditions; however, in vasectomized mice, the initial segment of the epididymis rather than the tubuli recti is the site where more TGC autoantigens drain into the blood capillaries to some degree (Hirai et al. 2010).

4.2.1.11 Modulation of EAO by Exogenously Administered Immune-Related Agents

Three different phases of EAO induction can be identified: the preclinical phase (until day 20 after the start of TGC immunization), the disease onset phase (from day 20 to day 25), and the disease developing phase (from day 25) (Itoh et al. 1995a).

To evaluate the role of endogenous IFN-gamma, mice immunized with TGC on days 0 and 14 received a single injection of anti-murine IFN-gamma monoclonal antibodies on day 15, 20, or 25. The results showed that the monoclonal antibody treatment on day 20 significantly suppressed both EAO and relevant DTH, while the treatment on day 15 or 25 did not influence them. Therefore, the EAO was prevented by eliminating the action of Th1 cytokine IFN-gamma with neutralizing monoclonal antibody, provided that the treatment is given at an optimal point during disease development. This also suggests that the critical immune reaction for this EAO is Th1 cytokine dependent (Itoh et al. 1998c). Maj et al. (2011a) reported that 17 beta-estradiol and IFN-tau, a type I interferon, interact in regulation of the immune response in EAO. The DTH against TGC was intensified after the administration of either IFN-tau or 17 beta-estradiol, but their co-administration had no effect. In regard to humoral immunity against TGC, the administration of IFN-tau increased IgG2a and decreased IgG1 levels of anti-TGC autoantibodies, whereas 17 beta-estradiol treatments abolished the augmenting effects exerted by the IFN-tau.

Knowing that the production and action of Th1 pro-inflammatory cytokines, including IFN-gamma, IL-2, and TNF, are often antagonized by type 2 cytokines, for example, IL-4, IL-5, IL-6, and IL-10, it is conceivable that an altered balance between these two cytokine subsets with relatively upregulated production or functions of Th1 cytokines favors development of EAO. On the contrary, Th2 cytokines may inhibit EAO. Actually, administration of recombinant IL-6 significantly reduced histological signs of EAO and appearance of DTH against TGC (Li et al. 2002). The inhibitory effect was seen even though the cytokine was administered for only 6 consecutive days from day 15 to day 20 during the preclinical phase. Since DTH to TGC were significantly reduced in mice that had received IL-6, IL-6 directly acts on T cells and macrophages or it acts by diminishing the production of Th1 cytokines such as IFN-gamma or TNF, which promote DTH responses.

In other experiments, exogenously administered recombinant murine IL-10, a well-known anti-inflammatory cytokine, paradoxically augmented severity of EAO when the mice had been administered for 6 consecutive days from days 15 to 20 after primary immunizations with TGC (Kaneko et al. 2003). It indicates that IL-10 with anti-inflammatory property also has pro-inflammatory functions capable of upregulating EAO processes in vivo. The precise mechanism by which IL-10 treatment advances EAO severity is not clear. IL-10, however, is known to induce cell adhesion molecules on endothelial cells in a manner similar to IL-1 beta and TNF-alpha (Vora et al. 1996), and this may have contributed to the orchitogenic response by favoring migration of inflammatory cells into the testicular parenchyma. The capacity of IL-10 to induce proliferation of $CD8^+$ T cell and augment the cytotoxic potency of $CD8^+$ T cells and NK cells (Hill and Sarvertnick 2002), especially in combination with other cytokines, may have contributed as well. It is also possible that the B cell stimulatory activity of IL-10 contributes to the exacerbation of EAO. Therefore, IL-10 may be a highly pleiotropic cytokine (Michell et al. 2004; Mannino et al. 2015).

Deoxyspergualin is one of the active metabolites of spergualin, an antibiotic originally obtained from culture filtrates from a strain of *Bacillus laterosporus*, and functions as an immunosuppressant (Schubert et al. 1987; Thomas et al. 1995). Both in vitro and ex vivo studies have shown that deoxyspergualin may suppress the production of IFN-gamma (Nicoletti et al. 1992, 1993, 1994, 1996). On the other hand, it was reported that reverse transcriptase-polymerase chain reaction showed that mRNA expressions of IL-3, IL-4, IL-5, IL-6, IFN-gamma, and stem cell factor were higher in deoxyspergualin-treated spleen cells than in control spleen cells (Zhu et al. 1994). In TGC-induced EAO model, the daily treatment with the immunosuppressant deoxyspergualin during days 15–20 effectively reduced both the incidence and severity of EAO lesions in a clearly dose-dependent fashion (Ablake et al. 2002). The deoxyspergualin also significantly reduced the degree of DTH against TGC. Considering that cyclosporine A is known to be toxic to TGC and Leydig cells (Seethalakshmi et al. 1987, 1990; Masuda et al. 2003), additional studies are required to demonstrate a lack of toxicity of TGC viability and function by deoxyspergualin.

4.2.1.12 Modulation of EAO by Environmental Chemicals and Pharmaceuticals

Epidemiological studies have shown that autoimmune diseases gradually increase with time (Hess 2002). This raises the question of whether pollutants have some adjuvant effect on the immune system without any antigenic specificity (Bigazzi 1994).

Cadmium, one of various environmental toxicants, is known to suppress systemic immunity and injure the testicular capillary endothelia with resultant necrosis of testicular tissues in mice and rats treated with high doses. It also became evident that cadmium can affect the integrity of the BTB, the endocrine function of Leydig cells, apoptosis of TGC, and systemic immunity, even on treatment with a low dose that does not induce the spermatogenic disturbance (Ogawa et al. 2012). With regard to the immune system, cadmium at low doses increased nonspecific antibody production, granulocyte function, and blood plasma levels of TNF-a and IL-6. In A/J mice, exposure to 3 mg cadmium/kg body weight did not affect the spermatogenic state. However, the BTB at the tubuli recti and the rete testis, but not the seminiferous tubules, was slightly weakened, and intra-testicular mRNA expressions of IL-6, TNF-alpha, and IL-1 beta were significantly increased by the cadmium treatment. Furthermore, immunization with TGC after the cadmium exposure significantly augmented the EAO severity (Ogawa et al. 2012). Cadmium at low doses may cause the release of cytokines that act on a variety of cells in terms of pro-inflammatory reaction. Therefore, exposure to a low dose of cadmium induces no significant disturbance of spermatogenesis; however, it does change the immunological micro-circumstances in the testis, resulting in increased susceptibility to TGC-induced EAO induction.

Di-(2-Ethylhexyl) phthalate has been used as a plastic plasticized for synthetic polymers and well-known toxicant as an endocrine disruptor. Exposure to di-(2-ethylhexyl) phthalate of high doses has been reported to induce the spermatogenic disturbance through oxidant stress and affect the immune system as an adjuvant. After exposure to doses of di-(2-ethylhexyl) phthalate of low doses in mice by giving daily food containing 0.01% or 0.1% di-(2-ethylhexyl) phthalate, significant spermatogenic disturbance was not induced; however, lymphocytes and macrophages significantly increased in number with the elevation of IL-10 and IFN-gamma mRNA expressions in the testes at 8 weeks (Kitaoka et al. 2013). Histochemical analyses involving horseradish peroxidase as a tracer showed that blood-borne horseradish peroxidase had faintly infiltrated into the lumen of a few seminiferous tubules beyond the BTB at 8 weeks. Furthermore, similar to the results using cadmium, exposure of di-(2-ethylhexyl) phthalate of low doses significantly increased a susceptibility to TGC-induced EAO (Hirai et al. 2015).

Tamoxifen is used to treat some types of breast cancer in men and women. It blocks the actions of estrogen and is also used for therapy in male infertility (AinMelk et al. 1987; Adamopoulos et al. 2003; Moein et al. 2012). Maj et al. (2011b) studied the antiestrogen effects of tamoxifen on estrogen receptor alpha level in immune cells and humoral specific response after immunization with TGC. The results showed that levels of estrogen receptor increased in various immune cells of TGC-immunized mice, and administration of tamoxifen decreased the level of their estrogen receptors. However, irrespective of tamoxifen treatment, the humoral response against TGC was similar between tamoxifen-treated and tamoxifen-untreated mice, suggesting that modulation of the level of estrogen receptor in immune cells is not directly related to specific autoantibody production.

4.2.2 EAO Induced by Immunization with Allogeneic TGC Alone

Susceptibility to EAO induction is variable among strains of inbred mice. However, the allogeneic TGC obtained from EAO low susceptible and resistant donor strains could also induce a high incidence of EAO by the twice immunization with the 1×10^7 TGC in highly susceptible mice (Tokunaga et al. 1993a, b). Therefore, autoimmunogenic TGC antigens for EAO induction are not specific to the susceptible strains such as C3H/He and A/J, and TGC of EAO-resistant mice have definite EAO-inducing autoantigens. It indicates that differences of genetic background of TGC-immunized mice, but not immunogenicity of TGC autoantigens of donors, are critical for EAO induction.

4.2.3 EAO Induced by Immunization with Xenogeneic TGC Alone

Previously, it was reported that DTH against allogeneic or xenogeneic TGC was elicited in mice immunized with syngeneic TGC (Yoshida et al. 1979). In guinea pigs that had been immunized with syngeneic, rat, and murine TGC, cross-reactivity was observed among TGC of the guinea pig, rat, or mouse at the levels of immunization with TGC and the DTH elicitation with TGC (Yoshida et al. 1981). Most recently, it was found that twice immunizations with rat TGC can induce murine EAO with no use of adjuvants (Qu et al. 2017). However, the immunization with guinea pig TGC failed to induce EAO in mice. It indicates that TGC autoantigens critical for EAO induction are not species specific. Interspecies common TGC antigens between the mouse and the rat should be important for EAO induction, but those between the mouse and the guinea pigs is not so. The DTH against to murine TGC was significantly elevated in mice immunized with murine or rat but not guinea pig TGC. Serum autoantibody to murine TGC determined by enzyme-linked immunosorbent assay was also significantly elevated in the same manner as the results of DTH. However, on reactions of immune sera with normal frozen sections of murine seminiferous tubules, autoantibodies were immunohistochemically detected in sera of mice immunized with TGC of all three animal species (Qu et al. 2017). In mice immunized with murine TGC, the serum autoantibodies preferentially reacted with immature spermatids. In contrast, in mice immunized with rat TGC, serum autoantibodies reacted with various typed TGC. On the other hand, in mice immunized with guinea pig TGC, the serum autoantibodies specifically reacted with the crescent-shaped acrosomes of mature spermatids and spermatozoa. This indicates that interspecies common antigens of immature rather than mature TGC is important for the EAO induction. By 2D gel electrophoresis, molecular masses around 55 and 70 kDa of murine TGC proteins were definitely detected with sera of mice immunized with murine or rat but not guinea pig TGC. The more detailed identification of common TGC antigens between the mouse and the rat will be needed in future.

4.2.4 EAO Induced by Repeated Intracutaneous Injections of Testicular Homogenate Alone

When the testicular homogenate is frequently injected over a long period of time without adjuvant, severe disturbance of spermatogenesis with little lymphocytic infiltration was found in guinea pigs (Bishop 1961). The significant lesions were induced after 100 days in guinea pigs which had received 40–95 injections of testicular homogenate at rate of 3 or 6 times per week.

4.2.5 EAO Induced by Abdominal Placement of Donor Testes

It was found that only one placement of a syngeneic donor testis connected with epididymis and vas deferens into the abdominal cavity or subcutaneous space was sufficient to induce EAO on the recipient mice with no use of any adjuvants (Terayama et al. 2011b). However, even with this protocol, the placement of a syngeneic testis + epididymis + vas deferens obtained from donor mice induced only orchitis without epididymo-vasitis. The serum autoantibodies were reactive with haploid germ cells existing throughout the testis, the epididymis, and the vas deferens. The phenomenon that reproductive organs other than the testes were free from autoimmune inflammation seems to be against the conventional idea that "the testis is an immune-privileged site." On the other hand, both epididymis and vas deferens appear resistant to inflammatory cell responses in spite of the placement of donor testis + epididymis + vas deferens. It is also noted that intraperitoneal placement of these organs rather than subcutaneous placement of them is effective in inducing severe EAO in the recipients.

References

Ablake M, Itoh M, Kaneko T, Iimura A, Nakamura Y, Meroni P, Nicoletti F. Short-term prophylaxis with deoxyspergualin prevents testicular autoimmunity in mice. Eur J Parmacol. 2002;450:209–12.

Adamopoulos DA, Pappa A, Billa E, Nicopoulou S, Koukkou E, Michopoulos J. Effectiveness of combined tamoxifen citrate and testosterone undecanoate treatment in men with idiopathic oligozoospermia. Fertil Steril. 2003;80:914–20.

AinMelk Y, Belisle S, Carmel M, Jean-Pierre T. Tamoxifen citrate therapy in male infertility. Fertil Steril. 1987;48:113–7.

Alexander NJ, Tung KSK. Immunological and morphological effects of vasectomy in the rabbit. Anat Rec. 1977;188:339–50.

Ansbacher R. Vasectomy: sperm antibodies. Fertil Steril. 1973;24:788–92.

Aoki A, Fawcett DW. Impermeability of Sertoli cell junctions to prolonged exposure to peroxidase. Andrologia. 1975;7:63–76.

Bigazzi PE. Autoimmunity and heavy metals. Lupus. 1994;3:449–53.

Bishop DW. Aspermatogenesis induced by testicular antigen uncombined with adjuvant. Proc Soc Exp Biol Med. 1961;107:116–20.

Bloembergen P, van Dijk H, Hofhuis FMA, van den Heiligenberg P, Willers JMN. Endotoxin-induced autoimmunity in mice. II. Reacting of LPS-hyporesponsive and C5-deficient animals. Int Arch Allergy Appl Immunol. 1988;86:370–4.

Coffman RL, Varkila K, Scott P, Chatelain R. Role of cytokines in the differentiation of CD4$^+$ T-cell subsets in vivo. Immubol Rev. 1991;123:189–207.

Davidson AP, von Dehn BJ, Schlafer DH. Adult-onset lymphoplasmacytic orchitis in a Labrador retriever stud dog. Top Companion Anim Med. 2015;30:31–4.

Dym M, Fawcett DW. The blood-testis barrier in the rat and the physiological compartmentation of the seminiferous epithelium. Biol Reprod. 1970;3:308–26.

Flickinger CJ, Howards SS, Bush LA, Baker LA, Herr JC. Temporal recognition of sperm autoantigens by IgM and IgG autoantibodies after vasectomy and vasovasostomy. J Reprod Immunol. 1994;27:135–50.

Flickinger CJ, Howards SS, Bush LA, Baker LA, Herr JC. Antisperm autoantibody responses to vasectomy and vasovasostomy in fisher and Lewis rats. J Reprod Immunol. 1995;28:137–57.

Flickinger CJ, Baran ML, Howards SS, Herr JC. Sperm autoantigens recognized by autoantibodies in developing rats following prepubertal obstruction of the vas deferens. J Andol. 1996;17:433–42.

Freund J, Lipton MM, Thompson GE. Aspermatogenesis in the guinea pig induced by testicular tissue and adjuvant. J Exp Med. 1953;97:711–26.

Fritz TE, Lombard LA, Tyler SA, Norris WP. Pathology and familial incidence of orchitis and its relation to thyroiditis in a closed beagle colony. Exp Mol Pathol. 1976;24:142–58.

Furbeth C, Hubner G, Thoenes GH. Spontaneous immune complex orchitis in brown Norway rats. Virchows Arch B Cell Pathol. 1989;57:37–45.

Hamilton DW. UDP-galactose:N-acetylglucosamine galactosyltransferase in fluids from rat rete testis and epididymis. Biol Reprod. 1980;23:377–85.

Herr JC, Flicjinger CJ, Howards SS, Yarbro S, Spell DR, Caloras D, Gallien TN. The relation between antisperm and testicular alterations after vasectomy and vasovasostomy in Lewis rats. Biol Reprod. 1987;37:1279–305.

Hess EV. Environmental chemicals and autoimmune disease: cause and effect. Toxicology. 2002;181:65–70.

Hill N, Sarvertnick N. Cytokines: promoters and dampeners of autoimmunity. Curr Opin Immunol. 2002;14:791–7.

Hirai S, Naito M, Terayama H, Qu N, Miura M, Shirakami G, Itoh M. Differences in abundance of blood and lymphatic capillaries in the murine epididymis. Med Mol Morphol. 2010;43:37–42.

Hirai S, Naito M, Terayama H, Qu N, Kuerban M, Musha M, Ikeda A, Miura M, Itoh M. The origin of lymphatic capillaries in murine testes. J Androl. 2012;33:745–51.

Hirai S, Naito M, Terayama H, Hatayama N, Qu N, Musha M, Itoh M. Serum autoantibodies in mice immunized with syngeneic testicular germ cells alone. Am J Reprod Immunol. 2013a;70:509–17.

Hirai S, Naito M, Terayama H, Qu N, Kuerban M, Musha M, Itoh M. Lymphangiogenesis in chronic inflammation in the testis. Andrology. 2013b;1:147–54.

Hirai S, Naito M, Kuramasu M, Ogawa Y, Qu N, Terayama H, Hatayama N, Itoh M. Low-dose di(2-ethylhexyl) phthalate (DEHP) exposure increases susceptibility to testicular autoimmunity in mice. Reprod Biol. 2015;15:163–71.

Hoffmann M. Serum from LPS nonresponder C3H/HeJ mice does not support the formation of functional EAC reagents. J Immunol. 1978;121:619–21.

Itoh M, Hiramine C, Koseto M, Hojo K. Enzyme-linked immunosorbent assay (ELISA) for detecting antisperm antibodies in mice with testicular autoimmunity. Am J Reprod Immunol. 1989;21:9–15.

Itoh M, Hiramine C, Hojo K. A new murine model of autoimmune orchitis induced by immunization with viable syngeneic testicular germ cells alone. I. Immunological and histological studies. Clin Exp Immunol. 1991a;83:137–42.

Itoh M, Hiramine C, Tokunaga Y, Mukasa A, Hojo K. A new murine model of autoimmune orchitis induced by immunization with viable syngeneic testicular germ cells alone. II. Immunohistochemical findings of fully-developed lesion. Autoimmunity. 1991b;10:89–97.

Itoh M, Mukasa A, Tokunaga Y, Hiramine C, Hojo K. New experimental model for adoptive transfer of murine autoimmune orchitis. Andrologia. 1991c;23:415–20.

Itoh M, Hiramine C, Mukasa A, Tokunaga Y, Fukui Y, Takeuchi Y, Hojo K. Establishment of an experimental model of autoimmune epididymo-orchitis mediated by T cell line in mice. Int J Androl. 1992a;15:170–81.

Itoh M, Mukasa A, Tokunaga Y, Hiramine C, Hojo K. Suppression of efferent limb of testicular autoimmune response by a regulatory $CD4^+$ T cell line in mice. Clin Exp Immunol. 1992b;87:455–60.

Itoh M, Hiramine C, Mukasa A, Tokunaga Y, Fukui Y, Takeuchi Y, Hojo K. Antigen non-specific tissue damage in T cell-mediated experimental autoimmune orchitis: preliminary characterization of a testis-specific T-cell line by using dermal tissue and cells. Andrologia. 1993;25:89–92.

Itoh M, Miyake M, Miki T, Takeuchi Y, de Rooij DG. Immunohistological localization of autoantigens detected by serum autoantibodies from mice with experimental autoimmune orchitis without using adjuvants. Arch Androl. 1994;32:45–52.

Itoh M, de-Rooij DG, Takeuchi Y. Mode of inflammatory cell infiltration in testes of mice injected with syngeneic testicular germ cells without adjuvant. J Anat. 1995a;187:671–9.

Itoh M, de-Rooij DG, Takeuchi Y. Histopathology of the seminiferous tubules in mice injected with syngeneic testicular germ cells alone. Arch Androl. 1995b;35:93–103.

Itoh M, de-Rooij DG, Jansen A, Drexhage HA. Phenotypical heterogeneity of testicular macrophages/dendritic cells in normal adult mice; an immunohistochemical study. J Reprod Immunol. 1995c;28:217–32.

Itoh M, Ueno M, Li XQ, Satriotomo I, Takeuchi Y. Topographical uptake of blood-borne horseradish peroxidase (HRP) in the murine testis at the light microscopic level. Int J Androl. 1998a;21:74–80.

Itoh M, Li XQ, Yano A, Xie Q, Takeuchi Y. Patterns of efferent lymphatics of the mouse testis. Int J Androl. 1998b;19:466–72.

Itoh M, Yano A, Xie Q, Iwahashi K, Takeuchi Y, Meroni PL, Nicoletti F. Essential pathogenic role for endogenous interferon-r (IFN-r) during disease onset phase of murine experimental autoimmune orchitis. I. In vivo studies. Clin Exp Immunol. 1998c;111:513–20.

Johnson AL, Howards SS. Intratubular hydrostatic pressure in testis and epididymis before and after vasectomy. Am J Phys. 1975;228:556–64.

Kaneko T, Itoh M, Nakamura Y, Iimura A, Hayashi S, Takahashi K, Stivala F, Bendtzen K, Nicoletti F. Proinflammatory effects of exogenously administered IL-10 in experimental autoimmune orchitis. Cytokine. 2003;22:50–3.

Kitaoka M, Hirai S, Terayama H, Naito M, Qu N, Hatayama N, Miyaso H, Matsuno Y, Komiyama M, Itoh M, Mori C. Effects on the local immunity in the testis by exposure to di-(2-ethylhexyl) phthalate (DEHP) in mice. J Reprod Dev. 2013;59:485–90.

Koji T, Hishikawa Y, Ando H, Nakanishi Y, Kobayashi N. Expression of Fas and Fas ligand in normal and ischemia-reperfusion testes: involvement of the Fas system in the induction of germ cell apoptosis in the damaged mouse testis. Biol Reprod. 2001;64:946–54.

Koji T. Male germ cell death in mouse testes: possible involvement of Fas and Fas ligand. Med Electron Microsc. 2001;34:213–22.

Kuerban M, Naito M, Hirai S, Terayama H, Qu N, Ikeda A, Musha M, Koji T, Itoh M. Involvement of Fas/Fas-L and Bax/Bcl-2 systems in germ cell death following immunization with syngeneic testicular germ cells in mice. J Androl. 2012;33:824–31.

Li L, Itoh M, Ablake M, Macri B, Bendtzen K, Nicoletti F. Prevention of murine experimental autoimmune orchitis by recombinant human interleukin-6. Clin Immunol. 2002;102:135–7.

Lustig L, Rival C, Tung KS. Autoimmune orchitis and autoimmune oophoritis. The autoimmune diseases. 5th ed. Amsterdam: Elsevier Academic Press; 2014. p. 1007–20.

Maj T, S-Awek A, Kaleta-Kuratewicz K, Che-Mo-Ska-Soyta A. 17 beta-estradiol and interferon tau interact in the regulation of the immune response in a model of experimental autoimmune orchitis. J Interf Cytokine Res. 2011a;31:825–37.

Maj T, Switala-Jelen K, Miazek A, Szafarowicz-Basta B, Kiczak L, Slawek A, Chelmonska-Soyta A. Effects of tamoxifen on estrogen receptor-alpha level in immune cells and humoral specific response after immunization of C3H/he male mice with syngeneic testicular germ cells (TGC). Autoimmunity. 2011b;44:520–30.

Mannino MH, Zhu Z, Xiao H, Bai Q, Wakefield MR, Fang Y. The paradoxical role of IL-10 in immunity and cancer. Cancer Lett. 2015;367:103–7.

Masuda H, Fujihira S, Ueno H, Kagawa M, Katsuoka Y, Mori H. Ultrastructural study on cytotoxic effects of cyclosporine a in spermiogenesis in rats. Med Electron Microsc. 2003;36:183–91.

Mealy K, Robinson B, Millette CF, Majzoub J, Wilmore DW. The testicular effects of tumor necrosis factor. Ann Surg. 1990;211:470–5.

Michell MD, Simpson KL, Keelan JA. Paradoxical proinflammatory actions of interleukin-10 in human amnion: potential roles in term and preterm labour. J Clin Endocrinol Metab. 2004;89:4149–52.

Moein MR, Tabibnejad N, Ghasemzadeh J. Beneficial effect of tamoxifen on sperm recovery in infertile men with nonobstructive azoospermia. Andrologia. 2012;44(Suppl 1):194–8.

Mukasa A, Itoh M, Tokunaga Y, Hiramine C, Hojo K. Inhibition of a novel model of murine autoimmune experimental autoimmune orchitis by intravenous administration with a soluble testicular antigen: participation of $CD8^+$ regulatory T cells. Clin Immunol Immunopahol. 1992;62:210–9.

Mukasa A, Hiramine C, Hojo K. Generation and characterization of a continuous line of $CD8^+$ suppressively regulatory T lymphocytes which down-regulates experimental autoimmune orchitis (EAO) in mice. Clin Exp Immunol. 1994;96:138–45.

Musha M, Hirai S, Naito M, Terayama H, Qu N, Hatayama N, Itoh M. The effects of adjuvants on autoimmune responses against testicular antigens in mice. J Reprod Develop. 2013;59:139–44.

Nagahori K, Hirai S, Terayama H, Qu N, Miyaso H, Li ZL, Naito M, Itoh M. Specific testicular proteins identified by sera of mice with autoimmune orchitis. 2017 (in preparation).

Naito M, Itoh M. Patterns of infiltration of lymphocytes into the testis under normal and pathological conditions in mice. Am J Reprod Immunol. 2008;59:55–61.

Naito M, Terayama H, Hirai S, Qu N, Kawata S, Itoh M. Histopathology of the tubuli recti at the start of experimental autoimmune orchitis in mice. Med Mo Morphol. 2009;42:230–5.

Naito M, Hirai S, Terayama H, Qu N, Kuerban M, Musha M, Kitaoka M, Ogawa Y, Itoh M. Post-inflammation stage of autoimmune orchitis induced by immunization with syngeneic testicular germ cells alone in mice. Med Mol Morphol. 2012a;45:35–44.

Naito M, Terayama H, Hirai S, Qu N, Lustig L, Itoh M. Experimental autoimmune orchitis as a model of immunological male infertility. Med Mol Morphol. 2012b;45:185–9.

Nashan D, Cooper TG, Knuth UA, Schulbeus P, Sorg C, Nieschlag E. Presence and distribution of leukocyte subsets in the murine epididymis after vasectomy. Int J Androl. 1990;13:39–49.

Natwar RK, Mann A, Sharma RK, Aulitzky W, Frick J. Effect of human gamma interferon on mice testis: a quantitative analysis of the spermatogenic cells. Acta Eur Fertil. 1995;26:45–9.

Nicoletti F, Meroni PL, Di-Marco R, Grasso S, Barcellini W, Borghi MO, Lunetta M, Mughini L, Menta R, Schorlemmer HU. The effects of deoxyspergualin on the development of diabetes in diabetes-prone BB rats. Scand J Immunol. 1992;36:415–20.

Nicoletti F, Borghi MO, Meroni PL, Barcellini W, Fain C, Di-Marco R, Menta R, Schorlemmer HU, Bruno G, Magro G. Prevention of cyclophosphamide-induced diabetes in the NOD/WEHI mouse with deoxyspergualin. Clin Exp Immunol. 1993;91:232–6.

Nicoletti F, DI-Marco R, Barcellini W, Borghi MO, Lunetta M, Mughini L, Meroni PL. Protection from experimental autoimmune thyroiditis in CBA mice with the novel immunosuppressant deoxyspergualin. Scand J Immunol. 1994;39:333–6.

Nicoletti F, Borghi MO, Barcellini W, Fain C, Beltrami B, Del-Papa N, Schorlemmer HU, Mottola L, Meroni PL. Immunosuppressive activity of 15-deoxyspergualin on normal and autoimmune peripheral blood mononuclear cells. Eur J Pharmacol. 1996;311:213–20.

Ogawa Y, Itoh M, Hirai S, Suna S, Naito M, Qu N, Terayama H, Ikeda A, Miyaso H, Matsuno Y, Komiyama M, Mori C. Cadmium exposure increases susceptibility to testicular autoimmunity in mice. J Appl Toxicol. 2012;33:652–60.

Pelletier RM, Yoon SR, Akpovi CD, Silvas E, Vitale ML. Defects in the regulatory clearance mechanisms favor the breakdown of self-tolerance during spontaneous autoimmune orchitis. Am J Physiol Regul Intergr Como Physiol. 2009;296:R743–62.

Pelletier RM, Akpovi CD, Chen L, Day R, Vitale ML. CX43 expression, phosphorylation, and distribution in the normal and autoimmune orchitic testis with a look at gap junctions joining germ cell to germ cell. Am J Physiol Regul Intergr Como Physiol. 2011;300:R121–39.
Qu N, Terayama H, Naito M, Ogawa Y, Hirai S, Kitaoka M, Yi SQ, Itoh M. Caput epididymitis but not orchitis was induced by vasectomy in a murine model of experimental autoimmune orchitis. Reproduction. 2008;135:859–66.
Qu N, Naito M, Terayama H, Hirai S, Li J, Ogawa Y, Kitaoka M, Itoh M. Developmental ontogeny of autoantigens associated with localized autoimmunity in murine testis and epididymis. J Reprod Immunol. 2010;87:45–51.
Qu N, Naito M, Terayama H, Hirai S, Musha M, Itoh M. Chronological changes of delayed-type hypersensitivity in mice immunized with testicular germ cells alone. Andrologia. 2014;46:556–63.
Qu N, Terayama H, Hirayanagi Y, Kuramasu M, Ogawa Y, Hayashi S, Hirai S, Naito M, Itoh M. Induction of experimental autoimmune orchitis by immunization with xenogeneic testicular germ cells in mice. J Repod Immunol. 2017;121:11–16.
Robinson R, Tung KSK, Meeker ND, Monson FG, Teuscher C. A murine model of spontaneous aspermatogenesis: linkage to H-2. J Reprod Immunol. 1994;26:251–60.
Schubert G, Stoffregen C, TImmermann W, Schang T, Thiede A. Comparison of the new immunosuppressive agent 15-deoxyspergualin and cyclosporine a after highly allogeneic pancreas transplantation. Transplant Proc. 1987;19:3978–89.
Scott P. IFN-gamma modulates the early development of Th1 and Th2 responses in a murine model of cutaneous leishmaniasis. J Immunol. 1991;147:3149–55.
Seethalakshmi L, Meron M, Malhotra RK, Diamond DA. Effect of cyclosporine a on male reproduction in rats. J Urol. 1987;138:991–5.
Seethalakshmi L, Flores C, Carboni AA, Bala R, Diamond DA, Menon M. Cyclosporine: its effects on testicular function and fertility in the prepubertal rat. J Androl. 1990;11:17–24.
Soramoto S, Hiramine C, Takenaka I, Hojo K. Murine experimental autoimmune orchitis (EAO) induced by syngeneic testicular germ cells (TC) alone: orchitogenic and lymphostimulatory activities of TC from mice at various ages. Clin Immunol Immunopathol. 1993;69:292–9.
Terayama H, Naito M, Qu N, Hirai S, Kitaoka M, Ogawa Y, Itoh M. Intra-testicular expression of mRNAs of both interferon gamma and tumor necrosis factor alpha is significantly increased in experimental autoimmune orchitis in mice. J Reprod Dev. 2011a;57:296–302.
Terayama H, Itoh M, Naito M, Hirai S, Qu N, Kuerban M, Musha M. Experimental model of autoimmune orchitis with abdominal placement of donor's testes, epididymides, and vasa deferentia in recipient mice. J Reprod Immunol. 2011b;90:195–201.
Terayama H, Naito M, Hirai S, Qu N, Katagiri C, Nagahori K, Hayashi S, Sasaki H, Moriya S, Hiramoto M, Miyazawa K, Hatayama N, Sakabe K, Matsushita M, Itoh M. Specific autoantigens identified by sera obtained from mice that are immunized with testicular germ cells alone. Sci Rep. 2016; doi:10.1038/srep35599.
Thomas F, Pittman K, Liung T, Cekada E. Deoxyspergualin is a unique immunosuppressive agent with selective utility in inducing tolerance to pancreas islet xenografts. Transplant Proc. 1995;27:417–9.
Tokunaga Y, Hiramine C, Itoh M, Muaksa A, Hojo K. Genetic susceptibility to the induction of murine experimental autoimmune orchitis (EAO) without adjuvant. I. Comparison of pathology, delayed type hypersensitivity, and antibody. Clin Immunol Immunopathol. 1993a;66:239–47.
Tokunaga Y, Hiramine C, Hojo K. Genetic susceptibility to the induction of murine experimental autoimmune orchitis (EAO) without adjuvant. II. Analysis on susceptibility to EAO induction using F1 hybrid mice and adoptive transfer system. Clin Immunol Immunopathol. 1993b;66:248–53.
Tokunaga Y, Terayama H, Naito M, Qu N, Hirai S, Ogawa Y, Yi SQ, Itoh M. Splenic cytokines in mice immunized with testicular germ cells. Int J Androl. 2007;31:471–6.
Tung KS, Ellis L, Teuscher C, Meng A, Blaustein JC, Kohno S, Howell R. The black mink (*Mustela vison*): a natural model of immunologic male infertility. J Exp Med. 1981;154:1016–32.

Tung KS, Ellis LE, Childs GV, Dufau M. The dark mink, a model of male infertility. Endocrinology. 1984;114:922–9.

Uhlen M, Oksvold P, Fagerberg L, Lundberg E, Jonasson K, Forsberg M, Zwahlen M, Kampf C, Wester K, Hober S, Wernerus H, Bjorling L, Ponten F. Towards a knowledge-based human protein atlas. Nat Biotechnol. 2010;28:1248–50.

Uhlen M, Fagerberg L, Hallstrom BM, Lindskog C, Oksvold P, Mardinoglu A, Sivertsson A, Kampf C, Sjostedt E, Asplund A, Olsson I, Edlund K, Lundberg E, Navani S, Szigyarto CA, Odeberg J, Djureinovic D, Takanen JO, Hober S, Alm T, Edqvist PH, Berling H, Tegel H, Mulder J, Rockberg J, Nilsson P, Schwenk JM, Hamsten M, von Feilitzen K, Forsberg M, Persson L, Johansson F, Zwahlen M, von Heijne G, Nielsen J, Ponten F. Tissue-based map of the human proteome. Science. 2015;347(6220):1260419.

Vora M, Romero LI, Karasek MA. Interleukin-10 induces E-selection on small and large blood vessel endothelial cells. J Exp Med. 1996;184:821–9.

Yoshida S, Nomoto K, Himeno K, Takeya K. Immune response to syngeneic or autologous testicular cells in mice. I. Augmented delayed footpad reaction in cyclophosphamide-treated mice. Clin Exp Immunol. 1979;38:211–7.

Yoshida S, Nomoto K, Himeno K, Sanui H. Delayed hypersensitivity to syngeneic or xenogeneic cells in guinea-pigs. Immunology. 1981;42:445–9.

Zhu X, Imamura M, Tanaka J, Han CW, Hashino S, Imai K, Asano M, Nakane A, Minagawa T, Kobayashi M. Effects of 15-deoxyspergalin in vitro and in vivo on cytokine gene expression. Transplantation. 1994;58:1104–9.

Testicular Autoimmunity by the Systemic Treatment with Immuno-Potentiating Agents in Experimental Animals

5

5.1 Introduction

Experimental autoimmune orchitis (EAO) can be induced by testicular antigens' immunization with simultaneous treatments with adjuvants such as complete Freund's adjuvant (CFA), *Bordetella pertussis antigens* (BP), other microbial agents, and some immune-stimulating chemical (Fig. 5.1). These immuno-potentiating agents may easily overcome the testicular immune privilege systemically and/or locally.

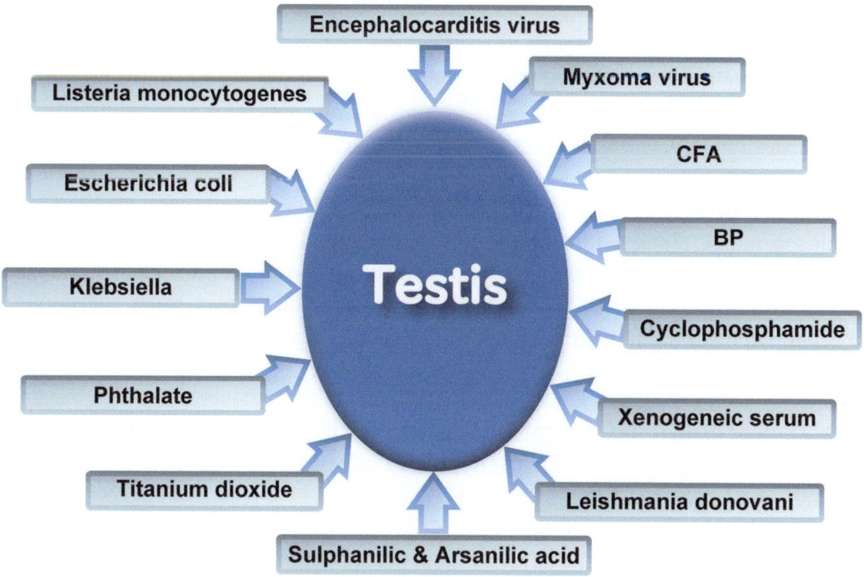

Fig. 5.1 Immuno-potentiating agents for stimulation of testicular inflammation. *CFA* complete Freund's adjuvant. *BP Bordetella pertussigens*

M. Itoh, *Testicular Autoimmunity*, DOI 10.1007/978-4-431-54460-9_5

5.2 Various EAO Models with the Aid of Immunopotentiators

5.2.1 EAO Induced by Treatment with Cyclophosphamide and the Following Immunization with TGC

Cyclophosphamide is an anticancer chemotherapy drug, which is classified as an alkylating agent. It has been used for therapy of Hodgkin's and non-Hodgkin's lymphoma, Burkitt lymphoma, chronic lymphocytic leukemia, chronic myelocytic leukemia, acute myelocytic leukemia, acute lymphocytic leukemia, T cell lymphoma (mycosis fungoides), and multiple myeloma. Its common side effect is low blood counts with increased risk for infection, anemia, and bleeding. Moreover, cyclophosphamide is also known to be toxic to male reproductive organs (Rezvangfar et al. 2008; Drumond et al. 2011). On the other hand, it appears that cyclophosphamide can eliminate $CD4^{+}CD25^{+}Foxp3^{+}$ Treg in experimental and clinical medicine (Yoshida et al. 1979; Brode et al. 2006; Audia et al. 2007; Cao et al. 2010) (Fig. 5.1). Indeed, cyclophosphamide-treated mice that received a single subcutaneous injection with TGC 2 days later developed EAO, whereas no such lesions were seen in TGC-immunized but cyclophosphamide-untreated mice (Sakamoto et al. 1985). Significant DTH against TGC and anti-TGC antibodies in sera were detected in EAO-affected mice. It is suggested that the mechanism that facilitated the EAO induction might be attributable to the elimination of endogenous cyclophosphamide-sensitive Treg (Sakamoto and Nomoto 1986). In mice that received cyclophosphamide on day 0 and TGC immunization on day 2, anti-TGC DTH is thought to play a key role in the induction of EAO. Actually, DTH against TGC was mildly induced by only one immunization with viable syngeneic TGC and was significantly augmented by cyclophosphamide pretreatment, and, furthermore, the DTH was suppressed by administration of cyclosporine A in a dose-dependent manner in mice that were cyclophosphamide pretreated and then immunized with TGC (Sakamoto et al. 1994). However, anti-TGC DTH was rather enhanced significantly in mice pretreated with cyclosporine A alone without any TGC immunization. Therefore, even though administration of cyclosporine A suppressed the specific DTH in TGC-immunized mice, administration of cyclosporine A alone rather eliminates some suppressive mechanism resulting in augmentation of anti-TGC DTH.

5.2.2 EAO Induced by Immunization with Testicular Antigens or Homogenate Emulsified in Complete Freund's Adjuvant (CFA)

CFA is most commonly used adjuvant in experimental research (Fig. 5.1). It is prepared from non-metabolizable oil containing killed *Mycobacterium tuberculosis* and designed to provide continuous release of antigens necessary for stimulating a strong, persistent immune response. CFA-induced peripheral inflammation evokes pro-inflammatory cytokines such as IL-1-beta, IL-6 TNF-alpha, and IFN-gamma

(Lapchak et al. 1992; Chuang et al. 1997; Raghavendra et al. 2004). The mycobacterial components in CFA activate CD4$^+$ T cells and signal them to assume a Th1 profile so that strong DTH against autoantigens develops (Billiau and Matthys 2001). On the other hand, immune effector cells induced by CFA exert an inhibitory effect on antigen-specific Th2 responses (Chuang et al. 1997).

Eyquem and Krieg (1965) produced bilateral EAO by injecting a small amount of CFA alone into the left testis in rats, guinea pigs, and monkeys. In left testes, infiltration of mononuclear cells, resorption of the inoculated product in the granulomata, spermatogenic disturbance, and exudation of fibrinoid products were induced. On the other hand, in the right testes, the spermatogenic disturbance was seen, but there was no inflammatory cell response and granulomata, implying the induction of sympathetic lesion.

Freund et al. (1953) discovered that subcutaneous injection of homologous testicular homogenate emulsified in CFA into guinea pigs is followed by inflammatory lesions of the testes and, finally, by the spermatogenic disturbance. It is generally assumed that CFA acts by prolonging the lifetime of injected autoantigen, by stimulating its effective delivery to the immune system, and by providing a complex set of signals to the innate compartment of the immune system, resulting in altered leukocyte proliferation and differentiation (Tung et al. 1971c; Billiau and Matthys 2001). Early events include rapid uptake of adjuvant components by macrophages and dendritic cells, enhanced phagocytosis, secretion of cytokines by mononuclear phagocytes, and transient activation and proliferation of CD4$^+$ T cells. The mycobacterial component in CFA also remodels the hemopoietic system, leading to a drastic expansion of Mac-1$^+$ immature myeloid cells. The effects of CFA cause the so-called ASIA (autoimmune/autoinflammatory syndrome induced by adjuvants), in which the injection of CFA accelerates various autoimmune manifestations (Bassi et al. 2012).

Studies on this EAO induced by testicular homogenate+CFA-immunization had been carried out using the guinea pigs because of the ease of disease induction in this species (Freund et al. 1953, Tung et al. 1971a, b, 1977; Hojo et al. 1980). Katsh (1964) found that testes from prepubertal guinea pigs failed to induce EAO lesions when incorporated in CFA, indicating that mature rather than immature TGC autoantigens is critical for EAO induction. In EAO-induced rats, both DTH and autoantibodies against testicular antigens were detected at different times with maximum levels at 50 days with significant decrease in CD8$^+$ T cells (Doncel et al. 1991; Doncel and Lustig 1991). Typical EAO was successfully transferred to naïve recipients with peritoneal exudate and lymph node cells from male and female donor guinea pigs preciously immunized with testicular antigens+CFA (Carlo et al. 1976). However, attempts to transfer EAO with circulating antibody from the immunized animals were not successful, supporting a cell-mediated basis for the immunologic events in EAO (Carlo et al. 1976). An important role of DTH to testicular antigen in both the induction and suppression of EAO has been also described (Tung et al. 1977; Hojo et al. 1980).

Bernard et al. (1975) found that immunization with homogenate of testicular antigens+CFA+saline induces EAO, while that with homogenate of testicular antigens+CFA+normal human serum failed to induce EAO, although the inhibitory components of normal serum have not yet been identified. They demonstrated that the capacity of antigen P purified from guinea pigs' spermatozoa to produce lesions of EAO could be inhibited by mixing antigen P with a small amount of normal human serum before immunization of animals. Characteristics of the serum inhibitory factors remain unsolved.

Chutna and Rychlikova (1964) reported that guinea pigs pretreated with testis antigens in incomplete Freund's adjuvant (non-metabolizable oils without killed *Mycobacterium tuberculosis*) were unresponsive to the sensitization for EAO. In the absence of *Mycobacterium tuberculosis*, T cell differentiation tends to assume a Th2 profile with strong antibody production only (Billiau and Matthys 2001). Later, Hojo and Hiramine (1982) and Hiramine and Hojo (1984a) investigated "antigen-specific" suppression of EAO in guinea pigs in a model made by subcutaneous injections with testicular antigens in incomplete Freund's adjuvant prior to EAO sensitization with testicular antigens in CFA. This suppressive state for EAO induction was adoptively transferable to normal syngeneic recipients with lymph node T cells taken from animals pretreated with testicular antigens+incomplete Freund's adjuvant, indicating the presence of specific Treg. The Treg suppressed DTH reaction to testicular antigens, but not anti-sperm antibody production in their recipients. Cyclophosphamide treatment 3 days before EAO sensitization abolished the preventive effect of pretreatment with testicular antigens+incomplete Freund's adjuvant. In another study, it was demonstrated that cyclosporine A administration for 2 weeks, starting on the day of testicular antigens+CFA-immunization, almost completely abrogated the EAO induction, DTH to testicular antigens, and also anti-sperm antibody response in guinea pigs (Hojo and Hiramine 1985). Transfer of lymphocytes taken from cyclosporine A-treated, EAO-suppressed guinea pigs into normal syngeneic recipients inhibited the EAO induction in an antigen-specific manner, indicating the induction of specific Treg by cyclosporine A. However, as far as guinea pig EAO is employed, it is impossible to describe in detail the suppression mechanism, such as the phenotype of Treg and related cytokines.

In the rat, EAO is also inducible by immunization with Sertoli cells+CFA (Tung and Fritz 1987), by immunization with basal lamina of the seminiferous tubules+CFA (Denduchis et al. 1975, 1979; Lustig et al. 1977, 1982, 1986), and by immunization with pachytene spermatocytes+CFA (Tung and Fritz 1987) (Fig. 5.2). This indicates that testicular cells other than spermatids and spermatozoa have a potential to induce EAO with the aid of CFA. It is also noted that male rats treated with CFA alone have reduced serum testosterone and elevated serum luteinizing hormone concentrations, showing the induction of testicular dysfunction (Clemens and Bruot 1989) (Fig. 5.3).

In the mouse, thymectomy in adult life prevented EAO induction or interfered with further development of established EAO (Vojtiskova and Pokorna 1964). On the contrary, neonatal thymectomy further enhanced severity of EAO by subsequent immunization with testicular antigens+CFA in the rat (Lipscomb et al. 1979). These two studies suggest an involvement of the thymus for both induction and suppression of EAO. In general, mice have been considered relatively resistant to testicular antigens+CFA-induced EAO in comparison with guinea pigs, but Feng et al. (1990) developed a protocol for transferring EAO to naïve recipient mice in this disease model. In that study, cell donors were balb/c mice immunized 12 days earlier with epididymal spermatozoa+CFA+bovine serum albumin (Figs. 5.1 and 5.2). As few as 3×10^6 sperm-specific T lymphocytes obtained from the immunized mice were

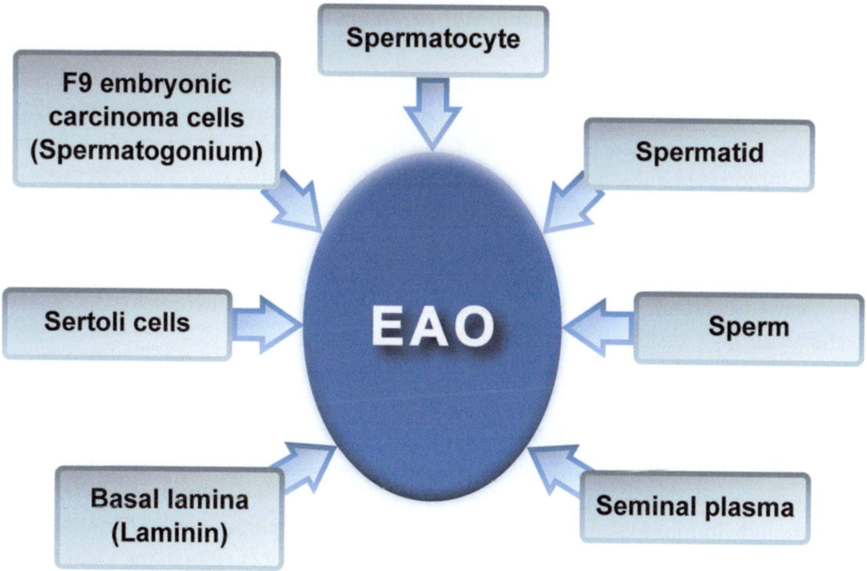

Fig. 5.2 Various sensitizing antigens by which EAO is inducible with the aid adjuvants

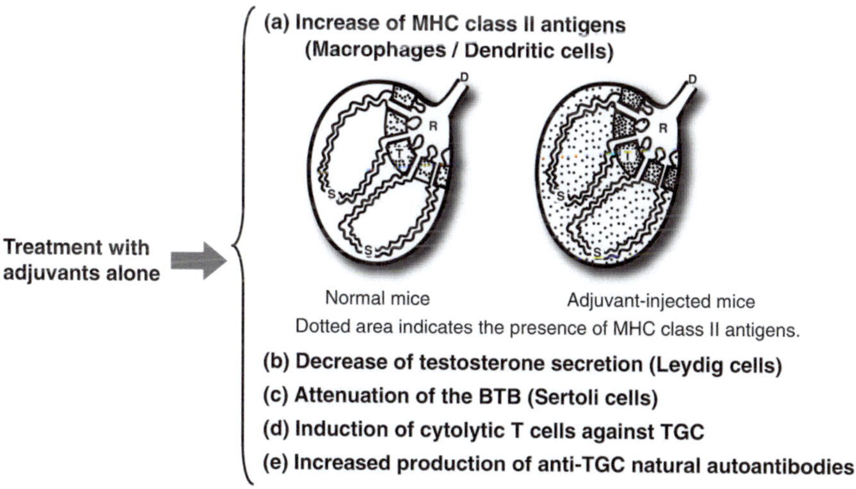

Fig. 5.3 Effects of adjuvants on the testis. *BTB*, blood-testis barrier. D, tubuli recti. *TGC*, testicular germ cells

able to transfer EAO. Later, Li et al. (2014) aimed to determine the role of Axl and Mer receptor tyrosine kinases in maintaining the systemic tolerance to TGC antigens. Axl and Mer double knockout ($Axl^{-/-}Mer^{-/-}$) mice developed severe EAO after a single immunization with TGC homogenates+CFA. This immunization protocol also induced mild EAO in Axl or Mer single-gene knockout mice. By contrast, the TGC homogenate+CFA-immunization failed to induce EAO in wild-type mice.

These results indicate that Axl and Mer receptors cooperatively regulate the systemic immune tolerance to TGC antigens. More recently, the roles of TLR2 and TLR4 in mediating the EAO induction were investigated in mice (Liu et al. 2015). Wild-type mice developed severe EAO after three immunizations with TGC antigens+CFA; however, TLR2- or TLR4-deficient mice showed relatively low susceptibility to EAO induction. It was demonstrated that TLR2 was crucial in mediating autoantibody production in response to the immunization. Notably, TLR2 and TLR4 double knockout mice were almost completely protected from EAO induction, implying that TLR2 and TLR4 cooperatively mediate EAO induction. However, it remains unclear whether TLR2 and TLR4 affect EAO induction locally in the testis or through systemic immunity.

Significant spermatogenic disturbance and appearance of anti-TGC autoantibodies were also observed in mice and guinea pigs after syngeneic, allogeneic, and xenogeneic immunization with mouse F9 embryonic carcinoma cells+CFA (Vojtiskova et al. 1983) (Fig. 5.2). This indicates that common cancer antigens between mice and guinea pigs may play a critical role for EAO induction in the both species.

Although immune T cells are most importantly required for EAO induction, Hiramine and Hojo (1984b) elucidated the participation of B cells in the local transfer system of EAO in the guinea pig. Proliferative response of EAO-inducing (orchitogenic) T cells was enhanced by the presence of B cells as well as macrophages (Hojo et al. 1980). Their study showed the requirement of B cells in the local adoptive transfer of EAO and suggested the possibility of cooperative interactions among T cells, B cells, and macrophages involved in the generation of the transferred EAO lesions. From this study, it was first demonstrated that B cells possess the antigen-presenting capability like macrophages and dendritic cells in the guinea pig EAO. However, the participation of humoral antibodies themselves has been the subject of controversy. Although typical EAO was successfully transferred to naïve recipients with peritoneal exudate and lymph node cells from male and female donor guinea pigs previously immunized with testicular antigens+CFA, attempts to transfer EAO with circulating antibody from the immunized animals were not successful (Carlo et al. 1976). In contrast, in testicular antigens+CFA-immunized guinea pigs and rats, passive transfer of antiserum against testicular antigens induced EAO (Tung et al. 1971b; Toullet and Voisin 1976; Lustig et al. 1977, 1978; Denduchis et al. 1979, 1985). In guinea pigs that had been injected into the recipient testis with immune sera from donors immunized with testicular homogenate+CFA, congestive vessels and exudation of polymorphonuclear cells were seen in the testis during the first week after the local injection. Leukocytes also appeared in the vicinity of the canaliculi of the rete testis (Mancini et al. 1974). This picture was accompanied by vacuolization of Sertoli cells and sloughing of TGC. Later, marked disturbance of spermatogenesis with a moderate infiltration of mononuclear cells between the seminiferous tubules and also in the interstitium of the rete testis and the epididymis was found (Chattopadhyay 1979). Injection of normal sera did evoke any histological changes in the recipient testis. The autoantibodies induced by testicular homogenate+CFA-immunization should include not only anti-TGC but also anti-Sertoli cell and anti-basal lamina of the seminiferous tubules antibodies (Fig. 5.4). It is known that the

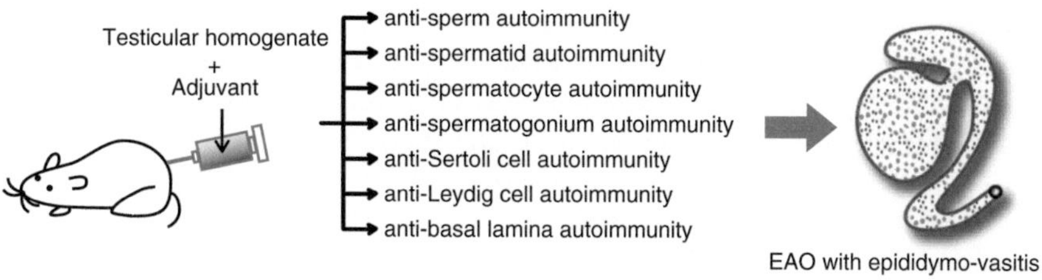

Fig. 5.4 Various immune responses induced by sensitization with testicular homogenates+adjuvants. D, ductuli efferentes. E, epididymis. T, testis. V, vas deferens. *Dotted areas* indicate the presence of the lymphocytic inflammation

laminins constitute the major non-collagenous components of basal lamina of the seminiferous tubules. When rabbit antibodies to laminin1 (IgG fraction) were injected into adult guinea pigs, thickening of the tubular limiting membrane, infolding in the basal lamina, deposits of immune complexes coincident with sloughing of pachytene spermatocytes and spermatids, and vacuolization of the Sertoli cells were induced. However, Sertoli cell tight junctions remained impermeable, and mononuclear cell infiltration in the testis was rare (Lustig et al. 2000). This indicates a possible participation of B cell lineage for EAO induction as well as T cells.

In EAO using animals immunized with testicular antigens+CFA, transfer of EAO with "immune RNA" was reported in guinea pigs. "Immune RNA" obtained from the lymphocytes of donor guinea pigs, which were immunized with testis antigens+CFA, was injected intraperitoneally into normal recipient guinea pigs (Fainboim et al. 1978). The transferred guinea pigs developed DTH to sperm antigens and EAO as seen in the "immune RNA" donor guinea pigs. In contrast, when the transfer was performed with RNA extracted from guinea pigs that were immunized with CFA alone, no specific DTH and EAO were observed. Furthermore, in cases of transfer with ribonuclease-treated "immune RNA," the recipient animals failed to have EAO lesions. "Immune RNA" may convert non-sensitized mouse peritoneal cells to a state of specific immunologic reactivity to testicular antigens. In an in vitro study, the "immune RNA" was incubated with normal guinea pig peritoneal exudate cells, which showed specific inhibition of migration when tested with the TGC antigen (Fainboim et al. 1979). In similar experiments, normal guinea pig peritoneal exudate cells, when incubated in vitro with "immune RNA" from "rats" immunized with testicular homogenate+CFA, recognized and responded to the TGC antigens specifically as assessed by the direct migration inhibition reaction (Sztein et al. 1980). This indicates the success of transfer of cell migration inhibition in vitro with not only syngeneic but also xenogeneic RNA in EAO. Therefore, "immune RNA" is able to cross the species barrier and sensitive to xenogeneic lymphoid cells. Sztein et al. (1980) also showed that the transferred antigen reactivity is directed against common testicular antigens present in rats, mice, and guinea pigs. The reaction would appear to be organ specific, kidney homogenate+CFA being unable to cause migration inhibition. EAO can be transferred by other "noncellular materials" (Pokorna 1969). In his study, male donor mice of C57BL/10 strain were immunized with testicular homogenate+CFA. On day 14, spleens and lymph nodes of the donors were taken, and their cell suspensions were prepared. The cell suspension was incubated at 56 C for 1 h, and cellular sediment was then centrifuged and the supernatant was used. EAO was induced in recipient mice that were intraperitoneally injected with "the prepared supernatant" in amount of 0.5 ml (Pokorna 1969). Furthermore, it was found that spleen cells and lymph node cells from non-immunized normal mice can also transfer EAO when the cells were incubated with "the prepared supernatant." The incubated cells from normal donors were washed three times with Hanks solution and injected intraperitoneally in amount of 0.5 ml containing 2×10^8 cells. The EAO-inducing supernatant exhibited cytotoxic complement-dependent activity on testicular cells and was partly inactivated by trypsin, whereas RNase and DNase did not influence their activity. Since the EAO transfer induced by "immune RNA" or the "noncellular supernatant" obtained from immune cells has not been further reexamined, the minute pathophysiology remains unclear.

In regard to testicular autoantigens, four glycoproteins (GP1, GP2, GP3, and GP4) rich in carbohydrate were isolated from guinea pig testes (Hagopian et al. 1975). The molecular weights of the glycoproteins were estimated to be 47,000, 105,000, and 13,000, respectively, for GP1, GP2, and GP4. GP3 showed two major bands, with molecular weights of 41,500 and 22,800. GP1, GP2, and GP4 were localized in the sperm acrosome (Fig. 5.2). Approximately, 5 mg each purified GP1, GP3, and GP4, and 3 mg of GP2 were isolated from 1000 g of wet guinea pig testes. In particular, both GP1 and GP4 are strongly orchitogenic (EAO-inducing) antigens, while GP2 and GP3 were inactive (Hagopian et al. 1975, 1976). A unique highly soluble aspermatogenic protein, AP1, was also isolated from guinea pig testes. Approximately 20 mg of AP1 were obtained from 5000 g of wet guinea pig testes (Jackson et al. 1975, 1976). This protein is localized on the outer surface of sperm acrosome and is a potent inducer of EAO (Fig. 5.2). Toullet and Voisin (1976) reported that three different autoantigens (S, P, and T), extracted and separated from guinea pig spermatozoa, give rise to EAO when injected with CFA. They also induce specific antibodies, such as anaphylactic (with S and P), complement-fixing (with P and T), spermotoxic (only with T), and precipitating and Arthus-inducing antibodies (only with P). Autoantigens S is present on proacrosomal granules, acrosomal granules, and acrosome and head cap of spermatozoa. Autoantigen P is present on the same formations except for the head cap. Autoantigen T is also localized on acrosomes and head caps but on their membranes as well as on the cytoplasmic membranes of spermatozoa and spermatids (Toullet et al. 1973). In particular, autoantigen S was detected on the acrosomal apparatus in not only guinea pigs but also rabbits, rats, and mice. Later, aspermatogenic polypeptides, AP2 and AP3, capable of inducing EAO in the guinea pig were purified from their testes and epididymides by sequential biochemical methods (Teuscher et al. 1983a, b). Approximately 80 mg of AP2 was obtained from 10^{10} cauda epididymal spermatozoa. AP2 has a molecular weight of 9500. Approximately 250 mg of AP3 were obtained from 500 g wet weight of the testes. AP3 appeared as a single band with a molecular weight of 12,500. Immunization with AP2+CFA or AP3+CFA induced severe EAO in 100% of the guinea pigs tested. Guinea pigs were immunized with a defined and highly potent aspermatogenic antigen, G75 m, and the following occurrence of EAO was correlated with cell-mediated immune response to G75 m (Meng and Tung 1983). Later, it was reported that the immunization of male guinea pigs with PH-20+CFA also reproducibly results in EAO induction (Tung et al. 1997). PH-20, a testis-specific protein first expressed in haploid TGC, is present on the posterior head plasma membrane and inner acrosomal membrane of mature guinea pig spermatozoa (Fig. 5.2). PH-20 is bifunctional, having a hyaluronidase activity that allows sperm to penetrate the cumulus layer and a separate activity required for binding of acrosome-reacted sperm to the zona pellucida. Remarkably, PH-20+CFA-induced EAO differed from testicular homogenate+CFA-induced EAO in two respects: (1) an absence of epididymitis with abscess and granulomata and (2) the deposit of antibodies on TGC within the seminiferous tubules and abnormal spermatozoa inside the cauda epididymis in PH-20-induced EAO lesions. The former suggests that crude testis antigens other than PH-20 are responsible for autoimmune epididymitis in testicular homogenate+CFA-immunized animals, and the latter suggests an active role of humoral immunity in PH-20-induced EAO pathogenesis. In addition, guinea pigs immunized with testicular acrosin with molecular weight of 34,000 + CFA also exhibited typical EAO (Falase et al. 1989).

5.2.3 EAO Induced by Immunization with Mixture Containing Testicular Homogenate and *Bordetella pertussis* (BP)

In vivo intoxication with BP elicits a variety of physiological responses including a marked leukocytosis, disruption of glucose regulation, adjuvant activity, alterations in vascular function, hypersensitivity to vasoactive agents, and upregulation of MHC class II molecules (Tonon et al. 2002; Gao et al. 2003) (Figs. 5.1 and 5.3). BP-induced lymphocytosis is associated with alteration in thymocyte subpopulations (Person et al. 1992b). BP primarily affects and depletes thymic T cells with an immature phenotype. However, in the periphery of BP-treated mice, the relative increase in the number of $CD4^+$ T cells is more than that of $CD8^+$ T cells. In regard to pro-inflammatory cytokines, BP treatment induced the release of IL-6, IL-12, and TNF-alpha (Mielcarek et al. 2001; Tonon et al. 2002).

EAO was induced in mice immunized with testicular homogenate+BP on day 0 and day 34 (Hargis et al. 1968). On day 50, the immunological aspermatogenesis was characterized by degenerating TGC, signet ring nuclei, abnormal mitotic figures, karyorrhexis, the presence of an eosinophilic coagulum, and multinucleate giant cells. There was moderate interstitial edema, but it is noted that accumulations and invasion of mononuclear cells were rare. Both Sertoli cells and Leydig cells appeared normal. BP enhances of the DTH as well as hypersensitivity of the immediate type. BP treatment alone in the absence of immunization with testicular homogenate induced systemic leukocytosis in mice with significant lymphocytic inflammation in the ductuli efferentes, epididymis, and prostate, but not in the testes (Itoh et al. 1995).

In vivo intoxication with BP elicits a variety of inflammatory responses, including vasoactive amine sensitization to histamine, serotonin, and bradykinin (Diehl et al. 2014). Histamine is genetically controlled by a locus controlling BP-induced histamine sensitization (Bphs). Furthermore, it was found that BP sensitizes mice to histamine independently of TLR4, a purported receptor for BP (Diehl et al. 2014). Therefore, Bphs on chromosome 6 may be critical in susceptibility to testicular homogenate+BP-induced EAO (Teuscher 1985, 1986; Sudweeks et al. 1993; Meeker et al. 1999; Ma et al. 2002; Gao et al. 2003).

5.2.4 EAO Induced by Immunization with Testicular Antigens or Homogenate Emulsified in CFA and the Following Intravenous Administration of BP

5.2.4.1 Induction of EAO

Previously, many investigators had a difficulty to reproduce murine EAO model by immunization with testis antigens+CFA or with testis antigens+BP. Bernard et al. (1978) were the first to develop active EAO model in mice by immunization with testicular homogenate emulsified in CFA followed by intravenous injection with BP. This EAO using both CFA and BP is reproducible and consistently accompanied by severe inflammation in the epididymis and the vas deferens (=epididymo-vasitis). They also first succeeded in adoptive transfer of murine EAO (=passive EAO) with immune T cells into T cell-deficient athymic nude recipient mice treated with BP. Therefore, an important role for T cells in mediation of murine EAO was demonstrated by this adoptive transfer experiment (Bernard et al. 1978). The inflammatory lesions composed of macrophages, lymphocytes, neutrophils, and eosinophils are mainly found in association with the spermatogenic disturbance and Leydig cell hyperplasia (Sato et al. 1981; Kohno et al. 1983). DTH against testicular antigens was detected early at day 7; it increased with time, reaching a maximum at day 80; and a good temporal relationship between DTH and histopathology was found (Doncel et al. 1989). In contrast, circulating specific autoantibodies were only present in approximately 60% of the animals with EAO, and no deposits of IgG or C3 in the seminiferous tubules were seen (Doncel et al. 1989). Later, Mahi-Brown et al. (1987, 1988) and Mahi-Brown and Tung (1989, 1990) have shown that activated T cells can successfully transfer of the EAO to thymus-bearing normal recipient mice. The donor mice used in the adoptive transfer experiment received an immunization schedule consisting of subcutaneous injection with whole testicular homogenate+CFA+BP. A successful transfer of EAO to naive recipient mice was done by performing an in vitro challenge of the donor $CD4^+$ T cells with testis antigens before the cell transfer (Tung et al. 1989). Later, EAO was shown to be induced by testis and sperm antigen-specific T cell clone that had been derived from testicular homogenate+CFA+BP-immunized mice (Yule and Tung 1993). Similar to other EAO models, MHC class II antigen-restricted $CD4^+$ T cells are the primary effectors; however, recent evidence suggests the involvement of $CD8^+$ T cells during the onset and maintenance of chronic EAO, in which Th17 cytokines are also involved in the pathogenesis of EAO (Jacobo et al. 2009, 2011a, b). At EAO onset, the number of $CD4^+$ and $CD8^+$ effector T cells dramatically increased in the testis, with the $CD4^+$ T cell subset predominating. As the severity of EAO progressed, CD4+ effector T cells declined in number, while the CD8+ effector T cell subset remained unchanged, suggesting their involvement in maintenance of the chronic phase of EAO (Doncel and Lustig 1991; Lustig et al. 1993; Jacobo et al. 2009). Mast cells increased tenfold in number, were more widely distributed throughout the interstitial tissue, and were partially degranulated (Iosub et al. 2006). Mielcarek et al. (2001) demonstrated that mast cells phagocytose BP and can process and present BP molecules to T lymphocytes. Furthermore, exposure of mast cells to BP induced the release of pro-inflammatory cytokines such as TNF-alpha and IL-6. In the seminiferous tubules, TGC death occurs through an apoptotic mechanism preceding TGC sloughing in an autocrine and/or paracrine way. Later lesions of EAO included granulomata formation and necrosis in the testis (Zhou et al. 1989).

EAO was also induced by immunization with laminin+CFA+BP in the rat (Lustig et al. 1977, 1982, 1986, 1987, 1989) (Fig. 5.2). Laminin has been characterized as the main non-collagenous glycoprotein of basal lamina of the seminiferous tubules and has been detected in a variety of cells, including Sertoli cells (Denduchis et al. 1975). The main components of basal lamina are type IV collagens, laminins, entactin/nidogen, and heparin sulfate proteoglycans. In this EAO, interstitial mononuclear cell infiltration was also seen in the epididymis. The testicular lesions were characterized by multiple foci of the seminiferous tubules with different degrees of sloughing of the germinal epithelium. In the basal lamina of the seminiferous tubules, splitting and focal thickenings of knob-like projections toward the epithelium was found (Lustig et al. 1982, 1987). The thickening and delamination of the basement membrane was consistently accompanied by vacuolization of the Sertoli cell cytoplasm. In vivo-bound rat IgG was detected along the walls of the seminiferous tubules as bright linear and dense reaction products on the basal lamina. High titers of circulating anti-laminin antibodies and a significant DTH to laminin were detected in the immunized rats. Leukocyte migration was also inhibited when the spleen cells of the immunized rats were incubated with laminins.

5.2.4.2 The Effects of CFA+BP Sensitization

The mycobacterial components within CFA signal T cells to assume a Th1 profile so that strong DTH against testicular autoantigens develops. In the absence of mycobacteria, T cell differentiation tends to assume a Th2 profile with strong antibody production only (Billiau and Matthys 2001). In the periphery of BP-treated mice, the relative increase in the number of CD4+ T cells is more than that of CD8+ T cells. As mentioned earlier, treatment with CFA and BP releases various pro-inflammatory cytokines involving IL-1-beta, IL-6, IL-12, TNF-alpha, and IFN-gamma in vivo (Lapchak et al. 1992; Chuang et al. 1997; Mielcarek et al. 2001; Tonon et al. 2002; Raghavendra et al. 2004). Considering that severe splenomegaly and lymphadenopathy was induced by CFA+BP treatment alone, various lymphocytic clones that are not specific to the testicular antigens should be also activated, resulting in enhancement of the immune responses and the breakdown of testicular immune privilege. Indeed, the employment of CFA and BP has proved to be instrumental in altering the completeness of BTB indirectly (Fig. 5.3), as well as in augmenting of DTH (Pelletier et al. 1981; Sewell et al. 1986; Adekunle et al. 1987). Foci of tubules with exfoliated TGC into the seminiferous tubular lumen or sloughing of the germinal epithelium was found in CFA+BP-injected mice and rats (Adekunle et al. 1987; Lustig et al. 1987). In particular, TNF at high concentrations are toxic to the spermatogenesis (Mealy et al. 1990). The presence of IL-6 made Sertoli cells in vitro to exhibit a redistribution of tight junction proteins, resulting in reduction of transepithelial electrical resistance (Perez et al. 2011, 2012). This indicates that IL-6 is also involved in downregulating BTB permeability.

The number of MHC class II antigen-bearing cells increased after the CFA+BP treatment even when immunization with testicular antigens was absent (Tung et al. 1987) (Fig. 5.3). Therefore, both CFA and BP also may affect histopathological pattern of autoimmune inflammation against the testicular antigens. Tung et al. (1987) have demonstrated that the tubuli recti, rete testis, and ductuli efferentes were predominant sites of inflammation in passive EAO (induced by transferring $CD4^+$ T cells isolated from the immunized donors into non-immunized, naïve recipients) but that active EAO (induced by immunization with testicular homogenate+CFA+BP) affected the peripheral seminiferous tubules under the tunica albuginea away from the tubuli recti and rete testis. The reason for the first involvement of the tubuli recti in passive model of EAO may be that the recipient mice were free from CFA+BP-induced upregulation of the distribution of antigen-presenting macrophages/dendritic cells throughout the testes (Fig. 5.2).

Sato et al. (1981) and Kohno et al. (1983) demonstrated minute histopathology of this EAO. In the EAO lesion, granular deposits of IgG were identified around seminiferous tubules. A focal degeneration and desquamation of both spermatogonia and Sertoli cells was induced prior to inflammatory cell responses. Yule et al. (1988) showed immune sera from mice immunized with testicular homogenate+CFA+BP and had reactivity with testicular cells of mice younger than 2 weeks of age. The autoantibodies bound to spermatogonia and spermatocytes were IgG1 but not IgG2 isotypes. Therefore, immunization with testicular homogenate+CFA+BP, but not with testicular homogenate alone, produced autoantibodies against diploid germ cells (spermatogonia and preleptotene spermatocytes) outside the BTB (Yule et al. 1988) (Fig. 5.4). Furthermore, it also became evident that immunization with testis homogenate+CFA+BP elicits not only immune responses against germ cells but also the responses against other testicular components such as Leydig cells, Sertoli cells, and basal lamina of the seminiferous tubules (Sato et al. 1981; Lustig et al. 1982) (Fig. 5.4). Namely, immunization with testicular homogenate+CFA+BP includes immune responses against spermatozoa, spermatids, spermatocytes, spermatogonia, Sertoli cells, Leydig cells, and basal lamina of the seminiferous tubules.

Recently, a new syndrome, namely, the "autoimmune/autoinflammatory syndrome induced by adjuvants" (ASIA), has been defined (Shoenfeld and Agmon-Levin 2011; Colafrancesco et al. 2014). In this syndrome, different conditions induced by various adjuvants such as infectious fragments, hormones, aluminum, silicone, and metal are included, and the syndrome is characterized by common signs and symptoms, resulting in boosting the immune response and triggering the development of autoimmune phenomena (Loyo et al. 2012; Cruz-Tapias et al. 2013;

Lujan et al. 2013). Therefore, CFA+BP treatment also may induce ASIA-like condition. Indeed, in CFA+BP-injected mice, both production of anti-TGC autoantibodies and development of cytolytic activity of T cells against TGC are inducible without the use of testicular antigens for sensitization (Ben et al. 1986; Musha et al. 2013) (Fig. 5.3). Moreover, reversibility of disease resistance to EAO was found by treatment with BP in EAO-resistant rats (Teuscher et al. 1989). Therefore, there is a possibility that EAO may be inducible with CFA+BP treatment alone if some optimal conditions such as longer injection periods and/or more frequent injections are devised.

5.2.4.3 Role of Antibodies

Demonstration of IgG in the testis after immunization with testicular homogenate+CFA+BP or in the recipient testis after transfer of sera from orchiectomized donor mice immunized with testicular homogenate+CFA+BP shows that autoantigens are present on TGC outside the Sertoli cell barrier. It suggests the existence of dynamic protective mechanisms against immune responses to the non-sequestered TGC in normal individuals (Yule et al. 1990). The IgG deposits in EAO lesions were characterized as antibodies bound to the spermatogonia and preleptotene spermatocytes and were detected as early as day 7 after immunization, 5–6 days before the onset of EAO (Tung and Teuscher 1995) (Fig. 5.4). Testis IgG deposits were also elicited by immunization with testis homogenate in incomplete Freund's adjuvant which does not elicit EAO. This IgG is absorbed from circulation by the testis, because the IgG is found only in the serum of mice orchiectomized before the immunization (Mahi-Brown et al. 1988). Thus the immune deposits alone are not sufficient to cause active EAO. The lack of pathogenicity by immunization with testis homogenate in incomplete Freund's adjuvant is probably related to the unique immunoglobulin subclass of the IgG deposits. Only IgG1 and IgG3 but not IgG2a or IgG2b were detected. This finding can explain lack of association of complement components in the deposits in testis. Actually, in the testis of mice immunized with testis homogenate, autoantibodies were detected as immune complexes around the damaged seminiferous tubules free of inflammatory cell response, although the pathogenic role of testicular immune complexes has not yet been explored. There is a possibility that binding of autoantibodies to the target antigen-bearing cells and tissues such as spermatogonia, spermatocytes, and basal lamina of the seminiferous tubular wall affects the physiological function of the seminiferous epithelium. To investigate it, autoantibodies against Sertoli cells and basal lamina of the seminiferous tubules can be obtained from animals immunized with testicular homogenate+CFA+BP. Lustig et al. (1978) found that EAO can be induced by passive transfer of an antiserum to seminiferous tubular basal lamina. The damage was characterized by foci of perivascular and peritubular infiltrates of mononuclear cells. Moreover, infolding, thickening, and rupture of the seminiferous tubular wall and vacuolization of Sertoli cells and spermatogenic disturbance were also seen. A linear deposit of immunoglobulins was detected along the basal lamina of seminiferous tubules and blood capillaries. Additionally, in the kidneys of recipients, a deposit of immunoglobulins along glomerular basement membrane, focal areas of mononuclear cell infiltrates, hypercellularity of glomeruli, and thickening of both glomerular capillary wall and Bowman's capsule were also found. Moreover, by using two kinds of monoclonal antibodies (IgM) against Sertoli cell and basal lamina of the seminiferous tubule that were derived from testicular antigens+CFA+BP-immunized mice, the spermatogenic disturbance was induced experimentally by intra-testicular injection of a set of these two monoclonal antibodies in mice (Ichinohasama et al. 1986) (Figs. 5.2 and 5.4). However, single injection of either monoclonal antibody failed to induce the lesion. This fact indicated that monoclonal antibody against Sertoli cells could reach the Sertoli cell to impair its function, which was otherwise inaccessible without coincidental action of monoclonal antibody against the basal lamina of the seminiferous tubules. The monoclonal antibody against the basal lamina appeared to alter the permeability of the BTB and lower its barrier effect. The most depressed spermatogenesis was frequently observed in testes 1 week after the second injection in mice that had been injected with a mixture of the two kinds of monoclonal antibodies twice at a 1-week interval. Immunohistochemically, the percentage of seminiferous tubules positive for anti-mouse IgM and anti-mouse complement appeared to parallel the impaired degree of spermatogenesis. It is important to note that there was no inflammatory cell infiltration. Neither congestion nor thrombosis of vessels nor ischemic changes was seen. The chronology of changes in the testes revealed that the spermatogenesis gradually recovered and became almost normal at 8 weeks after the second monoclonal antibody treatment. This suggests that humoral immunity is not so critical for producing chronic EAO.

5.2.4.4 Relevant Autoantigens

Immunization with allogeneic murine tissue homogenate of various organs emulsified in CFA accompanied by the injection of BP revealed that only testicular and epididymal homogenates of adult but not prepubertal mice are capable of eliciting EAO (Adekunle et al. 1987). Immunization of mice with xenogeneic testicular antigens+CFA+BP failed to elicit significant EAO, indicating that the major target autoantigens are highly species specific (Adekunle et al. 1987). Moreover, the use of allogeneic mouse testicular homogenate from EAO-resistant strains as sensitizing antigens exhibited similar potential for inducing significant EAO like in cases of the use of allogeneic testicular homogenates from EAO-susceptible strains. It suggests that immunoregulation against testicular antigens, but not autoimmunogenicity of testicular antigens, affect EAO sensitivity. However, testicular homogenates from NZB/B1NJ and MRL/MpJ$^{-/+}$ mice were significantly less potent at inducing autoimmune epididymitis as compared to other strains, indicating possible interstrain differences of relevant autoantigens for EAO induction (Adekunle et al. 1987).

By using SDS-polyacrylamide gel electrophoresis and immunoblotting by reaction of normal sera with normal testicular homogenates in mice, two immunoreactive bands corresponding to approximately 45 and 100 kDa were detected (Musha et al. 2013). These two natural autoantibodies were more definitely detected in CFA+BP-immunized mice with no use of testicular antigens. In immunohistochemical staining by reacting normal testicular sections with immune sera from CFA+BP-injected group, haploid TGC and other immature TGC near the basement membrane of seminiferous tubules were finely stained. Moreover, compared with the normal controls, one band of approximately 40 kDa was additionally detected by immune sera obtained from the CFA+BP-injected mice, indicating that treatment with CFA+BP alone can evoke autoimmune reactions against some testicular autoantigens despite the use of no testicular homogenate (Fig. 5.3). It may be due to CFA+BP-induced ASIA (autoimmune/autoinflammatory syndrome induced by adjuvants). In testicular homogenate+CFA+BP-induced EAO, two natural autoantibodies against testicular antigens corresponding to approximately 45 and 100 kDa were further definitely detected like in CFA+BP-immunized mice. Moreover, the serum samples of testicular homogenate+CFA+BP-immunized mice also reacted with eight additional testicular autoantigens of approximately 15, 22, 25, 40, 60, 75, 120, and 250 kDa.

Sperm-specific zonadhesin is a target autoantigen with an EAO-inducing (orchitogenic) polypeptide domain (Hardy and Garbers 1995; Wheeler et al. 2011) (Fig. 5.2). Zonadhesin is expressed on the acrosomal membrane of spermatid and sperm and can bind zona pellucida and inhibit interspecies gamete interaction (Tardif et al. 2010). Serum antibody reacted with the 340 kDa protein in sperm of wild type but not zonadhesin-null mice. It was next shown that mice immunized with recombinant zonadhesin+CFA+BP developed EAO. Two other murine testis-specific autoantigens (mAP1 and mAP2) for EAO induction were partially purified from mouse testis acetone powder (Teuscher et al. 1994). Dose-response bioassays revealed that mAP1 and mAP2 are most effective at eliciting active EAO by mixing with CFA+BP and passive EAO induced by transferring $CD4^+$ T cells isolated from the immunized donors into non-immunized, naïve recipients, respectively.

A proteomic approach using 2D SDS-PAGE and immunoblotting analysis with immune sera obtained from testicular homogenate+CFA+BP-injected mice identified 12 spots. Seven were subsequently identified by mass spectrometry as heat shock proteins (HSPs), including HSP60 and HSP70, disulfide isomerase ER-60, alpha-1 antitrypsin, heterogeneous nuclear ribonucleoprotein H1, sperm outer dense fiber major protein 2, and phosphoglycerate kinase 1, which are abundant in male TGC and characterized as testicular autoantigens for EAO (Fijak et al. 2005). HSP70 has been reported to promote antigen-presenting cell function and converts T cell tolerance to autoimmunity in vivo (Millar et al. 2003).

Laminin, a component of the basal lamina, was also shown to be important autoantigens for EAO induction, because immunization with laminin+CFA+BP induced EAO (Lustig et al. 1987) (Fig. 5.2). This indicates that immunologic injury specific to the basal lamina induces TGC depletion from the seminiferous epithelium in an antigen-nonspecific manner. Indeed, morphological alteration of the basal lamina of the seminiferous tubules in various pathological conditions including a varicocele, cryptorchid testes, hypogonadotropic hypogonadism, and irradiated testes have been reported. It has also been demonstrated that the basal lamina of the seminiferous tubules in the Japanese monkey is histologically changed when spermatogenetic activity decreases in the nonbearing season. These findings suggest a possibility that physiological condition of the basal lamina of the seminiferous tubules influences the activity of seminiferous tubules (Tainosho et al. 2011; Naito et al. 2012).

5.2.4.5 Pathophysiology of Leukocytic Infiltration and the Following Spermatogenic Disturbance

For EAO induction, interaction between blood capillary endothelial cells and circulating leukocytes are important, because the capillary endothelial cells play an essential role by facilitating leukocyte recruitment via their ability to express cell surface adhesion molecules. Rats with EAO showed a significant increase in the percentage of CD31$^+$ endothelial cells that upregulate the expression of CD106. The percentage of leukocytes expressing CD49d (CD106 ligand) also increases during EAO (Guazzone et al. 2012). The CD44 antigen is a cell surface glycoprotein involved in cell-cell interactions, cell adhesion, and migration. It functions as a hyaluronic acid receptor, and both lipopolysaccharide and TNF-alpha upregulate CD44-mediated hyaluronic acid binding. It is known that activated lymphocytes bind hyaluronic acid present on the endothelium, and this specific binding facilitates the rolling and extravasation of leukocytes into the inflammation site (Guazzone et al. 2005). By in vitro hyaluronic acid-binding assay, the level of peripheral blood mononuclear cell adhesion was higher in testicular antigens+CFA+BP-immunized rats compared to normal controls. By immunohistochemistry, a significant increase in the number of CD44$^+$ cells was detected in the testicular interstitium of rats with severe EAO, indicating that the CD44 molecules are involved in the homing of lymphocytes into the testis of rats with EAO (Guazzone et al. 2005). In the testis under physiological conditions, IL-1-beta is feebly produced; however, an upregulation of IL-1-beta, which may promote adhesion and migration of leukocytes, was also observed in the testis of rats immunized with testicular antigens+CFA+BP (Guazzone et al. 2009). Chemokines such as monocyte chemoattractant protein-1 and macrophage inflammatory protein-1 were also upregulated in the EAO lesion and therefore might induce attraction and extravasation of immune cells into the testicular interstitium. A significant increase of monocyte chemoattractant protein-1 was observed in the testicular fluid and in the conditioned medium obtained from cultures of testicular macrophages of rats with EAO (Guazzone et al. 2003). An increase in monocyte chemoattractant protein-1 expression was immunohistochemically observed in mononuclear cells, endothelial cells, Leydig cells, peritubular myoid cells, and Sertoli cells of rats with severe EAO. This indicates that this chemokine has an important role in recruiting immune cells to the testis in rats undergoing EAO.

CD4$^+$ T cells that secrete Th1 cytokines in vitro play the most important role for EAO induction (Yule and Tung 1993; Tung 1998). All orchitogenic T cell clones, derived from mice immunized with testicular homogenate+CFA+BP, expressed both CD4 and the alpha-beta TCR. When activated, they produced IL-2, IFN-gamma, and TNF-alpha, but not IL-4. EAO transfer was significantly and reproducibly attenuated when recipients were given neutralizing antibody to TNF-alpha but not IFN-gamma in vivo. Hence, TNF-alpha rather than IFN-gamma was shown to be required for amplification of the pathogenic T cell response (Tung and Teuscher 1995). Although TNF-alpha protects TGC from apoptosis at physiologically low concentrations in normal testes, it behaves as an apoptotic factor that induces TGC death under inflammatory conditions (Theas et al. 2008). Actually, spermatogenic disturbance was experimentally induced by injection of TNF into the rat testis through a direct effect on TGC and an indirect mechanism involving Leydig cells or Sertoli cell dysfunction (Mealy et al. 1990). On the contrary, there is a study demonstrating that TNF does not appear to be the principal cytokine involved in the pathogenesis of actively induced EAO (Teuscher et al. 1990c). In that study, the ability of TNF to function as a coadjuvant in eliciting active EAO was examined by treating the EAO-immunized mice with recombinant murine TNF or anti-TNF antibodies at various time points throughout both the induction and effector phase of the EAO process; however, the all treated mice failed to exhibit a markedly significant change in EAO outcome in comparison with EAO-sensitized mice without TNF or anti-TNF antibodies.

Ben et al. (1986) have shown a good correlation between the severity of testicular pathological changes and cytolytic activity of immune lymphocytes against TGC. They concluded that the cytolytic activity against TGC might be a major factor in the development of EAO, but they did not determine the phenotype of the lymphocytes responsible for the cytolytic function. They also demonstrated that spleen cells from CFA+BP-injected mice kill TGC in vitro in spite of no immunization with testicular homogenate+CFA+BP (Fig. 5.3). They hypothesized that CFA+BP treatment nonspecifically damages the BTB by which testis-specific cytotoxic T cell clones are stimulated and expanded. However, there is another possibility that the adjuvant treatment nonspecifically stimulates all immune cells to secrete various kinds of cytokines, which are toxic and injurious to the seminiferous epithelium. Ben et al. (1986) also suggested that EAO may be induced in mice with adjuvants alone if the optimal experimental procedures are used. If this hypothesis is correct, an anamnesis of tuberculosis or whooping cough could be one of causes for immunologic orchitis, like mumps orchitis.

Testicular macrophages in rats immunized with testicular homogenate+CFA+BP also secreted both IFN-gamma and TNF-alpha, like $CD4^+$ T cells (Suescun et al. 2003; Rival et al. 2008; Theas et al. 2008). Furthermore, IL-6 expression in testicular macrophages is also significantly increased in EAO (Rival et al. 2006a). In the rat EAO, the balance between $ED1^+$ macrophage (circulating monocytes arriving at the testis) and $ED2^+$ macrophage (resident macrophages in the testis) subsets can be disrupted under EAO conditions (Rival et al. 2008). The increased number of $ED1^+$ cells is maintained for long periods of time during chronic inflammation in EAO. What causes the persistent elevated macrophage numbers in the testis with EAO is still unclear. $ED1^+$ cells notably express IL-6 at high levels compared with $ED2^+$, suggesting the distinct roles of the two types of macrophages in mediating inflammatory responses. An in vitro study has shown that exogenous IL-6 induces TGC apoptosis (Theas et al. 2003). Therefore, the high production of IL-6 by testicular $ED1^+$ macrophages, the increased expression of IL-6 receptor in TGC, and the involvement of this cytokine in TGC apoptosis suggest a pathogenic role of IL-6 in EAO. Actually, IL-6 mRNA expression in murine testes also dramatically increased in testicular homogenate+CFA+BP-induced EAO (Musha et al. 2013).

Dendritic cells bearing CD80, CD86, and MHC class II antigens in EAO lesions have a mature immunogenic status and are able to induce immune responses to testicular antigens (Jacobo et al. 2011b). The mRNA expression level of IL-10 and IL-12p35 was significantly upregulated in enriched dendritic cell fraction in draining lymph nodes from the EAO-affected testis (Guazzone et al. 2011a). Furthermore, mRNA level of chemokine receptor for monocyte chemoattractant protein 3 was significantly increased, and the expression of chemokine receptor for monocyte chemoattractant protein-1 was decreased in isolated dendritic cells from rats with EAO (Rival et al. 2006b, 2007). In co-culture experiments, testicular dendritic cells isolated from EAO lesion significantly enhanced naïve T cell proliferation compared with control testicular dendritic cells (Rival et al. 2007). Therefore, testicular dendritic cells in control testis is not mature and functionally tolerogenic, while they reach a mature immunogenic state by IL-12 expression in EAO-affected testes and stimulate T cell proliferation prior imminent migration to the draining lymph nodes to amplify immune responses against testicular antigens (Rival et al. 2007). During EAO, elevated levels of high-mobility group box protein 1 were found. High-mobility group box protein 1 is a pro-inflammatory cytokine released from both monocytes and macrophages and functions as an immunostimulatory signal that induces dendritic cell maturation. This protein appears to be involved in regulating inflammatory reactions in EAO-affected testes, as blocking its action by ethyl pyruvate reduces the disease progression (Aslani et al. 2014). Therefore, high-mobility group box protein 1 could be one of promising targets in attenuating testicular damage caused by inflammatory reactions.

Mast cells are also involved in this EAO. They increased tenfold in number throughout the interstitial tissue and were partially degradated (Iosub et al. 2006). Protease-activated receptor 2 is known to be activated by mast cell tryptase. In EAO, protease-activated receptor 2 on testicular macrophages and peritubular cells was strongly upregulated. Isolated peritubular-like cells responded to protease-activated receptor 2 activation by increased mRNA expressions of monocyte chemoattractant protein-1, transforming growth factor-beta-2, and cyclooxygenase-2 in vitro. Indeed, expression of these three inflammatory mediators, together with nitric oxide-nitric oxide synthase, increased significantly in EAO-affected testes (Iosub et al. 2006; Jarazo-Dietrich et al. 2012). Furthermore, expression of these cytokines was upregulated after injection of recombinant tryptase in vivo. This suggests that mast cell tryptase contributes to pathogenic mechanisms of EAO.

The spermatogenic disturbance is characterized by apoptosis of TGC, which is mediated by the Fas/Fas ligand and Bax/Bcl-2 systems during EAO (Theas et al. 2003, 2006; Jacobo et al. 2012). Fas/Fas ligand system works through activation of caspase 8, whereas the Bax/Bcl-2 system works through activation of caspase 9; these activations eventually lead to activation of caspase 3, thereby resulting in TGC apoptosis. In testicular antigens+CFA+BP-immunized rats, real-time RT-PCR analyses revealed that Fas mRNA expression significantly increased compared with the control group. Most spermatocytes expressing Fas were apoptotic (Theas et al. 2003). The numbers of membrane Fas ligand-expressing $CD4^+$ and $CD8^+$ T cells were increased in the testis during EAO, but no expression of Fas ligand by macrophages was found (Jacobo et al. 2012). By Western blotting, an increase in soluble form of Fas ligand content was detected in the testicular fluid in EAO-affected testis (Jacobo et al. 2012). Since the soluble form of Fas ligand is able to enter the adluminal compartment of the seminiferous tubules, this molecule induces apoptosis of

Fas-bearing TGC. Indeed, many Fas-bearing TGC were also immunoreactive for Fas ligand (Theas et al. 2003). On the other hand, Bax was mainly expressed in spermatocytes and spermatids and Bcl-2 in TGC at the basal compartment of the seminiferous tubules. Bax-beta isoform content increased in EAO rat testis compared with controls, whereas content of Bax-alpha remained unchanged. However, Bax-alpha content decreased in the cytosol and increased in the mitochondrial and endoplasmic reticulum-enriched fractions of testis from EAO rats compared with controls. Bcl-2 content also increased in the EAO-affected testes. Therefore, extrinsic, mitochondrial and possibly endoplasmic reticulum pathways are inducers of TGC apoptosis in EAO and Bax and Bcl-2 proteins modulate this process (Theas et al. 2006).

During EAO, reduced expressions of occludin and delocalization of both claudin and tight junction protein 1 were detected. Rat Sertoli cells cultured in the presence of IL-6 exhibited a redistribution of tight junction proteins and reduced transepithelial electrical resistance, indicating the involvement of IL-6 in downregulating the BTB permeability (Perez et al. 2011, 2012). Th17 cells and their hallmark cytokine IL-17A were reported to be involved in the EAO development. The addition of IL-17A to normal rat Sertoli cell cultures induced a significant decline in transepithelial electrical resistance and a reduction of occluding expression and redistribution of occludin and claudin-11, altering the Sertoli cell tight junction barrier (Perez et al. 2013, 2014). Also in vivo, intra-testicular injection of recombinant rat IL-17A in rats induced increased the BTB permeability and delocalization of occludin and claudin-11.

5.2.4.6 Regulation of EAO

Substrains of balb/c mice differ in their susceptibility to EAO, with balb/cJ as a low responder and balb/cBy as a high responder. Between the two strains, reciprocal adoptive transfer of lymphocytes was examined. After the adoptive transfer of lymphocytes obtained from donor mice immunized with testicular homogenate+CFA+BP into the recipient mice, the recipients were immunized with testicular homogenate+CFA+BP 3 weeks later. The donor lymphocytes were consistently effective in transferring high susceptibility to EAO from balb/cBy (high responder) to balb/cJ (low responder). In the reverse experiments, resistance to EAO could be also transferred from balb/cJ (low) to balb/cBy (high) with donor lymphocytes (Mahi-Brown and Tung 1990). This suggests that susceptibility to EAO in balb/c mice depends on the T cell responses in the mice but not on differences at the level of the testis. Treatment of donor balb/cJ (low) spleen cells with cytotoxic monoclonal anti-Thy-1.2 or anti-CD4 antibodies+complements before transfer abrogates their ability to inhibit EAO, indicating that Treg are $CD4^+$ T cells (Teuscher et al. 1990a). In another study, the mechanistic basis for EAO resistance was examined using reciprocal bone marrow radiation chimeras generated between balb/cByJ (high) and balb/cJ (low) mice (Teuscher et al. 1985a, b, 1987a, 1990a). Recipient mice were lethally irradiated and received intravenous injections of 10^7 T cell-depleted donor bone marrow cells. Radiation chimera were made, balb/cByJ (high)→balb/cByJ (high), balb/cByJ (high)→balb/cJ (low), balb/cJ (low)→balb/

cByJ (high), and balb/cJ (low)→balb/cJ (low), and it was shown that all four chimeric constructs developed severe EAO following testicular homogenate+CFA+BP immunization. It is quite noted that balb/cJ (low)→balb/cJ (low) chimera also developed severe EAO after the immunization. This suggests that an active immunoregulatory mechanism by Treg rather than the lack of effector T cells and/or B cells with specific receptors for the orchitogenic autoantigens is responsible for disease resistance in balb/cJ mice. The characteristics of Treg were examined by pretreating balb/cJ mice (low) with either cyclophosphamide or low-dose whole-body irradiation 2 days prior to homogenate+CFA+BP immunization. It was found that the Treg relevant to EAO suppression are cyclophosphamide-sensitive and also low-dose radiation-sensitive T cell population (Teuscher et al. 1990a). Taken together, genetically controlled resistance to EAO in balb/cJ (low) mice may be associated with a mutation in an immunoregulatory locus of which effects appear to be mediated through a cyclophosphamide and low-dose radiation-sensitive $CD4^+$ Treg (Teuscher et al. 1990a).

There is a trial to induce EAO in severe combined immunodeficient (scid) mice (Wakabayashi et al. 1997). In this study, scid mice were reconstituted with fetal liver cells (including hematopoietic cells) from balb/c fetuses at gestation day 14. Untreated scid mice lacked both T and B cells, but their immune system had gradually developed later up to 9 weeks after the reconstitution with fetal liver cells. In the reconstituted mice, B cells started to appear at 2 weeks after the transfer of fetal liver cells and reached the level of normal balb/c mice at 5 weeks. Both $CD4^+$ and $CD8^+$ T cells started to appear at 5 weeks after the transfer and reached the level of normal balb/c mice at 7 weeks. EAO was induced by immunization with testicular antigens+CFA+BP in scid mice reconstituted with fetal liver cells 12 weeks before, as well as balb/c mice. There was no significant difference in the grade of EAO between the reconstituted scid mice and balb/c mice. As expected, untreated scid mice showed total absence of EAO.

EAO can be also inducible in transplanted testis under the renal capsule. Freshly prepared donor testis of 1-week-old balb/c mice was transplanted to orchiectomized adult balb/c mice under the renal capsule. Later, the transplanted mice were immunized with testicular homogenate+CFA+BP, and EAO was induced in the transplanted testes, although the severity of EAO in the transplanted testes was milder than that of the original testes of non-orchiectomized mice when immunized in the same manner (Wakabayashi et al. 1997).

In the transplanted testis of scid mice reconstituted with fetal liver cells, orchiectomy was performed at various stages of immunological development to test whether the orchiectomy influences the degree of EAO. In this experimental model, self-tolerance can be established by contact between testicular autoantigens and immune cells in the early developmental stage. The grade of EAO in the transplanted testis appeared significantly enhanced in scid mice that were orchiectomized 2–4 weeks before the transfer of fetal liver cells or 0–2 weeks after the cell transfer when compared to that of the transplanted testis in scid mice orchiectomized 12 weeks after the transfer of fetal liver cells. Therefore, the absence of testicular autoantigens during the early stage of immunological development might interfere with the establishment of sell-tolerance in the later stage and therefore enhance the degree of EAO. In other words, the presence of testicular autoantigens in the early development phase of the immune system may promote proper establishment of self-tolerance and accordingly ameliorated the grade of EAO.

In chronically inflamed testis during EAO, Foxp3-expressing $CD4^+$ and $CD8^+$ Treg were detected (Jacobo et al. 2009). At the onset of EAO, $CD4^+$ $Foxp3^+$ Treg were more abundant than $CD8^+$ $Foxp3^+$ Treg. Within $Foxp3^+$ Treg population, $CD25^-$ T cells were unexpectedly more than $CD25^+$ cells. $CD4^+$ $Foxp3^+$ Treg were also increased in draining lymph nodes from the testis in EAO-affected rats (Jacobo et al. 2015). Indeed, $CD4^+$ $CD25^-$ $Foxp3^+$ T cells from the draining lymph nodes of EAO-affected rats expressed transforming growth factor-beta and were able to suppress T cell proliferation more efficiently than those derived from lymph nodes of normal control rats.

5.2.4.7 The Effects of Exogenous Agents on EAO

Orchitogenic (EAO-inducing) T cell lines and clones derived from testicular homogenate+CFA+BP-immunized mice express CD4 and the alpha-beta TCR. When the lines and clones were activated, they produced IL-2, IFN-gamma, and TNF, but not IL-4. It is noted that the adoptive transfer of EAO by the orchitogenic clones was significantly and reproducibly attenuated when recipients were administered with neutralizing antibodies to TNF, but not neutralizing antibodies to IFN-gamma (Yule and Tung 1993).

In EAO lesion, an increased number of macrophages infiltrate the testicular interstitium concomitantly with progressive TGC degeneration and impaired steroidogenesis. Macrophages are the main producers of nitric oxide, and upregulation of nitric oxide-nitric oxide synthase system occurs in testicular homogenate+CFA+BP-immunized rats (Jarazo-Dietrich et al. 2012; Perez et al. 2013). Blockage of nitric oxide-nitric oxide synthase system by intraperitoneal injection with a competitive inhibitor, N(G)-nitro-L-arginine methyl ester, significantly reduced the incidence and severity of EAO and lowered testicular nitrite content (Jarazo-Dietrich et al. 2015). Furthermore, co-culture of control testicular fragments with testicular macrophages obtained from EAO-affected rats significantly increased TGC apoptosis, whereas addition of N(G)-nitro-L-arginine methyl ester lowered the apoptosis-inducing effects and reduced nitrite content (Jarazo-Dietrich et al. 2015). Therefore, nitric oxide secreted mainly by testicular macrophages could promote oxidative stress inducing the spermatogenic disturbance and interfering Leydig cell function.

Galectin-1, a prototype member of galectin family, is highly expressed in immune-privileged testis. A significant reduction in the incidence and severity of EAO was observed in mice that are genetically deficient in Galectin-1 when compared with wild-type mice. On the contrary, exogenous administration of recombinant Galectin-1 to wild-type mice undergoing EAO attenuated the severity of EAO (Perez et al. 2015). Therefore, a dual role of endogenous versus exogenous Galectin-1 was demonstrated in the control of EAO.

Recombinant human secretory leukocyte protease inhibitor inhibits mitogen-induced proliferation of human peripheral blood mononuclear cells. In experiments in which microspheres containing recombinant human secretory leukocyte protease inhibitor were administered subcutaneously during or after the EAO immunization, the treatment significantly decreased EAO incidence and severity (Guazzone et al. 2011b). In vivo DTH and ex vivo proliferative response to testicular antigens were also reduced by treatment with recombinant human secretory leukocyte protease inhibitor.

5.2.4.8 Immunogenetics of EAO

Segregation analysis employing a second-generation backcross population shows that resistance to both experimental allergic encephalomyelitis induced by immunization with spinal cord homogenate+CFA+BP and EAO is due to a mutation in a common immunoregulatory gene (Teuscher et al. 1998). Genes outside the MHC strongly influence susceptibility to testicular antigens+CFA+BP-induced EAO (Teuscher 1985, 1985b). Sublines of the balb/c (H-2^d) mice differ in EAO susceptibility (Teuscher et al. 1987a, b, 1988). balb/cByJ mice are highly susceptible to EAO (high responder), whereas balb/cJ mice are resistant (low responder). DBA/2 J mice, another H-2^d strain, are resistant to EAO, and (balb/cByJ × DBA/2 J) F1 mice are also resistant. This demonstrates that resistance to EAO is inherited as a dominant phenotype in this strain combination (Teuscher et al. 1985a, b; Teuscher 1985). Additionally, resistance can be adoptively transferred to susceptible balb/cByJ mice with primed spleen cells of (balb/cByJ × DBA/2 J) F1 mice (Meeker et al. 1995). In sharp contrast, EAO susceptibility is dominantly inherited in bidirectional (susceptible balb/cByJ × resistant balb/cJ)F1 hybrids.

The immune T cells obtained from testicular homogenate+CFA+BP-immunized balb/cByJ (high) mice were consistently effective in transferring EAO susceptibility to balb/cJ (low) mice. On the contrary, when spleen cells from balb/cJ (low) mice immunized with testicular homogenate+CFA+BP are transferred to balb/cByJ (high) mice, the recipients become resistant to EAO induction by testicular homogenate+CFA+BP immunization (Mahi-Brown and Tung 1990). Lymphocytes responsible for EAO suppression were isolated and typed as CD4$^+$T cells (Teuscher et al. 1990a). This indicates that resistance to EAO in balb/cJ (low) mice is mediated by CD4$^+$ Treg cells.

Further studies also demonstrated that autoimmune orchitis, epididymitis, and vasitis are immunogenetically distinct lesions controlled by both MHC-linked and non-MHC-linked genes (Roper et al. 1998). Mice with the H-2^s haplotype developed mainly orchitis, whereas mice of the H-2^k haplotype developed epididymitis and vasitis (Teuscher et al. 1990b). Unique loci were identified on chromosome 8 for orchitis, chromosome 16 for epididymitis, and chromosome 1 for vasitis and have been designated as Orch6, Epd1, and Vas1, respectively. This difference was also demonstrated using series of recombinant inbred lines derived from the EAO-susceptible C57BL/6 J (H-2^b) and the EAO-resistant C3H/HeJ (H-2^k) strains (Person et al. 1992a). This genetic study has identified four additional orchitis susceptible genes: Orch-1, which maps within H-2, Orch-2, Bphs, and Orch-3, which are genes that reside outside H-2, showing the polygenic control of EAO. Induction of testicular homogenate+CFA+BP-induced EAO requires the BP as an adjuvant. The Bphs locus controls the phenotypic expression of susceptibility to BP-induced histamine sensitization (Wardlaw 1970). Mice which possess a susceptible allele at this locus die from hypovolemic shock following histamine challenge. Therefore, susceptibility to the induction of EAO is associated with the locus controlling BP-induced sensitivity to histamine, which for histamine is a single bob-H-2-linked dominant autosomal (Teuscher 1985, 1986; Sudweeks et al. 1993; Meeker et al. 1999; Ma et al. 2002; Noubade et al. 2007). Orch-3 is the most important immunosuppressive locus controlling dominant resistance to EAO (Del Rio et al. 2012). Using congenic mapping, kinesin family member 1C was identified as a positional candidate for Orch-3. Furthermore, overexpression of the kinesin family member 1C-resistant allele in susceptible mice rendered mice EAO resistant. Additionally, failure to induce testicular homogenate+CFA+BP-induced EAO in C3H/He (H-2^k) mice was noted because of that this strain is highly susceptible to TGC-induced EAO (Itoh et al. 1991a, b, c). This indicates that controls of testicular antigen+CFA+BP-induced EAO and TGC-induced one are genetically different.

To investigate whether the frequency of natural Treg ($CD4^+CD8^-TCR^+Foxp3^+$ cells) in the lymph node is associated with resistance to EAO, the frequency of natural Treg in adult B10.S mice (EAO-resistant strain) was compared with that of adult SJL/J mice (EAO-susceptible strain) (Del Rio et al. 2011). The results showed that the frequency of natural Treg of B10.S mice was greater than that of SJL/J mice, correlating with susceptibility and resistance to EAO.

5.2.4.9 The Effect of Vasectomy on EAO

The effect of vasectomy followed by immunization with testicular antigens+CFA+BP 3 weeks later on EAO was investigated (Wheeler et al. 2011). Rapid cell apoptosis and necrosis of epididymal epithelium, persistent inflammation, and spermatic granulomata formation were induced in vasectomized mice; however, they did not have EAO in spite of immunization with testicular antigens+CFA+BP. Similar phenomenon was also found in another EAO model induced by immunization with TGC alone; mice receiving sham-vasectomy and the following TGC immunization had EAO; however, no EAO was found in the testes of any mice receiving vasectomy and the following TGC immunization (Qu et al. 2008). Vasectomized mice immunized with testicular antigens+CFA+BP developed sperm antigen-specific tolerance and exhibited resistance to induction of EAO but not experimental autoimmune encephalomyelitis. This organ-specific tolerance switches over to pathologic autoimmune state following concomitant $CD4^+CD25^+Foxp3^+$ Treg depletion; unilaterally vasectomized mice produce dominant autoantibodies to an orchitogenic antigen (zonadhesin) and develop $CD4^+$ T cell- and antibody-dependent bilateral EAO by testicular antigens+CFA+BP immunization. Thus, sperm antigens released from the post-vasectomy epididymal granulomata induce tolerance or autoimmunity depending on the balance of Treg and effector T cell responses. Approximately 65% of the testis-infiltrating T cells expressed CD4; among them, 20% had potential to produce IFN-gamma, and fewer than 2% produced IL-17. Importantly, $CD4^+$ T cells from mice with post-vasectomy EAO transferred severe EAO to syngeneic recipients. Notably, only the $CD4^+$ T cells from the testis-draining lymph nodes were pathogenic. This indicates that deviation of intrinsic Treg can influence the divergent tolerogenic versus autoimmune response to vasectomy.

5.2.4.10 The Immune-Endocrine Milieu in EAO

A significant increase in the number of Leydig cells was observed in rats with EAO. Most Leydig cells exhibited features of active steroid-secreting cells and closely associated with macrophages during EAO. Moreover, rats with EAO had significantly increased intra-testicular testosterone, and serum luteinizing hormone did not change in any immunized animals (Suescun et al. 1994). In vitro experiments, Leydig cells from rats with EAO exhibited an enhanced steroidogenic response to human chorionic gonadotropin (Suescun et al. 1997). An increase in testosterone production by Leydig cells incubated with macrophage-conditioned media from testicular, but not peritoneal, macrophages of rats with EAO was also observed (Suescun et al. 2000). In regard to the seminiferous epithelium of EAO-affected rats, serum levels of follicle-stimulating hormone in EAO-affected rats were two- to threefold higher than those of controls. Strong expressions of the inhibin-alpha subunit in Sertoli cells were observed in control rats; however, this subunit was undetectable or poorly detectable in rats with EAO. A significant decrease in circulating inhibin B, a product by Sertoli cells, was also observed in rats with EAO, so an inverse correlation between inhibin B and follicle-stimulating hormone were found (Suescun et al. 2001). This means that both circulating inhibin B levels and inhibin-alpha subunit expression in Sertoli cell cytoplasm closely correlate with the degree of damage of the seminiferous epithelium.

On the other hand, Fijak et al. (2011) reported decreased levels of testosterone and increased follicle-stimulating hormone concentrations in serum of rats with EAO. This indicates that the detrimental influence of EAO extends to the dysfunction of not only seminiferous epithelium (TGC and Sertoli cells) but also Leydig cells. Considering the immunosuppressive activity of testosterone, the effect of subcutaneous testosterone implants on EAO induction was examined in rats. In rats immunized with testicular homogenate+CFA+BP on days 0, 14, and 28, testosterone capsule were implanted subcutaneously on day 20. EAO incidence was significantly reduced in animals that had been treated with testosterone implants when compared with that in positive control animals receiving testicular antigens+CFA+BP immunization alone (Fijak et al. 2011). Expression of pro-inflammatory mediators such as monocyte chemoattractant protein-1, TNF-alpha, and IL-6 in the testis and secretion of Th1 cytokines such as IFN-gamma and IL-2 by mononuclear cells isolated from testicular draining lymph nodes were significantly decreased in testosterone-implanted rats. In the testis, testosterone implants prevented the accumulation of testicular macrophages and $CD4^+$ T cells with a strong concomitant increase of Treg ($CD4^+CD25^+Foxp3^+$ T cells), suggesting that testosterone play a role on the differentiation of Treg. Generation of $CD4^+CD25^+Foxp3^+$ Treg in Leydig cell-conditioned media was determined to investigate the influence of testosterone (Fijak et al. 2015). Leydig cell-conditioned media dose-dependently stimulated expression of transcription factor Foxp3 and secretion of IL-10 in splenic $CD4^+$ T cells, and these effects were abolished by addition of the anti-androgen flutamide. In isolated Sertoli and peritubular myoid cells, testosterone pretreatment suppressed the lipopolysaccharide-induced inflammatory response on TNF-alpha mRNA expression, while no effect was evident in testicular macrophages. Therefore, androgens can influence the immune system by the generation and functional differentiation of Treg under normal conditions and by direct effect on Sertoli cells and peritubular myoid cells during testicular inflammation.

balb/cByJ substrain mice are highly susceptible to the induction of EAO, whereas balb/cJ mice are resistant (Teuscher et al. 1985b, 1987a). However, these two substrains do not differ significantly from each other in their mean serum testosterone levels, suggesting that the EAO-resistant phenotype exhibited by balb/cJ mice is not a result of the immunosuppressive effects of testosterone (Steenstra et al. 1989).

5.2.5 EAO Induced by Immunization with Testicular Antigens and *Klebsiella* Lipopolysaccharide

EAO in mice is induced by repeated injection at intervals of 30 days of a mixture of syngeneic testis homogenate and *Klebsiella* 3 lipopolysaccharide as a potent adjuvant (Yokochi et al. 1990; Fujii et al. 1991) (Fig. 5.1). At 10 days after the second immunization, there was marked infiltration of neutrophils in the seminiferous tubules and the testicular interstitium, followed by destruction of the seminiferous tubules and the spermatogenic disturbance. At 20 days after the second immunization, infiltration with neutrophils was replaced by lymphocytes, plasma cells, and macrophages. After the tenth immunization, the EAO lesions at terminal stage were characterized by complete destruction of the tubular architecture of the testis and fibrosis. DTH against testicular antigens developed in the immunized mice. The antisera obtained from mice with EAO lesions defined several testicular antigens with molecular weights of 38, 86, 100, and >200 kDd. The acrosomal 86 kDa antigen is predominantly expressed in the testis, while the 100 kd antigen is dominant in the epididymal spermatozoa. These antigens were organ specific and exclusively present on the acrosome of spermatozoa, suggesting that these acrosomal antigens were highly relevant to EAO.

5.2.6 EAO Induced by Intraperitoneal Injection with Both TGC and *Listeria monocytogenes*

In mice that had received intraperitoneal injection with both TGC and virulent *Listeria monocytogenes*, specific DTH and proliferative response against TGC were observed, although the intraperitoneal injection with TGC alone or virulent *Listeria monocytogenes* alone did not induce such a significant response (Sonoda et al. 1997). Histologically, mice injected with both TGC and virulent *Listeria monocytogenes* had EAO lesions, but the mice injected with TGC alone or virulent *Listeria monocytogenes* alone did not (Fig. 5.1). This EAO was not caused by the direct invasion of virulent *Listeria monocytogenes* into the testis, because the bacteria were not detected in the EAO-affected testis. In contrast, the intraperitoneal co-injection with avirulent *Listeria monocytogenes* and TGC induced neither TGC-specific DTH nor proliferative response and thus failed to induce EAO.

5.2.7 EAO Induced by Adoptive Transfer of *Listeria monocytogenes*-Induced Macrophages with TGC Autoantigens

Listeria monocytogenes is a facultative intracellular pathogen that grows in the cytoplasm of infected host cells. *Listeria monocytogenes* is able to survive in the cytoplasm by escaping from phagosomes. Mac-1$^+$ peritoneal macrophages were obtained from mice that had been intraperitoneally inoculated with virulent or avirulent *Listeria monocytogenes* 4 days before. However, no viable bacteria were detected from the macrophage preparation in a colony-forming assay. After the preparation, 5×10^6 *Listeria monocytogenes*-induced peritoneal macrophages were transferred intraperitoneally to naïve syngeneic mice with TGC autoantigens. In mice injected with virulent *Listeria*-induced macrophages but not in those injected with avirulent *Listeria*-induced ones, EAO involving many testicular T cells was induced with specific DTH against TGC, although DTH against *Listeria* antigen was significantly and similarly induced by both virulent and avirulent *Listeria*-induced macrophages (Sonoda et al. 1997) (Fig. 5.1). The injection of virulent *Listeria*-induced macrophages in the absence of TGC autoantigens elicited neither TGC-specific DTH nor EAO, suggesting the importance of the coexistence. It was also noted that virulent *Listeria*-induced macrophages themselves did not directly damage testes.

The MHC class II expression was similarly upregulated on both virulent *Listeria*-induced and avirulent *Listeria*-induced macrophages. However, differing from the avirulent *Listeria*-induced macrophages, the virulent *Listeria*-induced macrophages expressed a high level of CD80 (B7–1) and CD86 (B7–2) molecules. CD80 is a protein found on activated monocytes that provides a costimulatory signal necessary for T cell activation and survival, and it works in tandem with CD86 to prime T cells. Therefore, macrophage activation by virulent *Listeria monocytogenes* is important, and the upregulation of B7 molecules by virulent *Listeria* infection may be a candidate of the mechanism for activation of autoreactive T cells. To investigate the mechanism of this EAO, functions of not only autoreactive T cells but also antigen-presenting cells which present autoantigens to effector T cells must be further studied.

5.2.8 EAO Induced by Immunization with Mouse F9 Embryonic Carcinoma Cells+CFA

T cells obtained from mice sensitized with mouse H-2-negative F9 embryonic carcinoma cells (derived from 129/Sv mice) and rechallenged in vitro with irradiated F9 stimulator cells differentiated into anti-F9 cytotoxic T cells, which can lyse syngeneic spermatogonia (Wagner et al. 1978). This confirmed the antigenic similarity between F9 embryonic carcinoma cells and spermatogonia. The spermatogenic disturbance accompanied by appearance of autoantibodies against TGC were observed after syngeneic, allogeneic, and xenogeneic immunization with mouse F9 embryonic carcinoma cells+CFA in 129/Sv mice, balb/c mice, and albino guinea pigs (Vojtiskova et al. 1983). This indicates that F9 embryonal carcinoma cells have orchitogenic antigens, which are common antigens among syngeneic, allogeneic, and xenogeneic animals (Fig. 5.2).

In guinea pigs, anti-F9 sera were produced by immunization with mouse F9 embryonic carcinoma cells+CFA. Short-term administration of the globulin fractions of the anti-F9 sera produced in guinea pigs resulted in a significant spermatogenic disturbance, suggesting a participation of not only cellular but also humoral autoimmunity in EAO lesion (Pokorna et al. 1984).

In another study, repeated intraperitoneal administration of F9 carcinoma cells to guinea pigs starting from birth prevented the induction of EAO by subsequent TGC+CFA-immunization, implying the induction of specific Treg by way of repeated and intraperitoneal exposure of F9 cells at neonatal period (Vojtiskova et al. 1984).

5.2.9 EAO Induced by Immunization with Chemically Modified Seminal Plasma+CFA

Seminal plasma is mixed fluid secreted from the testis, epididymis, prostate gland, seminal vesicle, and bulbourethral gland. It should include various autoantigens in male reproductive tract. For preparation of chemically modified seminal plasma, native semen samples were centrifuged to remove spermatozoa, and the proteins of the collected seminal plasma were coupled to diazonium derivatives of sulfanilic and arsanilic acid. Prepared seminal plasma materials incorporated with CFA were subcutaneously injected at 0, 30, and 50 days. Immunization with chemically modified seminal plasma+CFA induced EAO accompanied by the appearance of autoantibodies against the seminal plasma proteins as well as against testicular antigens in rabbits (Yantorno et al. 1971) (Fig. 5.2). The spermatogenic disturbance in atrophied seminiferous tubules was invariably observed, but the hyperplasia of Leydig cells, interstitial infiltration of leukocytes, and thickening of basement membrane of the seminiferous tubular wall were rare in the immunized rabbits. In contrast, when accessory gland extract was chemically modified and then used as the sensitizing materials instead of seminal plasma, the repeated immunization failed to induce EAO.

5.2.10 EAO Induced by Immunization of Fluid of Seminal Vesicles+CFA

Vulchanov (1969) has shown that immunization with seminal vesicular fluid induced EAO with epididymitis in guinea pigs with the aid of adjuvant (Fig. 5.2). Seminal vesicular fluid was collected directly from seminal vesicles of dissected donors and emulsified with CFA. Each animal received four injections of seminal vesicular fluid+CFA on days 0, 13, 29, and 32. In EAO lesion, the mononuclear cell infiltration of the testicular interstitium and the atrophy of the seminiferous tubules were observed, but the Sertoli cells seemed to be intact. This indicates that accessory sex glands also take part in inducing reproductive autoimmunity leading to EAO. The EAO resulting from immunization with seminal vesicular fluid antigens cannot be explained by autoantigens shared with spermatozoa since there was insignificant cross-reactivity between the antisera against seminal vesicular fluid and the spermatozoa. Autoantigens of seminal vesicle relevant to this EAO has not yet determined, but there remains a possibility of the presence of common antigens between the testicular proteins and the seminiferous vesicular fluid ones.

5.2.11 EAO Induced by Local Transfer of Lymphocytes Cultured with Testicular Cells in the Presence of Xenogeneic Sera

Normal lymph node cells of rats cultured with autologous dissociated testis cells form rosette-like aggregates and later undergo blast transformation and proliferation (Wekerle and Begemann 1976, 1977, 1978). Autoreactive T cells were induced by in vitro stimulation of rat T cells with autologous testicular cells in culture medium supplemented with horse serum. These stimulated lymphocytes caused EAO lesions in vivo, when injected locally into syngeneic recipients. It therefore appears that testicular self-antigens are recognized by clonally preformed autologous lymphocytes. However, instead of horse serum, supplementation of autologous serum into culture medium prevented in vitro-induced EAO. In particular, syngeneic serum is more effective than allogeneic one for prevention of EAO. Furthermore, autologous male serum is a markedly stronger inhibitor in EAO induction than syngeneic female serum (Wekerle and Begemann 1977). It indicates that syngeneic serum is an inhibitor for autoimmune reactions, and xenogeneic serum functions as an adjuvant (Fig. 5.1). The self-reactivity of individual rats of varying ages (3–26 months) was compared by testing the in vitro EAO responsiveness. In parallel, their reactivity to alloantigens and a polyclonal T lymphocyte activator (Con A) was monitored (Wekerle 1978; Kyewski and Wekerle 1978). The results showed a decrease in the alloantigen and the mitogen responsiveness in aged rats (from 20 months on) compared to young controls (3 months). In contrast, the self-reactivity was in all cases significantly increased in aged rats. It was also found that the increased EAO response was not dependent on age-dependent changes of the target autoantigens in the testis. Therefore, an age-dependent loss of Treg may play an active role in the pathogenesis of autoimmune diseases involving EAO in the aging organism.

EAO can be also induced by thymic lymphocytes autosensitized against syngeneic Sertoli cells in vitro (Tung and Fritz 1984) (Fig. 5.2). Thymic lymphocytes from normal rats were co-cultured with syngeneic Sertoli cell-peritubular cell preparations in the presence of xenogeneic or allogeneic serum. Local transfer of such lymphocytes into syngeneic rat testes resulted in EAO; however, thymic lymphocytes incubated with Sertoli cells in autologous or syngeneic serum did not elicit these changes. These in vitro experimental systems offer an approach for analysis of the cellular interactions at the beginning and during EAO and for the determination of the self-antigens involved.

5.2.12 EAO-Like Lesion Induced by Intraperitoneal Injection with Infectious Agents Other Than CFA or BP

As described above, CFA+BP treatment produces ASIA-like condition, in which both production of anti-TGC autoantibodies and development of cytolytic activity of T cells against TGC are inducible without the use of any testicular antigens for sensitization (Ben et al. 1986; Musha et al. 2013).

Lipopolysaccharide of *Escherichia coli* is also well known to trigger an autoinflammatory response in various organs involving the testis when administered intraperitoneally or intravenously (Sliwa et al. 2009) (Fig. 5.1). The blockage of cell divisions by lipopolysaccharide leaded to the degeneration of seminiferous epithelium and the decrease of number of spermatozoa in the lumen of seminiferous tubules. The number of testicular macrophages rose quickly, and it remained constant until day 28 after the administration of lipopolysaccharide (Sliwa et al. 2009). In next experiments, adult TCR alpha-beta$^{-/-}$, TCR gamma-delta$^{-/-}$, CD1d$^{-/-}$, and beta2m$^{-/-}$ mice and control mice were intraperitoneally injected with lipopolysaccharide. The animals were killed 24 h and 10 days post-lipopolysaccharide treatment. Histological changes in the testes such as disturbance of Leydig cell structure, blood vessel dilatation, and the spermatogenic disturbance were found only in control mice (Sliwa et al. 2014). Lack of either TCR alpha-beta^{+} CD8^{+} or TCR gamma-delta^{+} lymphocytes diminished the response of testicular macrophages to lipopolysaccharide, whereas the absence of CD1d-dependent NKT cell does not affect macrophage reactivity. Therefore, lack of TCR alpha-beta^{+} CD8^{+} and TCR gamma-delta^{+} lymphocytes ameliorate lipopolysaccharide-induced orchitis in mice.

Testicular inflammation and spermatogenic disturbance were also induced by intraperitoneal inoculation of *Leishmania donovani* in hamsters (Gonzalez et al. 1983) (Fig. 5.1). Lymphocytes and plasma cells infiltrates with macrophages containing *Leishmania* appeared in the testicular interstitium with progressive testicular atrophy. Amyloid deposits in the intertubular space and tubular basal lamina were identified, suggesting that testicular amyloidosis may have a pathogenic mechanism related to a dysfunction of plasma cells and stimulation of the reticuloendothelial system, due to the antigenic character of the parasite. However, intraperitoneal injection with *Listeria monocytogenes* alone did not induce testicular inflammation (Sonoda et al. 1997).

Testicular lesions were induced in mice by intraperitoneal injection with low dose of encephalomyocarditis virus (Yamanouchi-Ueno et al. 2004) (Fig. 5.1). The IFN-gamma and iNOS mRNAs expression in the testis and spleen was prominently elevated at 7 days postinoculation, although the expression level of TNF-alpha mRNA was not affected. Signals of viral RNA were clearly detected in degenerative seminiferous epithelium, which was surrounded by a small number of macrophages and a few CD4^{+} cells and CD8^{+} cells. At 35 days post-injection, marked atrophy of seminiferous epithelium composed of Sertoli cells alone was observed, and there were almost no infiltrating cells detected. In mice injected with high dose of encephalomyocarditis virus, prominent infiltration of neutrophils was observed in and around the affected seminiferous epithelium (Ueno et al. 1996, 1997).

Autoimmune responses against TGC antigens or other testicular antigens have not been investigated in animals treated with *Escherichia coli* lipopolysaccharide, encephalomyocarditis virus, and *Leishmania donovani*.

In rabbits injected intraperitoneally with a myxoma virus, systemic disease was evoked with viral replication to high titers in the testes (Fountain et al. 1997). In their testes, interstitial orchitis with the spermatogenic disturbance and impaired steroidogenesis was found (Fig. 5.1). Virus was localized within the interstitial cells, and anti-sperm autoantibodies were present in the serum as early as 5 days after the infection.

5.2.13 EAO-Like Lesion Induced by Exposure to Endocrine Disruptors

Phthalate has been used as a plastic plasticized for synthetic polymers and well-known toxicant as an endocrine disruptor. Exposure to mono- or di-(2-ethylhexyl) phthalate of high doses has been reported to induce the spermatogenic disturbance through oxidant stress and affect the immune system as an adjuvant (Fig. 5.1). After exposure to phthalate of low doses in mice by giving daily food containing di-(2-ethylhexyl) phthalate, lymphocytes and F4/80$^+$ macrophages involving MHC class II-positive cells were significantly increased with a slight disturbance of spermatogenesis in their testes (Kitaoka et al. 2013). In particular, lymphocytes accumulated around the tubuli recti. In the treated testes, both IL-10 and IFN-gamma mRNA expressions were elevated (Kitaoka et al. 2013), and a significant increase in monocyte chemoattractant protein-1 by peritubular myoid cells also occurred after phthalate exposure (Murphy et al. 2014). Histochemical analyses involving horseradish peroxidase as a tracer showed that a little blood-borne horseradish peroxidase had infiltrated into the lumen of a few seminiferous tubules beyond the BTB, and serum anti-TGC autoantibodies were produced in the phthalate-treated mice (Kitaoka et al. 2013; Hirai et al. 2015). In contrast, in mice treated with busulfan (an alkylating agent exhibiting testicular toxicity), severe spermatogenic disturbance was induced; however, there is no significant infiltration of lymphocytes into their testes, and significant serum anti-TGC autoantibodies were not detected (Qu et al. 2017).

Titanium dioxide nanoparticles as endocrine disruptors have been demonstrated to be able to cross the BTB and induce infiltration of inflammatory cells and apoptosis/necrosis of TGC and Sertoli cells (Hong et al. 2016) (Fig. 5.1). Furthermore, expressions of Tyro-3, Axl, and Mer were decreased, and expressions of TLR3, TLR4, IL-1-beta, IL-6, TNF-alpha, IFN-alpha, and IFN-beta were increased. Three members of a receptor tyrosine kinase family, including Tyro-3, Axl, and Mer, are collectively called as TAM receptors, which are essential for phagocytic removal of apoptotic cells and regulating immune response (Deng et al. 2016). Although analyses of autoimmune responses against testicular autoantigens have not been examined in titanium dioxide nanoparticle-treated mice, the testicular lesion may be associated with dysfunction of TAM/TLR3-mediated signal pathway (Sun et al. 2010).

References

Adekunle AO, Hickey WF, Smith SM, Tung KSK, Teuscher C. Experimental allergic orchitis in mice IV. Preliminary characterization of the major murine testis specific aspermatogenic autoantigen(s). J Reprod Immunol. 1987;12:49–62.

Aslani F, Schuppe HC, Guazzone VA, Bhushan S, Wahle E, Lochnit G, Lustig L, Meinhardt A, Fijak M. Targeting high mobility group box protein 1 ameliorates testicular inflammation in experimental autoimmune orchitis. Hum Reprod. 2014.; pii: deu320

Audia S, Nicolas A, Cathelin D, Larmonier N, Ferrand C, Foucher P, Fanton A, Bergoin E, Maynadie M, Arnould L, Bateman A, Lorcerie B, Solary E, Chauffert B, Bonnotte B. Increase of $CD4^{+}CD25^{+}$ regulatory T cells in the peripheral blood of patients with metastatic carcinoma: a Phase I clinical trial using cyclophosphamide and immunotherapy to eliminate $CD4^{+}CD25^{+}$ T lymphocytes. Clin Exp Immunol. 2007;150:523–30.

Bassi N, Luisetto R, Del Prete D, Ghirardello A, Ceol M, Rizzo S, Laccarino L, Gatto M, Valente ML, Punzi L, Doria A. Induction of 'ASIA' syndrome in NZB/NZWF1 mice after injection of complete Freund's adjuvant (CFA). Lupus. 2012;21:203–9.

Ben K, Alexander NJ, Huso N. In vitro cell-mediated and complement-mediated cytotoxicity to murine testicular cells. Am J Reprod Immunol. 1986;12:33–7.

Bernard CC, Toulett F, Lamoireux G. Inhibition by serum of autoimmune aspermatogenic orchitis. Aust J Exp Biol Med Sci. 1975;53:245–50.

Bernard CCA, Mitchell GF, Leydon J, Bargerbos A. Experimental autoimmune orchitis in T-cell-deficient mice. Int Arch Allergy appl Immunol. 1978;56:256–63.

Billiau A, Matthys P. Models of action of Freund's adjuvants in experimental models of autoimmune disease. J Leukoc Biol. 2001;70:849–60.

Brode S, Raine T, Zaccone P, Coole A. Cyclophosphamide-induced type-1 diabetes in the NOD mouse is associated with a reduction of $CD4^{+}CD25^{+}Foxp3^{+}$ regulatory T cells. J Immunol. 2006;177:6603–12.

Carlo DJ, Hagopian A, Jackson JJ, Limjuco GA, Eylar EH. Experimental allergic orchitis and aspermatogenesis. VI. Transfer of allegic orchitis with immune cells. J Immunol. 1976;116:619–22.

Cao Y, Zhao J, Yang Z, Cai Z, Zhang B, Zhou Y, Shen GX, Chen X, Li S, Huang B. $CD4^{+}Foxp3^{+}$ regulatory T cell depletion by low-dose cyclophosphamide prevents recurrence in patients wirh large condylomata acuminate after laser therapy. Clin Immunol. 2010;136:21–9.

Chattopadhyay U. Immunological induction of aspermatogenesis. J Steroid Biochem. 1979;11:687–93.

Chuang YH, Chiang BL, Chou CC, Hsieh KH. Immune effector cells induced by complete Freund's adjuvant exert an inhibitory effect on antigen-specific type 2 T helper responses. Clin Exp Allergy. 1997;27:315–24.

Chutna J, Rychlikova M. Prevention and suppression of experimental autoimmune aspermatogenesis in adult guinea pigs. Folia Biol. 1964;10:177–87.

Clemens JW, Bruot BC. Testicular dysfunction in the adjuvant-induced arthritic rat. J Androl. 1989;10:419–24.

Colafrancesco S, Perricone C, Priori R, Valesini G, Shoenfeld Y. Sjogren's syndrome: another facet of the autoimmune/inflammatory syndrome induced by adjuvants (ASIA). J Autoimmun. 2014;51:10–6.

Cruz-Tapias P, Agmon-Levin N, Israeli E, Anaya JM, Shoenfeld Y. Autoimmune (auto-inflammatory) syndrome induced by adjuvants (ASIA)—animal models as a proof of concept. Curr Med Chem. 2013;20:4030–6.

Del Rio R, Sun Y, Alard P, Tung KSK, Teuscher C. H2 control of natural T regulatory cell frequency in the lymph node correlates with susceptibility to day 3 thymectomy-induced autoimmune disease. J Immunol. 2011;186:382–9.

Del Rio R, McAllister RD, Meeker ND, Wall EH, Bond JP, Kyttaris VC, Tsokos GC, Tung KSK, Teuscher C. Identification of Orch3, a locus controlling dominant resistance to autoimmune orchitis, as kinesin family member 1C. PLoS Genet. 2012;8:1–9.

Denduchis B, Lustig L, Gonzalez NN, Mancini RE. Studies of the nature of extracellular components of rat seminiferous tubular wall. I. Isolation and chemical characterization of basement membrane. Biol Reprod. 1975;13:274–81.

Denduchis B, Lustig L, Gonzalez N, Puig RP. Isolation and immunological reactivity of soluble fractions from rat seminiferous tubule basement membrane. Arch Androl. 1979;2:233–40.

Denduchis B, Satz ML, Sztein MB, Puig RP, Doncel G, Lustig L. Multifocal damage of the testis induced in rats by passive transfer of antibodies prepared against non-collagenous fraction of basement membrane. J Reprod Immunol. 1985;7:59–75.

Deng T, Chen Q, Han D. The role of TAM receptor tyrosine kinases in the mammalian testis and immunoprivileged sites. Front Biosci. 2016;21:316–27.

Diehl SA, McElvany B, Noubade R, Seeberger N, Harding B, Spach K, Teuscher C. G proteins G-alpha-i1/3 are critical targets for Bordetella pertussis toxin-induced vasoactive amine sensitization. Infect Immun. 2014;82:773–82.

Doncel GF, Di Paola JA, Lustig L. Sequential study of the histopathology and cellular and humoral immune response during the development of an autoimmune in Wistar rats. Am J Reprod Immunol. 1989;20:44–51.

Doncel GF, Denduchis B, Lustig L. Testicular lesions and lymphocyte subpopulations in rats immunized with a soluble fraction of testicular homogenate. Int J Androl. 1991;14:468–78.

Doncel GF, Lustig L. Lymphocyte subsets in the lymph nodes of rats with autoimmune orchitis. Am J Reprod Immunol. 1991;25:35–40.

Drumond AL, Weng CC, Wang G, Chiarini-Garcia H, Eras-Garcia L, Meistrich ML. Effects of multiple doses of cyclophosphamide on mouse testes: accessing the germ cells lost, and the functional damage of stem cells. Reprod Toxicol. 2011;32:395–406.

Eyquem A, Krieg H. Experimental autosensitization of the testis. Ann N Y Acad Sci. 1965;124:270–8.

Fainboim L, Sztein MB, Serrate S, Mancini RE. Transfer of experimental allergic orchitis with immune RNA. Studies in vivo. Clin Exp Immunol. 1978;34:92–9.

Fainboim L, Sztein MB, Serrate S, Satz L. In vitro transfer of cellular immunity in experimental allergic orchitis by means of immune RNA. Immunology. 1979;38:311–6.

Falase EA, Adekunle AO, Neblett H, Teuscher C. Guinea pig testicular proacrosin-acrosin system: preliminary immunological characterization. J Reprod Immunol. 1989;15:241–56.

Feng ZY, Ming W, Li LD, Louis J, Fei WY. Adoptive transfer of murine autoimmune orchitis with sperm-specific T lymphoblast. Arch Androl. 1990;24:51–9.

Fijak M, Losub R, Schneider E, Linder M, Respondek K, Klug J, Meinhardt A. Identification of immunodominant autoantigens in rat autoimmune orchitis. J Pathol. 2005;207:127–38.

Fijak M, Schneider E, Klug J, Bhushan S, Hackstein H, Schuler G, Wygrecka M, Gromoll J, Meinhardt A. Testosterone replacement effectively inhibits the development of experimental autoimmune orchitis in rats: Evidence for a direct role of testosterone on regulatory T cell expansion. J Immunol. 2011;186:5162–72.

Fijak M, Damm LJ, Wenzel JP, Aslani F, Walecki M, Wahle E, Eisel F, Bhushan S, Hackstein H, Baal N, Shuler G, Konrad L, Rafiq A, O'Hara L, Smith LB, Meinhardt A. Influence of testosterone on inflammatory response in testicular cells and expression of transcription factor Foxp3 in T cells. Am J Reprod Immunol. 2015;10:1111.

Fountain S, Holland MK, Hinds LA, Janssens PA, Kerr PJ. Interstitial orchitis with impaired steroidogenesis and spermatogenesis in the testes of rabbits infected with an attenuated strain of myxoma virus. J Reprod Fertil. 1997;110:161–9.

Freund J, Lipton MM, Thompson GE. Aspermatogenesis in the guinea pig induced by testicular tissue and adjuvant. J Exp Med. 1953;97:711–26.

Fujii Y, Yokochi T, Nakashima I, Asai J, Kato N. A new mouse model for autoimmune orchitis. Med Microbiol Immunol. 1991;180:1–14.

Gao JF, Call SB, Fillmore PD, Watanabe T, Meeker ND, Teuscher C. Analysis of the role of Bphs/Hrh1 in the genetic control of responsiveness to pertussis toxin. Infect Immun. 2003:1281–7.

Gonzalez JL, Gallego E, Castano M, Rueda A. Testicular amyloidosis in hamsters experimentally infected with Leishmania donovani. Br J Exp Pathol. 1983;64:518–23.

Guazzone VA, Rival C, Denduchis B, Lustig L. Monocyte chemoattractant protein-1 (MCP-1/CCL2) in experimental autoimmune orchitis. J Reprod Immunol. 2003;60:143–57.

Guazzone VA, Denduchis B, Lustig L. Involvement of CD44 in leukocyte recruitment to the rat testis in experimental autoimmune orchitis. Reproduction. 2005;129:603–9.

Guazzone VA, Jacob P, Theas MS, Lustig L. Cytokines and chemokines in testicular inflammation: a brief review. Microsc Res Tech. 2009;72:620–8.

Guazzone VA, Hollwegs S, Mardirosian M, Jacob P, Hackstein H, Wygrecka M, Schneider E, Meinhardt A, Lustig L, FIjak M. Characterization of dendritic cells in testicular draining lymph nodes in a rat model of experimental autoimmune orchitis. Int J Androl. 2011a;34:276–89.

Guazzone VA, Guerrieri D, Jacobo P, Glisoni RJ, Chiappetta D, Lustig L, Chuluyan HE. Micro-encapsulated secretory leukocyte protease inhibitor decreases cell-mediated immune response in autoimmune orchitis. Life Sci. 2011b;89:100–6.

Guazzone VA, Jacobo P, Denduchis B, Lustig L. Expression of cell adhesion molecules, chemokines and chemokine receptors involved in leukocyte traffic in rats undergoing autoimmune orchitis. Reproduction. 2012;143:651–62.

Hagopian A, Jackson JJ, Carlo DJ, Limjuco GA, Eylar EH. Experimental allergic aspermatogenic orchitis. III. Isolation of spermatozoal glycoproteins and their role in allergic aspermatogenic orchitis. J Immunol. 1975;115:1731–43.

Hagopian A, Limjuco GA, Jackson JJ, Carlo DJ, Eylar EH. Experimental allergic aspermatogenic orchitis. IV. Chemical properties of sperm glycoproteins isolated from guinea pig testes. Biochim Biophys Acta. 1976;434:354–64.

Hardy DM, Garbers DL. A sperm membrane protein that binds in a species-specific manner to the egg extracellular matrix is homologous to von Willebrand factor. J Biol Chem. 1995;270:26025–8.

Hargis BT, Malkiel S, Berkelhammer J. Immunologically induced aspermatogenesis in the white mouse. J Immunol. 1968;101:374–5.

Hirai S, Naito M, Kuramasu M, Yuki O, Qu N, Terayama H, Hatayama N, Itoh M. Low-dose di(2-ethylhexyl) phthalate (DEHP) exposure increases susceptibility to testicular autoimmunity in mice. Reprod Biol. 2015;15:163–71.

Hiramine C, Hojo K. Adoptive transfer of suppression of experimental allergic orchitis with lymphoid cells from antigen-pretreated guinea pig. Clin Immunol Immunopathol. 1984a;30:202–13.

Hiramine C, Hojo K. Requirement of B lymphocytes in local adoptive transfer of experimental allergic orchitis by lymph node cells. Am J Reprod Immunol. 1984b;6:85–91.

Hojo K, Hiramine C, Ishitaki M. Lymphocytes proliferative response in vitro and its cellular dependency in guinea pigs with experimental autoimmune orchitis. J Reprod Fertil. 1980;59:113–23.

Hojo K, Hiramine C. Suppression of experimental allergic orchitis and cellular immune responses in guinea pig by pretreatment with testis antigen in incomplete Freund's adjuvant. Int Arch Allergy Appl Immunol. 1982;69:40–9.

Hojo K, Hiramine C. In vivo effects of cyclosporine A: abrogation of the induction of experimental allergic orchitis and sparing of the generation of suppressor cells. Int Arch Allergy Appl Immunol. 1985;78:63–70.

Hong F, Wang Y, Zhou Y, Zhang Q, Ge Y, Chen M, Hong J, Wang L. Exposure to TiO2 nanoparticles induces immunological dysfunction in mouse testis. J Agric Food Chem. 2016;64:346–55.

Ichinohasama R, Hirokawa K, Hatakeyama S. Spermatogenic disturbance induced in mice by combined local injection of monoclonal antibodies to Sertoli cell and to basal lamina of seminiferous tubules. Am J Reprod Immunol Microbiol. 1986;10:158–65.

Iosub R, Klug J, Fijak M, Schneider E, Frohlich S, Blumbach K, Wennemuth G, Sommerhoff CP, Steinhoff M, Meinhardt A. Development of testicular inflammation in the rat involves activation of proteinase-activated receptor-2. J Pathol. 2006;208:686–98.

Itoh M, Hiramine C, Hojo K. A new murine model of autoimmune orchitis induced by immunization with viable syngeneic testicular germ cells alone. I. Immunological and histological studies. Clin Exp Immunol. 1991a;83:137–42.

Itoh M, Hiramine C, Tokunaga Y, Mukasa A, Hojo K. A new murine model of autoimmune orchitis induced by immunization with viable syngeneic testicular germ cells alone. II. Immunohistochemical findings of fully-developed lesion. Autoimmunity. 1991b;10:89–97.

Itoh M, Mukasa A, Tokunaga Y, Hiramine C, Hojo K. New experimental model for adoptive transfer of murine autoimmune orchitis. Andrologia. 1991c;23:415–20.

Itoh M, Chen XA, Takeuchi Y, Miki T. Morphological demonstration of the immune privilege in the testis using adjuvants: tissue responses of male reproductive organs in mice injected with Bordetella pertussigens. Arch Histol Cytol. 1995;58:575–9.

Jackson JJ, Hagopian A, Carlo DJ, Limjuco GA, Eylar EH. Experimental allergic aspermatogenic orchitis. I. Isolation of a spermatozoal protein (AP1) which induces allergic aspermatogenic orchitis. J Biol Chem. 1975;250:6141–50.

Jackson JJ, Hagopian A, Carlo DJ, Limjuco GA, Eylar EH. Experimental allergic aspermatogenic orchitis. II. Some chemical properties of the AP1 protein of the sperm acrosome. Biochim Biophys Acta. 1976;427:251–61.

Jacobo P, Guazzone VA, Jarazo-Dietrich S, Theas MS, Lustig L. Differential changes in $CD4^+$ and $CD8^+$ effector and regulatory T lymphocyte subsets in the testis of rats undergoing autoimmune orchitis. J Reprod Immunol. 2009;81:44–54.

Jacobo PV, Perez CV, Theas MS, Guazzone VA, Lustig L. $CD4^+$ and $CD8^+$ T cells producing Th1 and Th17 cytokines are involved in the pathogenesis of autoimmune orchitis. Reproduction. 2011a;141:249–58.

Jacobo P, Guazzone VA, Theas MS, Lustig L. Testicular autoimmunity. Autoimmun Rev. 2011b;10:201–4.

Jacobo PV, Fass M, Perez CV, Jarazo-Dietrich S, Lustig L, Theas MS. Involvement of soluble Fas ligand in germ cell apoptosis in testis of rats undergoing autoimmune orchitis. Cytokine. 2012;60:385–92.

Jacobo P, Guazzone VA, Perez CV, Lustig L. $CD4^+$ $Foxp3^+$ regulatory T cells in autoimmune orchitis: phenotypic and functional characterization. Am J Reprod Immunol. 2015;73:109–25.

Jarazo-Dietrich S, Jacobo P, Perez CV, Guazzone VA, Lustig L, Theas MS. Up regulation of nitric oxide synthase-nitric oxide system in the testis of rats undergoing autoimmune orchitis. Immunobiology. 2012;217:778–87.

Jarazo-Dietrich S, Fass MI, Jacobo PV, Sobarzo CM, Lustig L, Theas MS. Inhibition of NOS-NO system prevents autoimmune orchitis development in rats: relevance of NO released by testicular macrophages in germ cell apoptosis and testosterone secretion. PLoS One. 2015;10:e0128709.

Katsh S. Adjuvants and aspermatogenesis in the guinea pig. Int Arch Allergy Appl Immunol. 1964;24:319–31.

Kitaoka M, Hirai S, Terayama H, Naito M, Qu N, Hatayama N, Miyaso H, Matsuno Y, Komiyama M, Itoh M, Mori C. Effects on the local immunity in the testis by exposure to di-(2-ethylhexyl) phthalate (DEHP) in mice. J Reprod Dev. 2013;59:485–90.

Kohno S, Munoz JA, Williams TM, Teuscher C, Bernard CC, Tung KS. Immunopathology of murine experimental allergic orchitis. J Immunol. 1983;130:2675–82.

Kyewski B, Wekerle H. Increase of T lymphocyte self-reactivity in aging inbred rats: in vitro studies with a model of experimental autoimmune orchitis. J Immunol. 1978;120:1249–55.

Lapchak PH, Guilbert LJ, Rabinovitch A. Tumor necrosis factor production is deficient in diabetes-prone BB rats and can be corrected by complete Freund's adjuvant: a possible immunoregulatory role of tumor necrosis factor in the prevention of diabetes. Clin Immunol Immunolathol. 1992;65:129–34.

Li N, Liu Z, Zhang Y, Cheng Q, Liu P, Cheng CY, Lee WM, Chen Y, Han D. Mice lacking Axl and Mer tyrosine kinase receptors are susceptible to experimental autoimmune orchitis induction. Immunol Cell Biol. 2014; doi:10.1038/icb.2014.97.

Lipscomb HL, Gardner PJ, Sharp JG. The effect of neonatal thymectomy on the induction of autoimmune orchitis in rats. J Reprod Immunol. 1979;1:209–17.

Liu Z, Zhao S, Chen Q, Yan K, Liu P, Li N, Cheng CY, Lee WM, Han D. Roles of Toll-like receptors 2 and 4 in mediating experimental autoimmune orchitis induction in mice. Biol Reprod. 2015;92:63. doi:10.1095/biolreprod.114.123901.

Loyo E, Jara LJ, Lopez PD, Puig AC. Autoimmunity in connection with a metal implant: a case of autoimmune/autoinflammatory syndrome induced by adjuvants. Autoimmun Highlights. 2012;4:33–8.

Lujan L, Perez M, Salazar E, Alvarez N, GImeno M, Pincrowski P, Irusta S, Santamaria J, Insausti N, Cortes Y, Figueras L, Cuartielles I, Vila M, Fantova E, Chapulle JL. Autoimmune/autoinflammatory syndrome induced by adjuvants (ASIA syndrome) in commercial sheep. Immunol Res. 2013;56:317–24.

Lustig L, Denduchis B, Mancini RE. Studies of the nature of extracellular components of rat seminiferous tubular wall. II. Immunological characterization of basement membrane antigen. Int J Fertil. 1977;22:16–23.

Lustig L, Denduchis B, Gonzalez NN, Puig RP. Experimental orchitis induced in rats by passive transfer of an antiserum to seminiferous tubule basement membrane. Arch Androl. 1978;1:333–43.

Lustig L, Satz ML, Sztein MB, Denduchis B. Antigens of the basement membrane of the seminiferous tubules induce autoimmunity in Wistar rats. J Reprod Immunol. 1982;4:79–90.

Lustig L, Satz ML, Denduchis B. Induction of multifocal leisons of the testis by passive transfer of immune cells. J Reprod Immunol. 1986;9:195–204.

Lustig L, Doncel GF, Berensztein Denduchis B. Testis lesions and cellular and humoral immune responses induced in rats by immunization with laminin. Am J Reprod Immunol. 1987;14:123–8.

Lustig L, Doncel GF, Berensztein E, Puig RP, Denduchis B. Experimental autoimmune orchitis. Medicina (B Aires). 1989;49:225–31.

Lustig L, Lourtau L, Perez R, Doncel GF. Phenotypic characterization of lymphocytic cell infiltrates into the testes of rats undergoing autoimmune orchitis. Int J Androl. 1993;16:279–84.

Lustig L, Denduchis B, Ponzio R, Lauzon M, Pelletier RM. Passive immunization with anti-laminin immunoglobulin G modifies the integrity of the seminiferous epithelium and induces arrest of spermatogenesis in the guinea pig. Biol Reprod. 2000;62:1505–14.

Ma RZ, Gao J, Meeker ND, Fillmore PD, Yung KSK, Watanabe T, Zachary JF, Offner H, Blankenhorn EP, Teuscher C. Identification of Bphs, an autoimmune disease locus, as histamine receptor H1. Science. 2002;297:620–3.

Mahi-Brown CA, Yule TD, Tung KSK. Adoptive transfer of murine autoimmune orchitis to naive recipients with immune lymphocytes. Cell Immunol. 1987;106:408–19.

Mahi-Brown CA, Yule TD, Tung KS. Evidence for active immunological regulation in prevention of testicular autoimmune disease independent of the blood-testis barrier. Am J Reprod Immunol Microbiol. 1988;16:165–70.

Mahi-Brown CA, Tung KSK. Activation requirements of donor T cells and host T cell recruitment in adoptive transfer of murine experimental autoimmune orchitis (EAO). Cell Immunol. 1989;124:368–79.

Mahi-Brown CA, Tung KSK. Transfer of susceptibility to experimental autoimmune orchitis from responder to non-responder substrains of BALB/c mice. J Reprod Immunol. 1990;18:247–57.

Mancini RE, Fainboim L, Alonso A. Effect of intratesticular injection of antisperm serum. Allergy. Clin Immunol. 1974;53:69–76.

Mealy K, Robinson B, Millette CF, Majzoub J, Wilmore DW. The testicular effects of tumor necrosis factor. Ann Surg. 1990;211:470–5.

Meeker ND, Hickey WF, Korngold R, Hansen WK, Sudweeks JD, Wardell BB, Griffith JS, Teuscher C. Multiple loci govern the bone marrow-derived immunoregulatory mechanism controlling dominant resistance to autoimmune orchitis. Proc Natl Acad Sci U S A. 1995;92:5684–8.

Meeker ND, Stafford AN, Lunceford JK, Avner P, Ma RZ, Teuscher C. Physical mapping of the autoimmune disease susceptibility locus, Bphs:co-localization with a cluster of genes from the TNF receptor superfamily on mouse chromosome 6. Mamm Genome. 1999;10:858–63.

Meng AL, Tung KS. Cell-mediated and humoral immune responses to aspermatogenic antigen in experimental allergic orchitis in the guinea-pig. J Reprod Fertil. 1983;69:279–88.

Mielcarek N, Hornquist EH, Johansson BR, Locht C, Abraham SN, Holmgren J. Interaction of Bordetella pertussis with mast cells, modulation of cytokine secretion by pertussis toxin. Cell Microbiol. 2001;3:181–8.

Millar DG, Garza KM, Odermatt B, Elford AR, Ono N, Li Z, Ohashi PS. Hsp70 promotes antigen-presenting cell function and converts T-cell tolerance to autoimmunity in vivo. Nat Med. 2003;9:1469–79.

Murphy CJ, Stermer AR, Richburg JH. Age- and species-dependent infiltration of macrophages into the testis of rats and mice exposed to mono-(2-ethylhexyl) phthalate (MEHP). Biol Reprod. 2014;91:18. doi:10.1095/biolreprod.113.115527.

Musha M, Hirai S, Naito M, Terayama H, Qu N, Hatayama N, Itoh M. The effects of adjuvants on autoimmune responses against testicular antigens in mice. J Reprod Develop. 2013;59:139–44.

Naito M, Hirai S, Terayama H, Qu N, Kuerban M, Musha M, Kitaoka M, Ogawa Y, Itoh M. Post-inflammation stage of autoimmune orchitis induced by immunization with syngeneic testicular germ cells alone in mice. Med Mol Morphol. 2012;45:35–44.

Noubade R, Milligan G, Zachary JF, Blankenhorn EP, del Rio R, Rincon M, Teuscher C. Histamine receptor H1 is required for TCR-mediated p38 MAPK activation and optimal IFN-gamma production in mice. J Clin Invest. 2007;117:3507–18.

Pelletier RM, Nemirovsky RC, Hugon JS. Effects of immunization with Freund's complete adjuvant and isologous spermatozoaon the seminiferous epithelium and blood-testis barrier in guinea pigs. Anat Rec. 1981;199:197–211.

Perez C, Sobarzo C, Jacobo P, Jarazo Dietrich S, Theas M, Denduchis B, Lustig L. Impaired expression and distribution of adherens and gap junction proteins in the seminiferous tubules of rats undergoing autoimmune orchitis. Int J Androl. 2011;34:e566–77.

Perez CV, Sobarzo CM, Jacobo PV, Pellizzari EH, Cigorraga SB, Denduchis B, Lustig L. Loss of occludin expression and impairment of blood-testis barrier permeability in rats with autoimmune orchitis: effect of interleukin-6 on Sertoli cell tight junctions. Biol Reprod. 2012;87:122. doi:10.1095/biolreprod.112.101709.

Perez CV, Theas MS, Jacobo PV, Jarazo-Dietrich S, Guazzone VA, Lustig L. Dual role of immune cells in the testis: Protective or pathogenic for germ cells? Spermatogenesis. 2013;3:e23870.

Perez CV, Pellizzari EH, Cigorrage SB, Galardo MN, Naito M, Lustig L, Jacob PV. IL17A impairs blood-testis barrier integrity and induces testicular inflammation. Cell Tissue Res. 2014;358:885–98.

Perez CV, Gomez LG, Gualdoni GS, Lustig L, Rabinovich GA, Guazzone VA. Dual roles of endogenous and exogenous galectin-1 in the control of testicular immunopathology. Sci Rep. 2015;5:12259. doi:10.1038/srep12259.

Person PL, Snoek M, Demant P, Woodward SR, Teuscher C. The immunogenetics of susceptibility and resistance to murine experimental allergic orchitis. Reg Immunol. 1992a;4:284–97.

Person PL, Korngold R, Teuscher C. Pertussis toxin-induced lymphocytosis is associated with alterations in thymocyte subpopulations. J Immunol. 1992b;148:1506–11.

Pokorna Z. Induction of autoimmune aspermatogenesis by noncellular cytophilic material. Folia Biol. 1969;15:173–80.

Pokorna Z, Vojtiskova M, Draber P. Induction of autoimmune damage to spermatogenesis in guinea pigs by passive transfer of anti-F9 mouse tetatocarcinoma stem cell serum fraction. Folia Biol. 1984;30:50–6.

Qu N, Terayama H, Naito M, Ogawa Y, Hirai S, Kitaoka M, Yi SQ, Itoh M. Caput epididymitis but not orchitis was induced by vasectomy in a murine model of experimental autoimmune orchitis. Reproduction. 2008;135:859–66.

Qu N, Hirayanagi Y, Kuramasu M, Nagahori K, Hayashi S, Hirai S, Hatayama N, Ogawa Y, Itoh M. Goshajinkigan completely recover the severe aspermatogenesis after busulfan treatment in mice. 2017 (in preparation).

Raghavendra V, Tanga FY, DeLeo JA. Complete Freund's adjuvant-induced peripheral inflammation evokes glial activation and proinflammatory cytokine expression in the CNS. Eur J Neurosci. 2004;20:467–73.

Rezvangfar M, Sadrkhanloy R, Ahmadi A, Shojaei-Sadee H, Rezvanfar M, Mohammadirad A, Salehnia A, Abdollahi M. Protection of cyclophosphamide-induced toxicity in reproductive tract histology, sperm characteristics, and DNA damage by an herbal source; evidence for role of free-radical toxic stress. Hum Exp Toxicol. 2008;27:901–10.

Rival C, Theas MS, Guazzone VA, Lustig L. Interleukin-6 and IL-6 receptor cell expression in testis of rats with autoimmune orchitis. J Reprod Immunol. 2006a;70:43–58.

Rival C, Lustig L, Iosub R, Guazzone VA, Schneider E, Meinhardt A, Fijak M. Identification of a dendritic cell population in normal testis and in chronically inflamed testis of rats with autoimmune orchitis. Cell Tissue Res. 2006b;324:311–8.

Rival C, Guazzone VA, von Wulffen W, Hackstein H, Schneider E, Lustig L, Fijiak M. Expression of co-stimulatory molecules, chemokine receptors and proinflammatory cytokines in dendritic cells from normal and chronically inflamed rat testis. Mol Hum Reprod. 2007;13:853–61.

Rival C, Theas MS, Suescun MO, Jacobo P, Guazzone V, Van Rooijen N, Lustig L. Functional and phenotypic characteristics of testicular macrophages in experimental autoimmune orchitis. J Pathol. 2008;215:108–17.

Roper RJ, Doerge RW, Call SB, Tung SK, Hickey EF, Teuscher C. Autoimmune orchitis, epididymitis, and vasitis are immunogenetically distinct lesions. Am J Pathol. 1998;152:1337–45.

Sakamoto Y, Himeno K, Sanui H, Yoshida S, Nomoto K. Experimental allergic orchitis in mice. I. A new model induced by immunization without adjuvants. Clin Immunol Immunopathol. 1985;37:360–8.

Sakamoto Y, Nomoto K. Suppression of delayed-type hypersensitivity to syngeneic testicular cells in mice: involvement of suppressor T cells which act at the induction stage. Cell Immunol. 1986;102:168–76.

Sakamoto Y, Matsumoto T, Kumazawa J. Suppressive effect of cyclosporine A on delayed-type hypersensitivity to syngeneic testicular cells. J Antibiot. 1994;47:708–14.

Sato K, Hirokawa K, Hatakeyama S. Experimental allergic orchitis in mice. Histopathological and immunological studies. Virchows Arch [Pathol Anat]. 1981;392:147–58.

Sewell WA, Moerloose PA, McKimm-Breschkin JL, Vadas MA. Pertussigen enhances antigen-driven interferon-r production by sensitized lymphoid cells. Cell Immunol. 1986;97:238.

Shoenfeld Y, Agmon-Levin N. 'ASIA'-Autoimmune/inflammatory syndrome induced by adjuvants. J Autoimmun. 2011;36:4–8.

Sliwa L, Macura B, Majewska M, Szczepanik M. Histological changes in seminiferous epithelium in testis of male mice induced by injection of lipopolysaccharide. Folia Med Cracov. 2009;50:107–17.

Sliwa L, Macura B, Majewska-Szczepanik M, Szczepanik M. Lack of TCRalphanbeta$^+$ CD8$^+$ and TCRgammadelta$^+$ lymphocytes ameliorates LPS induced orchitis in mice –preliminary histological observations. Folia Biol. 2014;62:67–71.

Sonoda KH, Matsuzaki G, Nomura A, Yamada H, Hamano S, Nakamura T, Mukasa A, Nomoto K. Macrophages activated by *Listeria monocytogenes* induce organ-specific autoimmunity. Immunology. 1997;92:274–83.

Steenstra R, Neblett H, Teuscher C. Serum testosterone levels in Balb/cByJ and Balb/cJ substrain mice: potential relationship with differential susceptibility to experimental autoimmune orchitis (EAO). Autoimmunity. 1989;2:285–9.

Sudweeks JD, Todd JA, Blankenhorn EP, Wardell BB, Woodward SR, Meeker ND, Estes SS, Teuscher C. Locus controlling Bordetella pertussis-induced histamine sensitization (Bphs), an autoimmune disease-susceptibility gene, maps distal to T-cell receptor beta-chain gene on mouse chromosome 6. Proc Natl Acad Sci U S A. 1993;90:3700–4.

Suescun MO, Calandra RS, Lustig L. Alteration of testicular function after induced autoimmune orchitis in rats. J Androl. 1994;15:442–8.

Suescun MO, Calandra RS, Lustig L. Increased testosterone production in vitro by Leydig cells from rats with severe autoimmune orchitis. Int J Androl. 1997;20:339–46.

Suescun MO, Calandra RS, Lustig L. Effect of testicular macrophage conditioned media from rats with autoimmune orchitis on Leydig cell function. Am J Reprod Immunol. 2000;43:116–23.

Suescun MO, Lustig L, Calandra RS, Groome NP, Campo S. Correlation between inhibin secretion and damage of seminiferous tubules in a model of experimental autoimmune orchitis. J Endocrinol. 2001;170:113–20.

Suescun MO, Rival C, Theas MS, Calandra RS, Lustig L. Involvement of tumor necrosis factor-alpha in the pathogenesis of autoimmune orchitis in rats. Biol Reprod. 2003;68:2114–21.

Sun B, Qi N, Shang T, Wu H, Deng T, Han D. Sertoli cell-initiated testicular innate immune response through toll-like receptor-3 activation is negatively regulated by Tyro3, Axl, and Mer receptors. Endocrinology. 2010;151:2886–97.

Sztein MB, Satz ML, Serrate SA. Transfer of cell migration inhibition in vitro with xenogeneic RNA in experimental autoimmune orchitis. J Clin Lab Immunol. 1980;3:39–43.

Tainosho S, Naito M, Hirai S, Terayama H, Qu N, Itoh M. Multilayered structure of the basal lamina of tubuli recti in normal mice. Med Mol Morphol. 2011;44:34–8.

Tardif S, Wilson MD, Wagner R, Hunt P, Gertsenstein M, Nagy A, Lobe C, Koop BF, Hardy DM. Zonadhesin is essential for species specificity of sperm adhesion to the egg zona pellucida. J Biol Chem. 2010;285:24863–70.

Teuscher C, Wild GC, Tung KSK. Experimental allergic orchitis: the isolation and partial characterization of an aspermatogenic polypeptide (AP3) with an apparent sequential disease-inducing determinants. J Immunol. 1983a;130:2683–8.

Teuscher C, Wild GC, Tung KS. Acrosomal autoantigens of guinea pig sperm. I. The purification of an aspermatogenic protein, AP2. J Immunol. 1983b;130:317–22.

Teuscher C, Smith SM, Goldberg EH, Shearer GM, Tung KSK. Experimental allergic orchitis in mice. I. Genetic control of susceptibility and resistance to induction of autoimmune orchitis. Immunogenetics. 1985a;22:323–33.

Teuscher C, Potter M, Tung KS. Differential susceptibility to experimental autoimmune orchitis in Balb/c substrains. Curr Top Microbiol Immunol. 1985b;122:181–8.

Teuscher C. Experimental allergic orchitis in mice, II: association of disease susceptibility with the locus controlling Bordetella pertussis-induced sensitivity to histamine. Immunogenetics. 1985;22:417–25.

Teuscher C. Association of Bordetella pertussis-induced hypersensitivity to serotonin with the H-2 gene complex. J Immunogeneti. 1986;13:51–5.

Teuscher C, Smith SM, Tung KSK. Experimental allergic orchitis in mice. III. Differential susceptibility in Balb/c sublines. J Reprod Immunol. 1987a;10:219–30.

Teuscher C, Blankenhorn EP, Hickey WF. Differential susceptibility to actively induced experimental allergic encephalomyelitis (EAE) and experimental allergic orchitis (EAO) among Balb/c substrains. Cell Immunol. 1987b;110:294–304.

Teuscher C, Blankenhorn EP, Hickey WF. Genetic analysis of Balb/cJ subline resistance to actively induced experimental allergic orchitis (EAO) and experimental allergic encephalomyelitis (EAE). Curr Top Microbiol Immunol. 1988;137:233–9.

Teuscher C, Zhou ZZ, Hickey WF. Actively induced experimental allergic orchitis in Lewis-resistant rats: reversibility of disease resistance by immunization with Bordetella pertussis. Cell Immunol. 1989;119:233–8.

Teuscher C, Hickey WF, Korngold R. Experimental allergic orchitis in mice. V. Resistance to actively induced disease in Balb/cJ substrain mice is mediated by $CD4^+$ T cells. Immunogenetics. 1990a;32:34–40.

Teuscher C, Gasser DL, Woodward SR, Hickey WF. Experimental allergic orchitis in mice. VI: Recombinations within the H-2S/H-2 interval define the map position of the H-2-associated locus controlling disease susceptibility. Immunogenetics. 1990b;32:337–44.

Teuscher C, Hickey WF, Korngold R. An analysis of the role of tumor necrosis factor in the phenotypic expression of actively induced experimental allergic orchitis and experimental allergic encephalomyelitis. Clin Immunol Immunopathol. 1990c;54:442–53.

Teuscher C, Meeker ND, Livingstone KD, Sudweeks JD, Griffith JS, Wardell BB, Hickey WF. Experimental allergic orchitis in mice. VII. Preliminary characterization of the aspermatogenic autoantigens responsible for eliciting actively and passively induced disease. J Reprod Immunol. 1994;26:233–49.

Teuscher C, Hickey WF, Grafer CM, Tung KS. A common immunoregulatory locus controls susceptibility to actively induced experimental allergic encephalomyelitis and experimental allergic orchitis in BALB/c mice. J Immunol. 1998;160:2751–7.

Theas MS, Rival C, Lustig L. Germ cell apoptosis in autoimmune orchitis: involvement of the Fas-FasL system. Am J Reprod Immunol. 2003;50:166–76.

Theas MS, Rival C, Dietrich SJ, Guazzone VA, Lustig L. Death receptor and mitochondrial pathways are involved in germ cell apoptosis in an experimental model of autoimmune orchitis. Hum Reprod. 2006;21:1734–42.

Theas MS, Rival C, Jarazo-Dietrich S, Jacobo P, Guazzone VA, Lustig L. Tumor necrosis factor-alpha released by testicular macrophages induces apoptosis of germ cells in autoimmune orchitis. Hum Reprod. 2008;23:1865–72.

Tonon S, Goriely S, Aksoy E, Pradier O, Del Giudice G, Trannoy E, Willems F, Goldman M, De Wit D. Bordetella pertussis toxin induces the release of inflammatory cytokines and dendritic cell activation in whole blood: impaired responses in human newborns. Eur J Immunol. 2002;32:3118–31125.

Toullet F, Voisin GA, Nemirovsky M. Histoimmunochemical localization of three guinea-pig spermatozoal autoantigens. Immunology. 1973;24:635–53.

Toullet F, Voisin GA. Passive transfer of autoimmune aspermatogenic orchiepididymitis (AIAO) by antispermatozoa sera. Influence of the type of autoantigen and of the class of antibody. Clin Exp Immunol. 1976;26:549–62.

Tung KS, Unanue ER, Dixon FJ. Pathogenesis of experimental allergic orchitis. I. Transfer with immune lymph node cells. J Immunol. 1971a;106:1453–62.

Tung KS, Unanue ER, Dixon FJ. Pathogenesis of experimental allergic orchitis. II. The role of antibody. J Immunol. 1971b;106:1463–72.

Tung KS, Unanue ER, Dixon FJ. Immunological events associated with immunization by sperm in incomplete Freund's adjuvant. Int Arch Allergy Appl Immunol. 1971c;41:565–74.

Tung KS, Leong C, McCarty T. Pathogenesis of experimental allergic orchitis. III. T lymphocyte requirement in local adoptive transfer by peritoneal exudate cells. J Immunol. 1977;118:1774–9.

Tung KS, Yule TD, Mahi-Brown CA, Listrom MB. Distribution of histopathology and Ia positive cells in actively induced and passively transferred experimental autoimmune orchitis. J Immunol. 1987;138:752–9.

Tung KS, Mahi-Brown CA, Yule TD. Immunologic mechanisms and target antigens in testicular autoimmunity. Ann N Y Acad Sci. 1989;564:267–80.

Tung KS, Teuscher C. Mechanisms of autoimmune disease in the testis and ovary. Hum Reprod Update. 1995;1:35 50.

Tung KS, Primakoff P, Woolman-Gamer L, Myles DG. Mechanism of infertility in male guinea pigs immunized with sperm PH-20. Biol Reprod. 1997;56:1133–41.

Tung KS. Autoimmune disease of the testis and the ovary. The autoimmune diseases. 3rd ed. Amsterdam: Academic Press, 1998. p. 687–704.

Tung PS, Fritz IB. Autoimmune orchitis can be induced by thymic lymphocytes autosensitized against syngeneic Sertoli cells in vitro. Biol Reprod. 1984;30:979–90.

Tung PS, Fritz IB. Histopathological changes in testes of adult inbred rats immunized against pachytene spermatocytes or Sertoli cells. Int J Androl Suppl. 1987;2:459–81.

Ueno A, Takeda M, Hirasawa K, Itagaki S, Doi K. Relation-ship between distribution of viral RNA and development of histopathological changes in encephalomyocarditis virus-induced orchitis in mice. Int J Exp Pathol. 1996;77:25–30.

Ueno A, Takeda M, Hirasawa K, Itagaki S, Doi K. Detection of viral RNA by electron microscopic in situ hybridization (ISH-EM) in the germinal epithelium of mice infected with encephalomyocarditis (EMC) virus. Exp Anim. 1997;46:79–81.

Vojtiskova M, Pokorna Z. Prevention of experimental allergic aspermatogenesis by thymectomy in adult mice. Lancet. 1964;1:644–5.

Vojtiskova M, Pokorna Z, Draber P. Autoimmune damage to spermatogenesis in rodents immunized with mouse F9 embryonic carcinoma cells. Proc Natl Acad Sci U S A. 1983;80:459–61.

Vojtiskova M, Pokorna Z, Draber P. Immunological tolerance to spermatogenic cell antigens induced by teratocarcinoma stem cell antigens. Folia Biol. 1984;30:290–5.

Vulchanov VH. Testicular damage and autoantibody formation in guinea-pigs immunized with homologous seminal vesicular fluid. In: Immunology and reproduction. London: International Planned Parenthood Federation; 1969. p. 136–47.

Wagner H, Starzinsk-Powitz A, Rollinghoff M, Golstein P, Jakob H. T-cell-mediated cytotoxic immune responses to F9 teratocarcinoma cells: cytolytic effector T cells lyse H-2-negative F9 cells and syngeneic spermatozoa. J Exp Med. 1978;147:251–64.

Wakabayashi A, Eishi Y, Nakamura K. Regulation of experimental autoimmune orchitis by the presence or absence of testicular antigens during immunological development in SCID mice reconstituted with fetal liver cells. Immunology. 1997;92:84–90.

Wardlaw AC. Inheritance of responsiveness to pertussis HSF in mice. Int Arch Allergy Appl Immunol. 1970;38:573–89.

Wekerle H, Begemann M. Experimental autoimmune orchitis: in vitro induction of an autoimmune disease. J Immunol. 1976;116:159–61.

Wekerle H, Begemann M. In vitro induction of experimental autoimmune orchitis:role of serum factors. Transplant Proc. 1977;9:775–8.

Wekerle H, Begemann M. In vitro induction of experimental autoimmune: characterization of a primary T lymphocyte response against self antigens. Eur J Immunol. 1978;8:294–302.

Wekerle H. Immunological T cell memory in the in vitro-induced experimental autoimmune orchitis. Specificity of the reaction and tissue distribution of the autoantigens. J Exp Med. 1978;147:233–50.

Wheeler K, Tardif S, Rival C, Luu B, Bui E, del-Rio R, Teuscher C, Sparwasser T, Hardy D, Tung KSK. Regulatory T cells control tolerogenic versus autoimmune response to sperm in vasectomy. Proc Natl Acad Sci U S A. 2011;108:7511–6.

Yamanouchi-Ueno A, Nakatyama Y, Doi K. Characteristics of testicular lesions in mice infected with a low dose of encephalomyocarditis (EMC) virus. Exp Mol Pathol. 2004;77:72–9.

Yantorno C, Debanne MT, Vottero-Cima E. Autoimmune orchitis induced by autoimmunization with seminal plasma in the rabbit. J Reprod Fertil. 1971;27:311–20.

Yokochi T, Ikeda H, Inoue Y, Kimura Y, Ito H, Fujii Y, Kato N. Characterization of autoantigens relevant to experimental autoimmune orchitis (EAO) in mice immunized with a mixture of syngeneic testis homogenate and Klebsiella O3 Lipopolysaccharide. Am J Reprod Immunol. 1990;22:42–8.

Yoshida S, Nomoto K, Himeno K, Takeya K. Immune response to syngeneic or autologous testicular cells in mice. I. Augmented delayed footpad reaction in cyclophosphamide-treated mice. Clin Exp Immunol. 1979;38:211–7.

Yule TD, Montoya GD, Russell LD, Williams TM, Tung KSK. Autoimmunogenic germ cells exist outside the blood testis barrier. J Immunol. 1988;141:1161–7.

Yule TD, Mahi-Brown CA, Tung KS. Role of testicular autoantigens and influence of lymphokines in testicular autoimmune disease. J Reprod Immunol. 1990;18:89–103.

Yule TD, Tung KSK. Experimental autoimmune orchitis induced by testis and sperm antigen-specific T cell clones: an important pathogenic cytokines is tumor necrosis factor. Endocrinology. 1993;133:1098–107.

Zhou ZZ, Zeng Y, Steenstra R, Hickey WF, Teuscher C. Actively-induced experimental allergic orchitis (EAO) in Lewis/NCR rats: sequential histo-and immunopathologic analysis. Autoimmunity. 1989;3:125–34.

Testicular Autoimmunity by Local Injury of the Testis in Experimental Animals

6

6.1 Introduction

Experimental autoimmune orchitis (EAO) can be induced by various local factors in the testis, without depending on systemic immunization with testicular antigens. The factors include traumatic injury, obstruction of germ cell transport, thermal injury, and foreign body injection, which induce a disruption of the BTB with the resultant exposure of TGC autoantigens to the immune system.

6.2 Various EAO Models by Local Injuries

6.2.1 EAO Induced by Traumatic Injury of Unilateral Testis

If the BTB is severely damaged, the autoimmunogenic TGC leaks out beyond the BTB, causing a continuous supply of autoantigens with the resultant testicular inflammation. Fainboim et al. (1976) reported immunologic response in the testes of guinea pigs after unilateral traumatic orchitis (Fig. 6.1). They found that foci showing the classical picture of EAO appeared in the contralateral testis. Later, in mice, Naito et al. (2009a) also demonstrated that rupture of one testis by a scissor induced EAO in the contralateral testis (=sympathetic EAO). Traumatic rupture of unilateral testis induced significant DTH against TGC (Sakamoto et al. 1995; Naito et al. 2009a). The DTH response to TGC by testicular trauma was induced without any active immunization with TGC and was further enhanced by treatment with cyclophosphamide before the trauma and was significantly suppressed by cyclosporine A (Sakamoto et al. 1995, 1998). The traumatized testes undergo early degeneration of the seminiferous epithelium followed by neutrophilic inflammation and later fibrosis with little lymphocytic infiltration. In the contralateral testes, EAO characterized by both lymphocytic inflammation and spermatogenic disturbance was induced.

M. Itoh, *Testicular Autoimmunity*, DOI 10.1007/978-4-431-54460-9_6

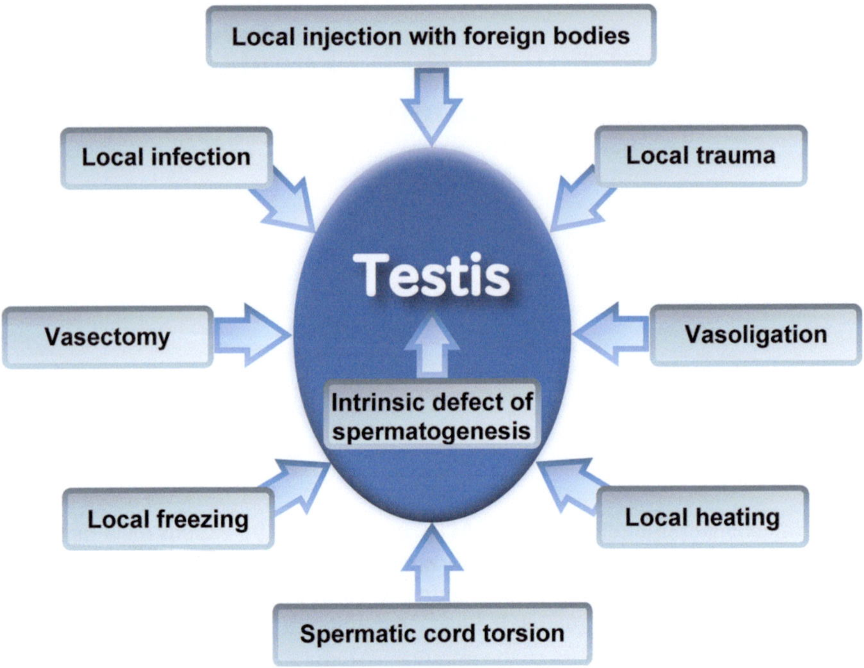

Fig. 6.1 EAO induced by testicular injuries followed by stimulation and proliferation of pathogenic T effector cells

In this sympathetic EAO model, adeno-associated virus-mediated human IL-10 gene transfer suppressed the disease development (Watanabe et al. 2005). A single intramuscular injection of IL-10 gene into mice with the testicular trauma significantly suppressed both EAO and DTH against TGC. In the EAO-suppressed mice, serum IL-10 peaked at 3 weeks after the injection, and numbers of IFN-gamma and IL-2-expressing cells in the spleen and testes were significantly fewer. The results are in contrast to the aggravating effect of exogenously administered IL-10 on TGC-induced EAO (Kaneko et al. 2003).

6.2.2 EAO Induced by Spermatic Cord Torsion of Unilateral Testis

Torsion of the spermatic cord results in vascular changes that can range from partial venous obstruction to complete occlusion of the testicular artery (Hirai et al. 2017). The damage of BTB undergoing experimental torsion of the spermatic cord also induced sympathetic EAO in the contralateral testis of rats and rabbits (Nagler and White 1982; Cerasaro et al. 1984; Rodriguez et al. 2006) (Fig. 6.1). In this model, animals were subjected to 720 degree unilateral spermatic cord torsion. In rats, the maximal degree of the spermatogenic disturbance was seen 30 days after torsion in the contralateral testis, in which T cells, mast cell, and macrophages increased in number. TNF-alpha concentration and the number of TNF receptor-positive TGC were also increased in the contralateral testis (Rodriguez et al. 2006). This contralateral EAO was prevented if splenectomy was performed on the rats with unilateral twisted testis (Nagler and White 1982). In rabbits, there were no differences of severity of contralateral EAO between animals that had received unilateral testis torsion alone and animals that had received detorsion at 36 h or 96 h. Salvaged unilateral testes after detorsion became atrophic and that detorsion did not protect the contralateral testis from EAO induction (Cerasaro et al. 1984). However, orchiectomy of the unilateral twisted testis appeared to protect the contralateral testis from EAO (Nagler and White 1982).

6.2.3 EAO Induced by Vasectomy or Vasoligation of Unilateral Testis

Vasectomy, a common male contraceptive approach, often results in immune responses to sperm antigens. In vasectomized animals and humans, the epididymis underwent epithelial cell apoptosis followed by necrosis, severe inflammation, and granuloma formation (spermatic granuloma) as a result of extravasated spermatozoa by vasectomy, creating a localized endogenous danger signal (Rival et al. 2013). In vasectomized rabbits, guinea pigs, monkeys, and mice, post-vasectomy EAO has been documented (Bigazzi et al. 1976; Tung 1978; Tonsy et al. 1979; Tung and Alexander 1980; Anderson and Alexander 1981) (Fig. 6.1). The post-vasectomy EAO is associated with deposition of IgG and complement on the basal lamina of the seminiferous tubules. These lesions are frequently accompanied by mononuclear cell infiltration and destruction of seminiferous epithelium. Some studies revealed the induction of both humoral and cellular autoimmune responses directed against sperm antigens after vasectomy (Ansbacher 1973; Alexander and Tung 1977; Herr et al. 1987; Nashan et al. 1990; McDonald and Halliday 1992; Flickinger et al. 1994, 1995, 1996). The post-vasectomy EAO is likely resulted from continuous stimulation by exposed sperm antigens coming from the inflamed epididymis. Indeed, testicular lymph and lymph nodes contained spermatozoa in men, rams, and boars after vasectomy (Ball et al. 1982; Ball and Setchell 1983). Such direct access of spermatozoa to lymph nodes is likely to provide a powerful stimulus to the development of anti-sperm autoimmunity.

In guinea pigs, EAO is developed 14 months after vasoligation. Furthermore, a similar histopathology was found in unoperated testes after unilateral vasoligation, and peritoneal exudate cells from vasoligated guinea pigs transferred identical lesions to syngeneic recipients (Tung 1978). Blood flow or lymphatic drainage in the testis and epididymis may be changed by vasectomy or vasoligation (Itoh et al. 1998a). It is known that the ducts of the caput epididymis are the sites of absorption of various materials leaving the testis. Therefore, vasectomy or vasoligation may allow the epididymal ducts to absorb testis-secreting materials, including autoantigens of mature spermatids, more strongly and to leak or excrete some of the absorbed autoantigens to the outside of the ducts. Actually, Johnson and Howards (1975, 1976, 1977) reported the leakage of epididymal spermatozoa from the caput epididymal ducts after vasectomy in guinea pigs and hamsters. It was also found that the levels of IFN-gamma, IL-6, and IL-10 in the epididymides strikingly increased with vasectomy alone (Qu et al. 2008).

Serum autoantibodies from vasectomized rats bound autoantigens of approximately 86 kDa, 63 kDa, 43 kDa, and 20 kDa of sperm extract and autoantigens of approximately 76 kDa, 60 kDa, and 42 kDa of testicular extracts (Handley et al. 1988). Immunohistochemically, autoantigens of 63 kDa and 43 kDa were synchronously expressed in the cytoplasm of spermatids (Handley et al. 1991). On immunization with syngeneic TGC alone, EAO is induced in mice with no involvement of autoimmune epididymitis (Itoh et al. 1991a, b). In contrast, autoimmune epididymitis with no EAO can be induced in vasectomized mice by immunization with TGC (Qu et al. 2008). The appearance of autoantigens relevant to EAO or autoimmune epididymitis was investigated by reaction of each immune serum with testicular and epididymal extracts from normal mice of various ages by immunoblotting. The results showed that the antisera obtained from mice with TGC-induced EAO lesions specifically defined testicular antigens with molecular weights of 15 kDa, 40 kDa, 75 kDa, and >200 kDa from 4 weeks of age, but the antisera obtained from mice with autoimmune epididymitis induced by vasectomy+TGC-immunization strongly defined testicular antigens of 25 kDa from 5 weeks of age and epididymal antigens of 25 kDa from 8 weeks of age (Qu et al. 2010). This suggests that vasectomy changes the target autoantigens in TGC-induced autoimmunity.

It has been demonstrated that autoreactive lymphocytes could preferentially gain access to the tubuli recti and the rete testis where BTB is incomplete. (Dym and Fawcett 1970; Aoki and Fawcett 1975; Itoh et al. 1995a, b, 1998b). Indeed, a focal lymphocytic infiltration was faintly and occasionally found in vasectomized mice (personal observation). However, vasectomy may increase the hydrostatic pressure in the epididymal ducts rather than the tubuli recti and the rete testis. This may result in possible leakage of more germ cell autoantigens into the epididymal interstitium, followed by autoimmune epididymitis (Qu et al. 2008). Therefore, ligation of ductuli efferentes rather than vasectomy may affect the integrity of BTB. The permeability of Sertoli cell tight junctions to lanthanum, a blood-borne tracer, has been compared in rats after ligation of the vas deferens and after ligation of the ductuli efferentes (Neaves 1978). In vasectomized rats, lanthanum penetrated only short distance into the Sertoli cell tight junctions; thereby, the BTB prevented diffusion of lanthanum into the adluminal compartment of the seminiferous epithelium. In contrast, lanthanum completely penetrated many Sertoli cell tight junctions and occupied intercellular spaces of the adluminal compartment in rats that had received ligation of the ductuli efferentes. Therefore, ligation of the ductuli efferentes is very effective in eliciting change in the BTB. A later study demonstrated the breakdown of the BTB by ligation of the ductuli efferentes is reversible (Tao et al. 2000). Clinically, a spermatocele refers to the cystic accumulation of semen in the male reproductive tract because of the blockade of the germ cell flow. Considering that the spermatocele is thought to be caused by narrowing of the lumen of the excurrent

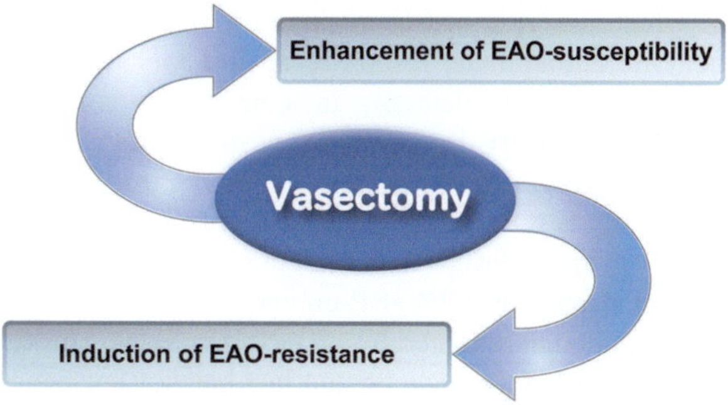

Fig. 6.2 Dual effects of vasectomy on EAO

duct with resultant cystic dilatation of the duct, the ductuli efferentes should be most vulnerable to the lumen occlusion. Actually, a senile change of the seminiferous epithelium, which releases agglutinated germ cells into the lumen of the seminiferous tubules, occupied the very narrow lumen of the ductuli efferentes with TGC, resulting in the blockade of TGC flow at the rete testis (Itoh et al. 1999). Therefore, occlusion of the ductuli efferentes may also break down the BTB, increasing susceptibility to EAO.

It is also noted that there are still conflicting reports on the immunological long-term effects of vasectomy. Vasectomized males represent a population whose immune potential may be compromised by leakage of sperm into the blood vascular system. Diminished T cell function after vasectomy has been reported in rhesus monkeys (Wilson et al. 1979), but none was revealed in mice (Anderson and Alexander 1981). The effect of vasectomy on EAO was investigated in the neonatal thymectomy model, in which neonatal thymectomy on day 3 induces multiple organ-localized autoimmune diseases involving EAO. The incidence of EAO was found to increase when day 3-thymectomized mice received vasectomy on day 60 after birth (Taguchi and Nishizuka 1981) (Fig. 6.2). Kojima and Spencer (1983) also reported that vasectomy increased the incidence of testicular atrophy in day 3-thymectomized mice.

Qu et al. (2008) demonstrated that vasectomized mice became resistant to active EAO induction; mice receiving sham-vasectomy and the following TGC immunization had EAO with no epididymitis. In sharp contrast, no EAO was found in the testes of any mice receiving vasectomy and the following TGC immunization. Instead, caput epididymitis involving infiltration of $CD4^+$ T cells, $CD8^+$ T cells, B cells, and macrophages was induced in them with striking elevation of the epididymal tissue levels of both IL-6 and IL-10 mRNA (Qu et al. 2008). Therefore, vasectomy suppressed EAO and alternatively induced caput epididymitis (Fig. 6.2). Later, in other studies, it was demonstrated that vasectomized mice did not develop any post-vasectomy EAO lesion. Instead, they became resistant to EAO induction by testicular antigens+CFA+BP-immunization but are sensitive to experimental autoimmune encephalomyelitis (Wheeler et al. 2011) (Fig. 6.2). This testis-specific tolerance is long lasting and has continued for at least 12–16 months; however, the specific tolerance in vasectomized mice switched over to pathologic autoimmunity following concomitant depletion of $CD4^+$ $CD25^+$ $Foxp3^+$ Treg, unilaterally vasectomized mice of which the Treg had been simultaneously depleted developed both cellular and humoral autoimmune responses against meiotic TGC antigens, resulting in post-vasectomy EAO bilaterally in spite of no active immunization with testicular antigens+CFA+BP. However, this post-vasectomy EAO did not occur in unilaterally vasectomized mice when Treg depletion was delayed by 1 week. Therefore, post-vasectomy EAO depends on a rapid "natural" Treg depletion just after vasectomy. However, the delayed Treg depletion at week 1 allowed active EAO induction by testicular antigens+CFA+BP-immunization at week 3 in unilaterally vasectomized mice, although unilaterally vasectomy alone showed resistance to this active EAO. Therefore, a dynamic and fine balance between tolerance and autoimmunity was demonstrated in this disease model. Moreover, tolerance was blunted in unilaterally vasectomized mice that are genetically deficient in PD-ligand1. The PD-1 receptor and its cognate PD-ligand1 are one of the major inhibitory ligand-receptor pairs that are highly expressed on Treg. The interaction of PD-1 and PD-ligand1 on T cells and antigen-presenting cells is critical for peripheral tolerance and autoimmunity prevention (Riella et al. 2012). Similar to the wild-type vasectomized mice, PD-1 knockout mice that had been unilaterally vasectomized exhibited the resistance to active EAO by immunization with testicular antigens+CFA+BP. In contrast, PD-ligand1 knockout mice that had been unilaterally vasectomized were sensitive to this active EAO. Since previous studies have demonstrated that PD-ligand1 is required for the generation of "induced" Treg and maintenance of Foxp3 expression (Riella et al. 2012), the findings suggest the involvement of "induced" Treg on suppression of active EAO in vasectomized mice. Therefore, there may be two types of Treg in vasectomized mice, in which preexisting "natural" Treg may prevent post-vasectomy EAO, whereas "vasectomy-induced Treg" may maintain post-vasectomy tolerance (Rival et al. 2013).

6.2.4 EAO Induced by Heating Injury of Unilateral Testis

Testis heating suppresses spermatogenesis which is marked by TGC loss via apoptotic pathways. Recent studies demonstrated that heat triggers autophagy and apoptosis in TGC (Zhang et al. 2012). EAO is induced in the untreated contralateral testis by unilateral heating injury in the guinea pig (Rapaport et al. 1969; Fernandez-Collazo et al. 1972) (Fig. 6.1). This sympathetic EAO is accompanied by humoral response and DTH against TGC. In thermally injured left testis, congested vessels, interstitial infiltration of both polymorphonuclear and mononuclear cells, and their infiltration into lumen of the seminiferous tubules were observed. Later, a fibrotic reaction appeared, followed by sclerosis of the testis. In the contralateral right testis, the lesions consisted of seminiferous tubules with sloughing of TGC, vacuolization of Sertoli cells, and mononuclear infiltration in the interstitial tissue, but no alteration in Leydig cells was observed (Fernandez-Collazo et al. 1972).

It is known that the environmental temperature in the abdominal cavity or inguinal canal is 2 degrees higher than in the scrotum and is the reason for the damage to an undescended testis. It is noted that experimental unilateral cryptorchidism induces pathologic changes leading to the spermatogenic disturbance in "both" testes. A high non-physiological environmental temperature makes the BTB permeable by immune cells. In the model of experimental unilateral testicular cryptorchidism using azathioprine as an immunosuppressant, the total number of spermatogonia in the ectopic as well as in the contralateral orthotopic testis increased significantly (Mengel and Zimmermann 1982).

The effect of 43 C warming on cell junctions in the seminiferous epithelium was examined. Expressions of adherence junction-associated molecules, such as N-cadherin and beta-catenin, and tight junction-associated molecule zonula occludens protein 1 were significantly reduced in 24–48 h after heat treatment, indicating to disruption of the BTB (Chen et al. 2008). Analyses using chromium Cr^{51}-EDTA as a tracer also revealed that the BTB was less effective during the period of spermatogenic disruption following local 43 C heating of the testis (Setchell et al. 1996).

6.2.5 EAO Induced by Freezing Injury of Unilateral Testis

Unilateral multiple in situ freezing of the rabbit testis was shown to be an effective antigenic stimulus as evidenced by production of tissue-specific antibodies against testicular antigens (Ablin et al. 1971). In the unilateral testes receiving cryoinjury, coagulation necrosis is evidenced by homogenous eosinophilia of the tubular and vascular elements. Around the tubules, a moderate and diffuse fibroblastic-histiocytic infiltration, as well as a perivascular cuff of lymphocytes, was recognized. Histological studies of testicular biopsies of the contralateral testis of frozen animals revealed modest to extensive alterations consisting of degenerative changes in the seminiferous tubules accompanied by interstitial edema, interstitial hyperplasia, and the spermatogenic disturbance (Ablin 1972; Ablin and Soanes 1972). Mild to moderate interstitial mononuclear cell infiltration was also induced in the contralateral testis following the unilateral cryoinjury, indicating the induction of sympathetic EAO (Zappi et al. 1973, 1974) (Fig. 6.1).

6.2.6 EAO Induced by Local Injection with Turpentine into Unilateral Testis and Intradermal Injection with CFA

Turpentine is a fluid produced by the distillation of resin obtained from live trees. It can cause a local and prolonged inflammation when injected into the target tissues. In the guinea pigs that had received local injection with turpentine into unilateral testis and intradermal injection with CFA, histological examination of the locally injected unilateral testis showed a large central core of coagulation necrosis, in which the outlines of the seminiferous tubules remained visible (Boughton and Spector 1963). Beyond the area of necrosis, the testis showed a zone of inflammatory cell infiltration, with fibrosis, extensive degeneration of the seminiferous tubules, and the interstitial edema. On the other hand, contralateral testis showed a patchy tubular degeneration among a great bulk of normal tubular zone on day 7 (Fig. 6.1). In the affected tubules, there were no spermatozoa or spermatids, and primary and secondary spermatocytes were disintegrating. The spermatogonia were relatively less affected, and the primary damage appeared to be in the spermatocytes. The Sertoli cells seemed unaffected, as did the interstitial tissues. In contrast, in animals receiving intra-testicular turpentine without intradermal CFA injection, contralateral testis showed no tubular degeneration. Furthermore, in animals that had received intradermal injection with CFA without intra-testicular turpentine, the testes were macroscopically and microscopically normal (Boughton and Spector 1963).

6.2.7 EAO Induced by Local Injection with CFA into Unilateral Testis

Eyquem and Krieg (1965) produced bilateral EAO by injecting a small amount of CFA alone into the left testis in rats, guinea pigs, and monkeys (Fig. 6.1). In CFA-injected unilateral testes, infiltration of mononuclear cells, resorption of the inoculated product in the granuloma, spermatogenic disturbance, and exudation of fibrinoid products were induced. In the contralateral testes, the spermatogenic disturbance was noted, but there was no apparent inflammatory cell response and granuloma. Boughton and Spector (1963) also tried similar experiments in guinea pigs; however, little damage in CFA-injected left testis and no detectable pathological changes in the contralateral testis were found.

6.2.8 EAO Induced by Bilateral CFA Injection into Epididymides

CFA was injected into cauda epididymides bilaterally in rats, in which the cauda was heavily infiltrated with polymorphonuclear leukocytes, lymphocytes, plasma cells, and macrophages (Tonsy et al. 1979). The cellular inflammatory infiltrate was also present in the regions of the corpus and caput epididymides. Furthermore, there was marked testicular degeneration. The testicular interstitium was infiltrated with lymphocytes, plasma cells, and macrophages, which seemed to be crossing the wall of the seminiferous tubules. Multinucleated large macrophages were also noted in the seminiferous tubules. The basal lamina of the seminiferous tubules was externally thickened. There was almost complete absence of all TGC except for Sertoli cells. Occasionally, some tubules were distended with large numbers of spermatozoa and no other immature TGC. Sera of the injected rats were all positive for anti-sperm autoantibodies.

6.2.9 EAO Induced by Intra-testicular Infection with Bacteria

Infection is a candidate of a trigger of autoimmune diseases that occur in the natural course of the diseases. Guinea pigs were inoculated into the testis with viable *Listeria monocytogenes*, *Escherichia coli*, *Pseudomonas aeruginosa*, or *Staphylococcus aureus* (Sanui et al. 1982, 1983). DTH skin reactions against TGC were carried out 1 week later and significantly detected only when guinea pigs were locally injected with *Listeria monocytogenes*. The DTH reactions involved many lymphocytes, macrophages, and basophils with some neutrophils and eosinophils at subdermal tissue and were specific for TGC since the significant DTH reaction could not be detected by the elicitation with sheep red blood cells as sensitizing antigens. Significant anti-TGC DTH reaction was not detected when guinea pigs were injected with *Listeria monocytogenes* intravenously or subcutaneously. However, the local injection of viable *Listeria monocytogenes* into unilateral testis induced EAO in the contralateral testis and epididymis (=sympathetic EAO) in guinea pigs (Fig. 6.1). The pathological changes in the contralateral testis were characterized by the severe spermatogenic disturbance and severe interstitial infiltration of mononuclear cells. In a small number of animals, polymorphonuclear leukocytes were detected in or around the seminiferous tubules. Mononuclear cells also invaded into some seminiferous tubules; however, basophils were not detected in the EAO lesion. In the rete testis, massive infiltration of mononuclear cells was observed. In the lumens of the rete testis, degenerated and desquamated TGC and macrophages phagocytosing many spermatozoa were found. Most seminiferous tubules were empty or sometimes contain a central mass of degenerated TGC. However, Sertoli cells still remained a normal appearance. Moreover, hypertrophic Leydig cells with eosinophilic cytoplasm appeared prominent when inflammatory cell infiltration was subsided (Sanui et al. 1982, 1983).

Listeria monocytogenes are facultative intracellular pathogens that grow in the cytoplasm of infected host cells. The virulent strain of *Listeria monocytogenes* is able to survive in the cytoplasm by escaping from phagosomes. In the sites of local infection with *Listeria monocytogenes* in the unilateral testis, apparent destruction of architecture of the seminiferous tubules was seen, and enhancement of both cellular and humoral immune responses was expected due to adjuvant effects of the bacterial components. *Listeria monocytogenes* was not detected in the EAO-affected contralateral testis, liver, or spleen during the period of experiments, showing that the bacterial growth was limited to the inoculated unilateral testis. These data show a possibility that the macrophages/dendritic cells accumulate in virulent *Listeria monocytogenes*-infected site and then uptake, process, and present TGC autoantigens released from the damaged testis with the infection (Sanui et al. 1982, 1983). On the other hand, avirulent *Listeria monocytogenes*, which lacks the expression of listeriolysin O, failed to induce any anti-TGC immune responses and sympathetic EAO even when inoculated at a high dose into the testis.

The unilateral testicular inoculation of virulent *Listeria monocytogenes* in mice also induced specific DTH response against TGC and caused sympathetic EAO (Fig. 6.1). A unilateral infection of *Listeria monocytogenes* into the testis of mice induced not only *Listeria*-specific T cells but also autoreactive T cells that can transfer EAO into naïve mice (Mukasa et al. 1995, 1997, 1998; Matsuzaki et al. 1997). In mice unilaterally infected with *Listeria monocytogenes*, the contralateral testis developed inflammatory lesion without detectable microorganisms, providing evidence for an autoimmune phenomenon, like in the guinea pig model. This model therefore gives the opportunity to investigate to two types of inflammation in one mouse: a bacterial-induced reaction and an autoimmunity-induced inflammatory reaction. The EAO can be adoptively transferred to naïve syngeneic mice by intravenous injection with TGC-specific T cell clones that were derived from spleens of the intra-testicular *Listeria*-infected mice. All EAO-inducing clones expressed both CD4 and TCR alpha-beta and showed proliferative response to TGC but did not cross-react to the *Listeria* antigen. They produced both IFN-gamma and TNF-alpha when stimulated with TGC, but IL-2, IL-4, and IL-10 were undetectable. Therefore, alpha-beta T cells play a central pathogenic role in causing EAO, as in other EAO models.

The TGC-specific T cells transferred EAO without histological changes in the liver and kidney. Therefore, the orchitogenic T cell clones recognize testis-specific antigens that are not expressed by other organs, although the antigenic molecules have not yet been identified. Furthermore, the increased number of gamma-delta T cells was found in both infected and sympathetic EAO-affected testes. The gamma-delta T cell ratio in infiltrated T cells in testes reached up to 20–30% in whole T cells. Surprisingly, when gamma-delta T cells were depleted, inflammation in both sides was significantly augmented. Thus, gamma-delta T cells in this model may function as Treg in the disease progress and may have some immunoregulatory control on alpha-beta T cells (Mukasa et al. 1997, 1998). It was also shown that the gamma-delta T cells reduced alpha-beta pathogenic T cell function through cytokines. The negative regulatory role of gamma-delta T cells in inflammation may be due to the production of IL-10 or transforming growth factor-beta, which is known to exert a suppressive function on alpha-beta T cells.

There is little information about whether sympathetic orchitis accompanied by cellular and humoral immune responses against TGC can be experimentally induced by other local infection in the testis. In mice, intra-seminiferous tubular injection of live *Escherichia coli* in unilateral testis resulted in that the bacteria actively propagated and reached a maximal level in a day but started to decrease after day 5 and completely disappeared within 2 months. The expression of macrophage inflammatory protein-2 and TNF-alpha became evident in testicular macrophages as early as 1–3 h. Neutrophils were first accumulated in the testicular interstitium at 9–12 h, and the spermatogenic disturbance was observed on day 1 and seemed unrecoverable and irreversible even after the bacteria were eliminated (Nagaosa et al. 2009). However, the spermatogenic disturbance was not evident in the contralateral testis. Additionally, in mice that received intra-testicular injection with lipopolysaccharide or dead *Escherichia coli*, the spermatogenic disturbance was not evident (Nagaosa et al. 2009).

Intra-testicular injection of bacterium Calmette-Guerin (BCG) induced reversible inhibition of spermatogenesis (Das et al. 1982; Torgersen et al. 1982). The local injection weakened the BTB and thus gave immunocompetent cells access to the tubular lumen. Individual Sertoli cells degenerated and separated from spermatocytes and spermatids. In the induction phase, the interstitium was full of inflammatory cells; however, full recovery of spermatogenesis was observed after 120 days. Therefore, EAO-like feature was not observed.

Experimental syphilitic orchitis was induced by intra-testicular injection of *Treponema pallidum* in rabbits. Phagocytosis of the organisms by testicular macrophages occurs during the reactive phase, followed by polymorphonuclear cell infiltration, DTH reaction by specific T cells, infiltration of plasma cells, and severe spermatogenic disturbance (Sell et al. 1982; Wicher et al. 1983). However, when mononuclear cells infiltrating rabbit testes infected with *Treponema pallidum* were co-cultured with peripheral blood lymphocytes, lymphocytic proliferation stimulated with concanavalin A was suppressed (Wicher and Wicher 1984), indicating the induction of immunosuppressive microenvironment in the testis.

In those experiments using *Escherichia coli*, BCG, and *Treponema pallidum*, it remains unclear whether autoimmune responses against TGC antigens or other testicular antigens are induced or not. However, in experimentally induced epididymo-orchitis by local injection of *Escherichia coli* into the right ductus deferens in the rat, both the infected testis and contralateral testis showed similar histopathological changes characterized by the inflammatory cell infiltration, the spermatogenic disturbance, and the interstitial fibrosis (Demir et al. 2007). There is a possibility that bacterial lipopolysaccharide induces endotoxemia, resulting in systemic inflammation-induced oxidative stress on steroidogenesis and spermatogenesis (Metukuri et al. 2010). A significant induction of stress response proteins such as heat shock protein (HSP)-60, high-mobility group box protein 1 (HMGB1), and HMGB2 may affect the testis after lipopolysaccharide injection. This induction of acute stress is closely followed by a significant reduction in Bcl/Bax ratio along with leakage of cytochrome c from mitochondria and increased caspase three activity levels in the testis. These stress response proteins and mitochondrial dysfunction may be involved in lipopolysaccharide-induced TGC death in the seminiferous epithelium.

6.2.10 EAO Induced by Intra-testicular Infection with Virus

It has been reported that autoimmune orchitis occurs spontaneously in the mink, beagle dog, and aging rat. (Fritz et al. 1976; Tung et al. 1981, 1984; Furbeth et al. 1989; Robinson et al. 1994). Actually, most cases of spontaneous autoimmune orchitis are supposed to be associated with a viral infectious disease of unknown origin (Fig. 6.1). Although several possible mechanisms of autoimmune induction by viral infection, which includes molecular mimicry and massive release of autoantigens, have been proposed, mechanisms that link infections to autoimmune diseases are not yet clarified. The pathogens are thought to induce orchitis by disrupting the mechanisms of testicular immune privilege rather than through a direct cytopathologic effect (Lustig and Tung 2006). Clinically, viral orchitis, induced by mumps or human immunodeficiency virus infection, can lead to male sterility.

Experimentally, the effects of testicular infection with Sendai virus, a virus related to mumps virus, were investigated in rats (Melaine et al. 2003). At 5–24 h post-injection of Sendai virus into the testes, a rapid and massive infiltration of leukocytes was induced in the interstitium. The virus does not appear to induce TGC transformation and may not be directly toxic to spermatogenesis. Interestingly, viral proteins were restricted to the cytoplasm of infiltrated leukocytes, although resident macrophages were unaffected by Sendai virus. However, the virus replicated in Leydig cells and peritubular myoid cells in vitro inhibited testosterone secretion and induced production of the chemokines (monocyte chemotactic protein-1, regulated on activation normal T cell expressed and secreted protein, growth-related oncogene-alpha, and IFN-gamma-inducible protein-10) that recruit leukocytes to the testis (Le Goffic et al. 2002). At present, it is not yet clear whether Sendai virus-induced orchitis is of autoimmune origin or not. In mice that had received intra-testicular inoculation with cytomegalovirus, pathological manifestations in mice pretreated with cyclophosphamide were severer than those observed in immunocompetent mice infected with the virus alone (Tebourbi et al. 2001, 2002). The typical cellular inclusions of the virus were present in interstitial spaces; however, the TGC were never directly infected in immunocompetent mice. Nonetheless, in mice pretreated with cyclophosphamide and then infected with the virus, definitive spermatogenic disturbance was obtained, suggesting that immune-depressed state deteriorate testicular injury indirectly.

6.2.11 EAO Induced by Intrinsic Disorder in the Testis

Mutations at the T/t complex in the mouse contain multiple genetic factors that affect specific events of differentiation during embryonic development and spermatogenesis (Bennett 1981). Specific biochemical and morphological defects of TGC such as spermatids and spermatozoa were found in mice with mutant alleles of the T/t complex (Scully and Shur 1988; Hui et al. 2006). The testes in affected mice are characterized by accumulations of lymphocytes and occasional plasma cells between the seminiferous tubules (Dooher et al. 1981) (Fig. 6.1). Although lymphocytes were rarely observed within the seminiferous epithelium, extensive degeneration of TGC was observed within affected tubules. Sertoli cells phagocytosed degenerating TGC at all stages of differentiation. In vitro co-culture of syngeneic T/tw18 spleen cells and TGC revealed that TGC from sterile T/tw18 mice failed to activate Treg; consequently, the syngeneic spleen cells displayed a vigorous proliferative response to testicular autoantigens. On the other hand, TGC from younger, fertile T/tw18 males behaved like TGC from normal mice. They activated Treg and, thereby, abrogated proliferation of spleen cells in vitro co-culture. This indicates that genetic factors associated with chromosome 17 are responsible for the failure of protection of TGC in maintained normal tolerance to TGC autoantigens in vivo; EAO is an extreme manifestation of the inability of the defective TGC to initiate Treg activation.

As another spontaneous EAO, a malfunction of the clearance mechanisms for apoptotic TGC debris arising from imbalances in phagocyte receptors or cytokines acting on Sertoli cells was identified in the mink (Akpovi et al. 2006; Pelletier et al. 2009, 2011, 2015). This imbalance constitutes a major factor leading to breakdown of self-tolerance against TGC autoantigens with the resultant EAO, in which excess anti-sperm antibody production, spermatogenic disturbance, and leukocytic infiltration were seen. The EAO serum specifically reacted with the postacrosomal region, the mid and end piece of mink sperm, whereas normal mink serum did not. Western blot analyses revealed that EAO serum reacted specifically to 23 and 50 kDa proteins. The number of apostain-labeled apoptotic cells was significantly higher in orchitic tubules compared with normal tubules. TNF-alpha and IL-6 serum levels were increased during EAO. Fas localized in TGC, Sertoli cells, and the lamina propria of the tubules and Fas ligand were on TGC. Furthermore, Fas co-localized with Fas ligand in residual bodies, giant cells, and infiltrating leukocytes in orchitic tubules.

The transcription factor E-twenty-six-variant gene 5 (ETV5) is essential for spermatogonial stem cell renewal, as the targeted deletion of the ETV5 gene in mice results in only the first wave of spermatogenesis and a Sertoli-cell-only phenotype (Morrow et al. 2007). The relative importance of ETV5 to the maintenance of the spermatogonial stem cells niche in neonatal Sertoli and TGC can be evaluated by reciprocal spermatogonial stem cells transplants between wild-type and $ETV5^{-/-}$ hosts and donors. It appeared that ETV5 is needed in both Sertoli cells and TGC for normal spermatogenesis. Furthermore, $ETV5^{-/-}$ recipients displayed EAO-like lesion characterized by increased interstitial inflammation, fibrosis, and tubular involution after transplantation of spermatogonial stem cells obtained from wild-type donors (Morrow et al. 2007). Interstitial cellularity was greatly increased and consisted of a mixture of fibrosis, macrophages, and plasma cells. Thickened basal lamina and occasional inflammatory cell infiltration were seen in partially atrophied tubules, while the presence of other tubules could only be identified by a swirl of connective tissue. Both cellular and humoral immune responses have been not yet determined in these mice, and it is yet unknown whether this widespread inflammation in the $ETV5^{-/-}$ recipient mice is due to intrinsic factors or extrinsic factors related to the transplant procedure. However, the BTB is actually abnormal and incomplete in the $ETV5^{-/-}$ mice. ETV5 may also mediate the immune response to transplant trauma, as IL-6 is decreased in $ETV5^{-/-}$ Sertoli cells. Among many physiologic roles of IL-6, this cytokine can act as an inflammatory or anti-inflammatory cytokine, depending on local tissue environment and balance of intracellular signaling cascade molecules. Therefore, intrinsic factors would involve ETV5 loss, which affect the physical integrity of the BTB and interstitial inflammation.

EAO is also induced by conditional knockout of the androgen receptor in Sertoli cells.

Androgens are required for male sexual differentiation, testicular descent, masculinization, and spermatogenesis. Androgen receptors in Sertoli cell are required for progression of spermatogenic cells through meiosis and spermatid differentiation. Sertoli cell-specific ablation of the androgen receptor in mice decreases expression of claudin-3, an androgen-regulated gene and component of Sertoli cell tight junctions, and increases the permeability of the BTB (Meng et al. 2005, 2011). In testes of mutant mice with Sertoli cell-specific androgen receptor ablation, the ultrastructure of Sertoli cell tight junctions is defective and testicular IgG levels are elevated, and the interstitium becomes populated with macrophages, neutrophils, plasma cells, and eosinophils, and their sera contain autoantibodies against TGC. Taken together, Sertoli cell-specific deletion of the androgen receptor may result in loss of testicular immune privilege, leading to EAO. Suppressed levels of androgen signaling may be one of the contributing factors in idiopathic male infertility. claudin-11 is a protein constitutively expressed by Sertoli cells, and both claudin-3 and claudin-11 proteins contribute to the integrity of Sertoli cell tight junctions. Knockdown of claudin-11 in Sertoli cells also results in male sterility, but in contrast to Sertoli cell-specific androgen receptor mutants, sterility is not immune mediated, as anti-TGC autoantibodies are undetected in the sera and testes of claudin-11$^{-/-}$ mice, and testes show no evidence of inflammatory cell infiltration. Furthermore, in contrast to that spermatogenesis proceeds through meiosis and early spermatid differentiation in Sertoli cell-specific androgen receptor mutant mice, spermatogenesis in claudin-11$^{-/-}$ male mice does not proceed beyond meiosis. Therefore, spermatogenic arrest in Sertoli cell-specific androgen receptor mutant mice may be best explained by the increased permeability of the BTB resulting from disruption of claudin-3 expression, and the BTB disorder may promote accessibility to TGC antigens that are no longer immunologically sequestered in the mutant mice.

References

Ablin RJ, Soanes WA, Bronson P. Autoantibodies to rabbit testes as a consequence of in situ freezing. Folia Biol Praha. 1971;17:429–31.

Ablin RJ. Experimental autoimmune aspermatogenic orchitis. J Allergy Clin Immunol. 1972;50:128.

Ablin RJ, Soanes WA. Experimental production of autoimmune aspermatogenic orchitis in the rabbit in consequence of in situ freezing of the testis. Eur Surg Res. 1972;4:98–106.

Akpovi CD, Yoon SR, Vitale ML, Pelletier RM. The predominance of one of the SR-BI isoforms is associated with increased esterified cholesterol levels not apoptosis in mink testis. J Lipid Res. 2006;47:2233–47.

Alexander NJ, Tung KSK. Immunological and morphological effects of vasectomy in the rabbit. Anat Rec. 1977;188:339–50.

Anderson DJ, Alexander NJ. Antisperm antibody titers, immune complex deposition and immunocompetence in long-term vasectomized mice. Clin Exp Immunol. 1981;43:99–108.

Ansbacher R. Vasectomy: sperm antibodies. Fertil Steril. 1973;24:7888–792.

Aoki A, Fawcett DW. Impermeability of Sertoli cell junctions to prolonged exposure to peroxidase. Andrologia. 1975;7:63–76.

Ball RY, Naylor CPE, Mitchinson MJ. Spermatozoa in an abdominal lymph node after vasectomy in a man. J Reprod Fertil. 1982;66:715–6.

Ball RY, Setchell BP. The passage of spermatozoa to regional lymph nodes in testicular lymph following vasectomy in rams and boars. J Reprod Fertil. 1983;68:145–53.

Bennett D. The T/t-complex in the mouse: mutations that impair differentiation. Prog Clin Biol Res. 1981;66:375–9.

Bigazzi PE, Kosuda LL, Hsu KC, Andres GA. Immune complex orchitis in vasectomized rabbits. J Exp Med. 1976;143:382–404.

Boughton B, Spector WG. Auto-immune testicular lesions induced by injury to the contralateral testis and intradermal injection of adjuvant. J Pathol Bacteriol. 1963;86:69–74.

Cerasaro TS, Nachtsheim DA, Otero F, Parsons CL. The effect of testicular torsion on contralateral testis and the production of antisperm antibodies in rabbits. J Urol. 1984;132:577–9.

Chen M, Cai H, Yang JL, CL L, Liu T, Yang W, Guo J, XQ H, Fan CH, ZY H, Gao F, Liu YX. Effect of heat stress on expression of junction-associated molecules and upstream factors androgen receptor and Wilms' tumor 1 in monkey Sertoli cells. Endocrinology. 2008;149:4871–82.

Das RP, Mustafa AS, Talwar GP. Atrophy of seminiferous tubules of mouse testes after intratesticular injection of BCG and their regeneration. Arch Androl. 1982;9:245–50.

Demir A, Turker P, Onol FF, Sirvanci S, Findik A, Tarcan T. Effect of experimentally induced *Escherichia coli* epididymo-orchitis and ciprofloxacin treatment on rat spermatogenesis. Int J Urol. 2007;14:268–72.

Dooher GB, Artzt K, Bennett D, Hurtenbach U. Observations on autoimmune orchitis in sterile mice carrying a recessive lethal mutation at the T/t complex exhibiting spontaneous allergic orchitis. J Reprod Fertil. 1981;62:505–11.

Dym M, Fawcett DW. The blood-testis barrier in the rat and the physiological compartmentation of the seminiferous epithelium. Biol Reprod. 1970;3:308–26.

Eyquem A, Krieg H. Experimental autosensitization of the testis. Ann N Y Acad Sci. 1965;124:270–8.

Fainboim L, Barreara CN, Mancini RE. Immunologic and testicular response in guinea pigs after unilateral traumatic orchitis. Andrologia. 1976;8:243–8.

Fernandez-Collazo E, Thierer E, Mancini RE. Immunologic and testicular response in guinea pigs after unilateral thermal orchitis. J Allergy Clin Immunol. 1972;49:167–73.

Flickinger CJ, Howards SS, Bush LA, Baker LA, Herr JC. Temporal recognition of sperm autoantigens by IgM and IgG autoantibodies after vasectomy and vasovasostomy. J Reprod Immunol. 1994;27:135–50.

Flickinger CJ, Howards SS, Bush LA, Baker LA, Herr JC. Antisperm autoantibody responses to vasectomy and vasovasostomy in Fisher and Lewis rats. J Reprod Immunol. 1995;28:137–57.

Flickinger CJ, Baran ML, Howards SS, Herr JC. Sperm autoantigens recognized by autoantibodies in developing rats following prepubertal obstruction of the vas deferens. J Andol. 1996;17:433–42.

Fritz TE, Lombard LA, Tyler SA, Norris WP. Pathology and familial incidence of orchitis and its relation to thyroiditis in a closed beagle colony. Exp Mol Pathol. 1976;24:142–58.

Furbeth C, Hubner G, Thoenes GH. Spontaneous immune complex orchitis in brown Norway rats. Virchows Arch B Cell Pathol. 1989;57:37–45.

Handley HH, Flickinger CJ, Herr JC. Post-vasectomy sperm autoantigens in the Lewis rat. Biol Reprod. 1988;39:1239–50.

Handley HH, Herr JC, Flickinger CJ. Localization of post-vasectomy sperm autoantigens in the Lewis rat. J Reprod Immunol. 1991;20:205–20.

Herr JC, Flickinger CJ, Howards SS, Yarbro S, Spell DR, Caloras D, Gallien TN. The relation between antisperm and testicular alterations after vasectomy and vasovasostomy in Lewis rats. Biol Reprod. 1987;37:1279–305.

Hirai S, Hatayama N, Naito M, Nagahori K, Kawata S, Hayashi S, Qu N, Terayama H, Shoji S, Itoh M. Pathological effect of arterial ischaemia and venous congestion on rat testes. Sci Rep. 2017;7(1):5422.

Hui L, Lu J, Han Y, Pilder SH. The mouse T complex gene Tsga2, encoding polypeptides located in the sperm tail and anterior acrosome, maps to a locus associated with sperm motility and sperm-egg interaction abnormalities. Biol Reprod. 2006;74:633–43.

Itoh M, Hiramine C, Hojo K. A new murine model of autoimmune orchitis induced by immunization with viable syngeneic testicular germ cells alone. I. Immunological and histological studies. Clin Exp Immunol. 1991a;83:137–42.

Itoh M, Hiramine C, Tokunaga Y, Mukasa A, Hojo K. A new murine model of autoimmune orchitis induced by immunization with viable syngeneic testicular germ cells alone. II. Immunohistochemical findings of fully-developed lesion. Autoimmunity. 1991b;10:89–97.

Itoh M, de-Rooij DG, Jansen A, Drexhage HA. Phenotypical heterogeneity of testicular macrophages/dendritic cells in normal adult mice; an immunohistochemical study. J Reprod Immunol. 1995a;28:217–32.

Itoh M, de-Rooij DG, Takeuchi Y. Mode of inflammatory cell infiltration in testes of mice injected with syngeneic testicular germ cells without adjuvant. J Anat. 1995b;187:671–9.

Itoh M, Li XQ, Yano A, Xie Q, Takeuchi Y. Patterns of efferent lymphatics of the mouse testis. Int J Androl. 1998a;19:466–72.
Itoh M, Ueno M, Li XQ, Satriotomo I, Takeuchi Y. Topographical uptake of blood-borne horseradish peroxidase (HRP) in the murine testis at the light microscopic level. Int J Androl. 1998b;21:74–80.
Itoh M, Li XQ, Miyamoto K, Takeuchi Y. Degeneration of the seminiferous epithelium with ageing is a cause of spermatocele? Int J Androl. 1999;22:91–6.
Johnson AL, Howards SS. Intratubular hydrostatic pressure in testis and epididymis before and after vasectomy. Am J Phys. 1975;228:556–64.
Johnson AL, Howards SS. Intratubular hydrostatic pressure in testis and epididymis before and after vasectomy in the guinea pig. Biol Reprod. 1976;14:371–6.
Johnson AL, Howards SS. Hyperosmolality in intraluminal fluids from hamster testis and epididymis: a micropuncture study. Science. 1977;195:492–3.
Kaneko T, Itoh M, Nakamura Y, Iimura A, Hayashi S, Takahashi K, Stivala F, Bendtzen K, Nicoletti F. Proinflammatory effects of exogenously administered IL-10 in experimental autoimmune orchitis. Cytokine. 2003;22:50–3.
Kojima A, Spencer CA. Genetic susceptibility to testicular autoimmunity: comparison between postthymectomy and postvasectomy models in mice. Biol Reprod. 1983;29:195–205.
Le Goffic R, Mouchel T, Aubry F, Patard JJ, Ruffault A, Jegou B, Samson M. Production of the chemokines monocyte chemotactic protein-1, regulated on activation normal T cell expressed and secreted protein, growth-related oncogene, and interferon-gamma-inducible protein-10 is induced by the Sendai virus in human and rat testicular cells. Endocrinology. 2002;143:1434–40.
Lustig L, Tung KS. Orchitis and Male Infertility. The autoimmune diseases. 4th ed. Amsterdam: Elsevier Academic Press; 2006. p. 841–7.
Matsuzaki G, Sonoda KH, Mukasa A, Yamada H, Nakamura T, Ikebe H, Hamano S, Nomoto K. The characterization of testicular cell (TC)-specific T-cell clones induced by intratesticular *Listeria monocytogenes* infection: TC-specific T cells with atypical cytokine profile transfer orchitis. Immunology. 1997;91:520–8.
McDonald SW, Halliday J. Cell-mediated immune response after vasectomy in rats. J Reprod Fertil. 1992;96:529–35.
Melaine N, Ruffault A, Dejucq-Rainsford N, Jegou B. Experimental inoculation of the adult rat testis with Sendai virus: effect on testicular morphology and leukocyte population. Hum Reprod. 2003;18:1574–9.
Meng J, Holdcraft RW, Shima JE, Griswold MD, Braun RE. Androgens regulate the permeability of the blood-testis barrier. Proc Natl Acad Sci U S A. 2005;102:16696–700.
Meng J, Greenlee AR, Taub CJ, Braun RE. Sertoli cell-specific deletion of the androgen receptor compromises testicular immune privilege in mice. Biol Reprod. 2011;85:254–60.
Mengel W, Zimmermann FA. Immunologic aspects of cryptorchidism. Urol Clin North Am. 1982;9:349–51.
Metukuri MR, Reddy CM, Reddy PR, Reddanna P. Bacterial LPS-mediated acute inflammation-induced spermatogenic failure in rats: role of stress response proteins and mitochondrial dysfunction. Inflammation. 2010;33:235–43.
Morrow CM, Hostetler CE, Griswold MD, Hofmann MC, Murphy KM, Cooke PS, Hess RA. ETV5 is required for continuous spermatogenesis in adult mice and may mediate blood testes barrier function and testicular immune privilege. Ann N Y Acad Sci. 2007;1120:144–51.
Mukasa A, Hiromatsu K, Matsuzaki G, O'Brien R, Born W, Nomoto K. Bacterial infection of the testis leading to autoaggressive immunity triggers apparently opposed responses of alpha-beta and gamma-delta T cells. J Immunol. 1995;155:2047–56.
Mukasa A, Lahn M, Pflum EK, Born W, O'Brien RL. Evidence that the same gamma delta T cells respond during infection-induced and autoimmune inflammation. J Immunol. 1997;159:5787–94.
Mukasa A, Yoshida H, Kobayashi N, Matsuzaki G, Nomoto K. Gamma-delta T cells in infection-induced and autoimmune-induced testicular inflammation. Immunology. 1998;95:395–401.

Nagaosa K, Nakashima C, Kishimoto A, Nakanishi Y. Immune response to bacteria in seminiferous epithelium. Reproduction. 2009;137:879–88.

Nagler HM, White R. The effect of testicular torsion on the contralateral testis. J Urol. 1982;128:1343–8.

Naito M, Sakamoto Y, Terayama H, Hirai S, Qu N, Aota Y, Itoh M. Effect of unilateral testicular rupture on histopathology and germ cell delayed-type hypersensitivity in C3H/He and A/J mice. J Reprod Immunol. 2009a;81:55–61.

Nashan D, Cooper TG, Knuth UA, Schulbeus P, Sorg C, Nieschlag E. Presence and distribution of leukocyte subsets in the murine epididymis after vasectomy. Int J Androl. 1990;13:39–49.

Neaves WB. Permeability of Sertoli cell tight junctions to lanthanum after ligation of ductus deferens and ductuli efferentes. J Cell Biol. 1978;59:559–72.

Pelletier RM, Yoon SR, Akpovi CD, Silvas E, Vitale ML. Defects in the regulatory clearance mechanisms favor the breakdown of self-tolerance during spontaneous autoimmune orchitis. Am J Phys Regul Integr Comp Phys. 2009;296:R743–62.

Pelletier RM, Akpovi CD, Chen L, Day R, Vitale ML. CX43 expression, phosphorylation, and distribution in the normal and autoimmune orchitic testis with a look at gap junctions joining germ cell to germ cell. Am J Phys Regul Integr Comp Phys. 2011;300:R121–39.

Pelletier RM, Akpovi CD, Chen L, Kumar NM, Vitale ML. Complementary expression and phosphorylation of Cx46 and Cx50 during development and following gene deletion in mouse and in normal and orchitic mink testes. Am J Phys Regul Integr Comp Phys. 2015;309:R255–76.

Qu N, Terayama H, Naito M, Ogawa Y, Hirai S, Kitaoka M, Yi SQ, Itoh M. Caput epididymitis but not orchitis was induced by vasectomy in a murine model of experimental autoimmune orchitis. Reproduction. 2008;135:859–66.

Qu N, Naito M, Terayama H, Hirai S, Li J, Ogawa Y, Kitaoka M, Itoh M. Developmental ontogeny of autoantigens associated with localized autoimmunity in murine testis and epididymis. J Reprod Immunol. 2010;87:45–51.

Rapaport FT, Sampath A, Kano K, McCluskey RT, Milgrom F. Immunological effects of thermal injury. I: Inhibition of spermatogenesis in guinea pigs. J Exp Med. 1969;130:1411–25.

Riella LV, Paterson AM, Sharpe AH, Chandraker A. Role of PD-1 pathway in the immune response. Am J Transplant. 2012;12:2575–87.

Rival C, Wheeler K, Jeffrey S, Qiao H, Luu B, Tewalt EF, Engelhard VH, Tardif S, Hardy D, del Rio R, Teuscher C, Tung K. Regulatory T cells and vasectomy. J Reprod Immunol. 2013;100:66–75.

Robinson R, Tung KSK, Meeker ND, Monson FG, Teuscher C. A murine model of spontaneous aspermatogenesis: linkage to H-2. J Reprod Immunol. 1994;26:251–60.

Rodriguez MG, Rival C, Theas MS, Lustig L. Immunohistopathology of the contralateral testis of rats undergoing experimental torsion of the spermatic cord. Asia J Androl. 2006;8:576–83.

Sakamoto Y, Matsumoto T, Mizunoe Y, Haraoka M, Sakumoto M, Kumazawa J. Testicular injury induces cell-mediated autoimmune response to testis. J Urol. 1995;153:1316–20.

Sakamoto Y, Matsumoto T, Kumazawa J. Cell-mediated autoimmune response to testis induced by bilateral testicular injury can be suppressed by cyclosporin A. J Urol. 1998;159:1735–40.

Sanui H, Yoshida S, Himeno K, Nomoto K. Delayed hypersensitivity to syngeneic testicular cells induced by intratesticular bacterial infection in guinea-pigs. Immunology. 1982;46:635–42.

Sanui H, Yoshida S, Himeno K, Nomoto K. Experimental allergic orchitis induced by unilateral intratesticular bacterial infection in guinea-pigs. Immunology. 1983;49:45–51.

Scully NF, Shur BD. Stage-specific increase in cell surface galactosyltransferase activity during spermatogenesis in mice bearing t alleles. Dev Biol. 1988;125:195–9.

Sell S, Baker-Zander S, Powell HC. Experimental syphilitic orchitis in rabbits. Ultrastructural appearance of Treponema pallidum during phagocytosis and dissolution by macrophages in vivo. Lab Investig. 1982;46:355–64.

Setchell BP, Tao L, Zupp JL. The penetration of chromium-EDTA from blood plasma into various compartments of rat testes as an indicator of function of the blood-testis barrier after exposure of the testes to heat. J Reprod Fertil. 1996;106:125–33.

Taguchi O, Nishizuka Y. Experimental autoimmune orchitis after neonatal thymectomy in the mouse. Clin Exp Immunol. 1981;46:425–34.
Tao L, Zupp JL, Setchell BP. Effect of efferent duct ligation of the function of the blood-testis barrier in rats. J Reprod Fertil. 2000;120:13–8.
Tebourbi L, Courtot AM, Duchateau R, Loeuillet A, Testart J, Cerutti I. Experimental inoculation of male mice with murine cytomegalovirus and effect on offspring. Hum Reprod. 2001;16:2041–9.
Tebourbi L, Emile JF, Cerutti I. Cyclophosphamide-immunodepressed FVB/N mice: potentiating the effects of testicular cytomegalovirus infection. Intervirology. 2002;45:119–24.
Tonsy MHE, Rose NR, Rehewy ME, Hafez ESE. Effect of Freund's complete adjuvant on the immune response of vasectomized rats. Arch Androl. 1979;2:323–9.
Torgersen HM, Rovan E, Steiner M, Frick J, Adam H. BCG-induced orchitis: structural changes during the degeneration of seminiferous tubules of rats and rabbits. Urol Res. 1982;10:97–104.
Tung KS. Allergic orchitis lesions are adoptively transferred from vasoligated guinea pigs to syngeneic recipients. Science. 1978;201:833–5.
Tung KS, Alexander NJ. Monocytic orchitis and aspermatogenesis in normal and vasectomized rhesus macaques (Masasa mulatta). Am J Pathol. 1980;101:17–29.
Tung KS, Ellis L, Teuscher C, Meng A, blaustein JC, Kohno S, Howell R. The black mink (*Mustela vison*): a natural model of immunologic male infertility. J Exp Med. 1981;154:1016–32.
Tung KS, Ellis LE, Childs GV, Dufau M. The dark mink, a model of male infertility. Endocrinology. 1984;114:922–9.
Watanabe M, Kashiwakura Y, Kusumi N, Tamayose K, Nasu Y, Nagai A, Shimada T, Daida H, Kumon H. Adeno-associated virus-mediated human IL-10 gene transfer suppresses the development of experimental autoimmune orchitis. Gene Ther. 2005;12:1126–32.
Wheeler K, Tardif S, Rival C, Luu B, Bui E, del-Rio R, Teuscher C, Sparwasser T, Hardy D, Tung KSK. Regulatory T cells control tolerogenic versus autoimmune response to sperm in vasectomy. Proc Natl Acad Sci U S A. 2011;108:7511–6.
Wicher K, Wicher V, Nakeeb SM, Dubiski S. Studies of rabbit testes infected with Treponema pallidum. I Immunopathology. Br J Vener Dis. 1983;59:349–58.
Wicher V, Wicher K. Studies of rabbit testes infected with Treponema pallidum. III. Immunosuppressive activity of infiltrating mononuclear cells. Br V Vener Dis. 1984;60:1–7.
Wilson BJ, Porter G, Goldstein A. Reduced T cell reactivity in vasectomized rhesus monkeys: association with histocompatibility type. Fertil Steril. 1979;31:434–40.
Zappi E, Nemirovsky M, Shulman S. Contralateral epididymo-orchitis after cryo-injury to the male rabbit gonad. Immunology. 1973;25:891–903.
Zappi E, Nemirovsky M, Shulman S. Cellular and humoral responses of autosensitized rabbits to a testis cryo-injury. Immunology. 1974;26:477–88.
Zhang M, Jiang M, Bi Y, Zhu H, Zhou Z, Sha J. Autophagy and apoptosis act as partners to induce germ cell death after heat stress in mice. PLoS One. 2012;7:e41412. doi:10.1371/journal.pone.0041412.

Testicular Autoimmunity by Alteration of the Immune System in Experimental Animals

7

7.1 Introduction

Experimental autoimmune orchitis (EAO) is not confined to animals that received artificial exposure to TGC autoantigens experimentally but occurs spontaneously in some animals with abnormal condition of immune system.

Historically, Miller (1961) is the first to demonstrate that the thymus is the most important organ for adoptive (acquired) immunity. He found that mice thymectomized on day 0 or 1 after birth had tended to be affected by some infectious diseases and die within 2–4 months. Later, Nishizuka and Sakakura (1969) found that mice thymectomized on day 3 after birth had gonadal dysgenesis without suffering from any infection, and the following studies showed that the gonadal dysgenesis is of autoimmune origin (Hattori and Brandon 1979; Lipscomb et al. 1979; Taguchi et al. 1980; Taguchi and Nishizuka 1981; Nishizuka 1982). This paradoxical discovery dramatically developed subsequent study of "thymus and autoimmunity" without the use of active immunization procedure.

The normal immune system is provided with a subset of tissue-specific Treg that are involved in the maintenance of self-tolerance. If the clonal balance of $CD4^{+}$ T cell subsets is tipped in favor of pathogenic (effector) T cells, multiple organ-localized autoimmune diseases involving EAO could ensue with no active immunization with testicular antigens or artificial testicular injury (Taguchi and Nishizuka 1987; Taguchi et al. 1990, 1994). In this situation, loss of Treg may occur through aberrant T cell development, or EAO-inducing T cells can be activated by non-testicular peptides that cross-react with testicular autoantigens at the level of the TCR (Tung and Teuscher 1995). Endogenous superantigens are recognized by TCR in a V beta-specific manner. V beta 11-positive T cells that recognize the endogenous superantigen of MHC class II and endogenous retroviral peptides might be involved. They are greatly reduced in the thymus and peripheral lymphoid tissues, most likely as a result of clonal deletion. However, V beta 11-positive T cells are normally undeleted and enriched in the thymus and spleen during neonatal period (Smith et al. 1989, 1991, 1992). Furthermore, the relative number of V beta

M. Itoh, *Testicular Autoimmunity*, DOI 10.1007/978-4-431-54460-9_7

11-positive cells was significantly higher in neonatally thymectomized adult mice than in normal adult mice. Therefore, normal murine T cells include pathogenic autoreactive T cells, which are controlled by thymus-derived regulatory cells under normal condition. It has been shown that elimination of a peripheral CD4$^+$ subpopulation expressing the CD5 molecule at high levels or the CD45RB/C molecules at low levels elicited spontaneous activation/expansion of autoreactive T cells from the remaining CD4 population, leading to the development of multiple organ-localized autoimmune diseases. Later, it appeared that CD25 expression appears to be more specific for the CD4$^+$ cells with autoimmune-preventive activity than CD5^{high} or CD45RB/C^{low} expression. CD25$^+$ T cells, which are CD5^{high} and CD45RB/C^{low}, constitute approximately 10% of peripheral CD4$^+$ cells and less than 1% of CD8$^+$ cells in normal unimmunized mice. Therefore, most Treg expresses CD4$^+$ and a high level of CD5 and CD25 (Sakaguchi et al. 1995; Itoh et al. 1999). Nowadays, it became evident that Foxp3 is a specific marker of CD4$^+$CD25$^+$Treg, which are composed of naturally occurring Treg and inducible Treg. Furthermore, a revival of CD8$^+$ suppressor T cells (CD8$^+$ Treg) involved in prevention and inhibition of pathogenic autoimmune response has been also noted (Tang et al. 2005; Smith and Kumar 2008; Filaci et al. 2011).

7.2 Various EAO Models by Immune-Alteration

7.2.1 EAO Induced by Neonatal Thymectomy

Vojtiskova and Pokorna (1964) found that thymectomy of adult mice prevented induction of EAO by testicular antigens+CFA-immunization. Later in the rat, neonatal thymectomy at 3 days of age led to the development of EAO without any active immunization in about 65% of Lewis rats (Hattori and Brandon 1979; Lipscomb et al. 1979) (Fig. 7.1). This is in contrast to classically induced experimental autoimmune model systems, where previous investigators have reported that thymectomy lessens or prevents induction of autoimmune disease. This difference should be related to the timing of thymectomy. Thymectomy after puberty when

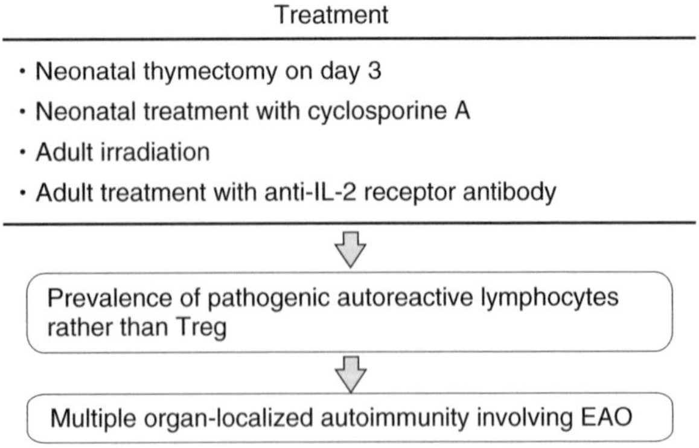

Fig. 7.1 EAO induced by acquired manipulation of the immune system in mice

autoimmunogenic haploid TGC are already present in the testis may be effective in reduction of pathogenic effector T cells rather than Treg; however, thymectomy before appearance of haploid TGC in the testis during neonatal period failed to develop Treg ontogenically. In about 20–30% of susceptible strains of mice that were thymectomized neonatally on day 3, a mild EAO occurred along with other organ-localized autoimmune diseases such as thyroiditis and gastritis, without any artificial immunization (Taguchi and Nishizuka 1981). It is noteworthy that in this post-thymectomy EAO, epididymitis and vasitis consistently occurred prior to the development of EAO in mice. However, neonatal thymectomy on day 7 after birth could not induce any organ-localized autoimmunity involving EAO and survived well until a natural death. This indicates that thymectomy around day 3 is critical for disturbance of immune regulation. The EAO lesion resulted in testicular atrophy and was characterized by disappearance of mature sperms, formation of multinuclear giant cells in the seminiferous tubules, and infiltration of lymphocytes in the testicular interstitium. Deposition of IgG, IgA, IgM, and C3 were also identified on the basal lamina of both seminiferous tubules and epididymal ducts. Serum autoantibodies in the neonatally thymectomized mice exclusively bound to acrosomes of mature spermatozoa, but not to round and oval spermatids. It seems, therefore, that the testicular autoimmunity following neonatal thymectomy on day 3 may be directed predominantly to acrosomal proteins of mature spermatozoa within epididymal ducts, rather than to immature TGC within seminiferous tubules.

The effect of vasectomy on EAO was also investigated in the post-thymectomy model. The incidence of EAO was found to increase when day 3-thymectomized mice received vasectomy on day 60 after birth (Taguchi and Nishizuka 1981). Kojima and Spencer (1983) also reported that vasectomy increased the incidence of testicular atrophy in day 3-thymectomized mice. Interestingly, in day 3-thymectomized males and females, the incidence of autoimmune inflammation is apparently higher in the ovary than in the testis. While approximately 95% female thymectomized animals develop autoimmune oophoritis, only 20–30% male thymectomized animals develop EAO in (C57BL6 × A/J)F1 mice. However, the prevalence of EAO increased to over 90% when day 3-thymectomized mice were vasectomized later. This indicates that testis is a relatively privileged organ against autoimmune attack compared with the ovary, but the vasectomy disrupts the immune privileged circumstance.

Later, Tung et al. (1987a, b) reexamined the findings of post-neonatal thymectomy model by Taguchi and Nishizuka (1981). They found epididymo-vasitis in 70–90% of (SWR/J × A/J)F_1, 50% of (C57BL6 × A/J)F_1, and 64% of balb/cBy mice after day 3-thymectomy, whereas orchitis occurred in approximately 20% in these strains. In some mice, epididymo-vasitis also developed after not only day 3 but also day 7 thymectomy. It may be that the time window of neonatal thymectomy for induction of autoimmune epididymo-vasitis is wider than that for EAO. In day 3-thymectomized mice, the incidences of inflammation in the vas deferens, the cauda, the corpus, and the caput of the epididymis were almost equal. At 5–7 weeks, polymorphonuclear leukocytes dominated and were replaced by lymphocytes and macrophages between 8 and 18 weeks. The inflammatory cells were distributed in perivascular and peritubular spaces, and they rarely invaded epithelial cell linings. Maximal incidence of epididymitis preceded immune complex deposition, which is probably a consequence of tissue injury. Immune complexes were found in less than 25% of day 3-thymectomized mice during the first 11 weeks, when the epididymo-vasitis reached its peak incidence. Later, at 12–14 weeks, the frequency of immune complexes rose to 70%. Typically, linear deposits of mouse IgG were detected along the basal lamina of epididymal ducts and seminiferous tubules. However, differing from findings by Taguchi and Nishizuka (1981), deposits of IgA, IgM, and C3 were absent. In the testis, inflammatory cells infiltrate focally, and invasion of lymphocytes and macrophages into the seminiferous tubules with extensive disturbance of spermatogenesis was rare. Granular deposits of IgG and C3 were detected only in 30% of day 3-thymectomized mice. In regard to serum autoantibodies, a positive and significant correlation was found between the levels of autoantibodies against testicular autoantigens and EAO occurrence (Tung et al. 1987a, b). In contrast, there was no correlation between the autoantibodies levels and occurrence of autoimmune epididymo-vasitis. Furthermore, there was no correlation between autoantibodies against acrosome of epididymal spermatozoa and occurrence of EAO or autoimmune epididymitis. Although Taguchi and Nishizuka (1981) specifically found autoantibodies against acrosome of elongated spermatids and epididymal spermatozoa, Tung et al. (1987a, b) demonstrated autoantibodies against (1) large granular speckles in nuclei of epithelial cells of the caput and corpus epididymal ducts, (2) fine spikes at the luminal surface of epithelial cells in corpus epididymal ducts, (3) ring-shaped antigens surrounding basal cells in corpus epididymal ducts, and (4) linear antigens surrounding Sertoli cell nuclei. Additionally, unusual autoantibodies reactive with vascular smooth muscle were also found.

EAO with autoimmune epididymitis in day3-thymectomized mice could be prevented by injection of adult normal spleen cells on day 4 (Taguchi and Nishizuka 1981). The most effective donor source was of normal male. Spleen cells from normal females and day 0-orchidectomized donors were less effective for EAO prevention, and spleen cells of day 3-thymectomized male and female donors failed to prevent EAO, indicating that tolerance for autoantigens relevant to this EAO is ontogenically regulated. It also became apparent that spleen cells from normal males had adequate Treg for prevention of EAO but that spleen cells from day 3-thymectomized males have little Treg. Normally, the neonatal repertoire is enriched in peripheral autoreactive T cells in immature system of immunoregulation. Since neonatal thymectomy should affect the T cell repertoire in the neonate, followed by decline of Treg and prevalence of autoreactive T cells, this could explain why autoimmune diseases occur spontaneously in day 3-thymectomized mice. Indeed, V beta 11-positive autoreactive T cells have been found to be enriched in adult I-E$^+$ day 3-thymectomized mice (Smith et al. 1989, 1991, 1992; Jones et al. 1990). Therefore, if the regulatory balance between the expansion of the autoreactive neonatal T cell repertoire and the relatively late ontogeny of Treg is tipped in favor of autoreactive T cell activity, EAO could occur. Testicular autoantigens in developing testis may leak latently for expansion of autoreactive T cells after puberty. There is another possibility that immune responses against some antigens with molecular mimicry can cause EAO through pathogenic T cell activation. In other words, the activation of testis-specific T cells by non-testicular peptides that mimic the target autoantigens cause enrichment of the EAO-inducing autoreactive T cells.

A previous study suggested that H-2-linked genes play little role in determining autoimmune disease outcome in neonatally thymectomized mice (Kojima and Prehn 1981). Studies using recombinant inbred strains showed that EAO susceptibility was not associated with the H-2 haplotype but appeared to be influenced by a minor histocompatibility locus and inherited as a recessive trait. In addition, the disease pathology was strictly controlled by the genetic background of the mice that carried the T cell receptor transgene. On the other hand, Del Rio et al. (2011) reported that H-2 control of natural Treg frequency in the lymph node correlates with susceptibility to day 3-thymectomy-induced autoimmunity. Quantitative trait loci on chromosome 17 (H-2) and also chromosomes 1, 2, 3, 7, and 16 control day 3-thymectomy-induced autoimmunity, and quantitative differences in the frequency of natural Treg in the lymph nodes, but not spleen or thymus, are present between the disease-resistant and disease-susceptible strains of mice. Using H-2-congenic mice, the observed difference in frequency of lymph node natural Treg is chiefly controlled by H-2 on chromosome 17. This indicates the existence of a lymph node-specific, H-2-controlled mechanism regulating the prevalence of natural Treg is critical for EAO in day 3-thymectomy model.

7.2.2 EAO Induced by Treatment with Cyclosporine A

Cyclosporine A, a fungal metabolite, may depress the synthesis of certain cytokines that support T cell growth, or may affect thymopoiesis or deplete the thymic stromal cells, especially in the medulla. Cyclosporine A abrogated $CD4^{+}CD8^{-}$ and $CD4^{-}CD8^{+}$ thymocytes and also affected thymic epithelial cells (Hiramine et al. 1989a, b). Therefore, it may destroy mature thymocytes or block the maturation of immature thymocytes. Depletion of thymic stromal cells in the medulla may interfere with the proliferation/differentiation of thymocytes (Hiramine et al. 1989b). Cyclosporine A has been routinely used in fields of transplantation immunology for establishment of nearly permanent immunologic tolerance to allografts; however, treatment with cyclosporine A paradoxically causes multiple organ-localized autoimmune diseases in balb/c mice later in life when the cyclosporine A (10 mg/kg body weight per day) was administered daily for 1 week to newborn (Fig. 7.1). Although the incidences of autoimmune gastritis and oophoritis were 20% and 10%, respectively, in mice that had received neonatal cyclosporine A treatment, EAO was not observed. However, daily treatment with cyclosporine A from day 1 day to day 6 after birth followed by thymectomy on day 7 increased the incidences of gastritis (95%) and oophoritis (58%) and also developed EAO (36%), thyroiditis (30%), insulitis (13%), adrenitis (9%), and sialadenitis (22%). Cyclosporine A does not appear to induce de novo production of forbidden clones by interfering with clonal deletion mechanism in the thymus. It is likely that

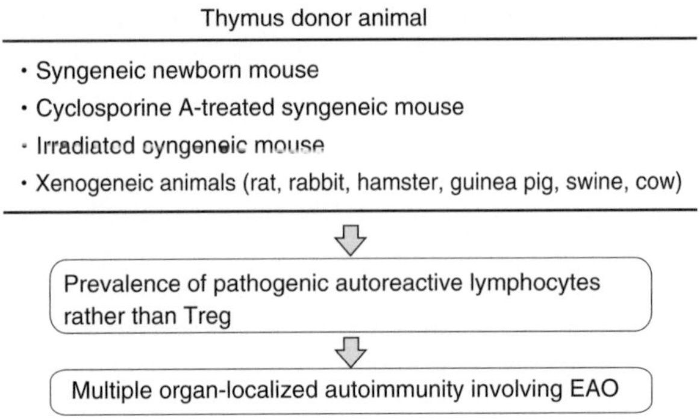

Fig. 7.2 EAO induced by thymus transplantation in congenitally athymic nu/nu mice

cyclosporine A would eventually affect the education of Treg in the thymus, as the formation of autoimmune lesions can be prevented by injection of splenic T cells from normal mice (Sakaguchi and Sakaguchi 1989, 1992). By the fact that cyclosporine A caused organ-localized autoimmune diseases involving EAO in mice when the drug was administered to newborns for a limited period, it is suggested that cyclosporine A primarily affects the neonatal thymus and interferes with the thymic production of Treg that regulates the expansion of autoreactive T cells. On the other hand, administration of cyclosporine A to adult mice failed to induce autoimmune disease presumably by that a sufficient number of Treg had been already produced and prevailed before starting cyclosporine A treatment, and cyclosporine A could not effectively eliminate them already delivered in the periphery. To investigate whether neonatal but not adult thymus is critical for cyclosporine A-induced autoimmunity or not, engrafting of the thymus from cyclosporine A-treated euthymic (nu/+) mice into syngeneic, athymic nude (nu/nu) mice was performed (Sakaguchi and Sakaguchi 1988). Athymic nude mice were engrafted with either one thymus from 7-day-old nu/+ mice treated daily with cyclosporine A (10 mg/kg body weight per day) for 1 week from the day of birth, or one thymic lobe from the adult mice administered daily with cyclosporine A (20 mg/kg per day) for 2 weeks. When examined histologically 3 months later, multiple organ-localized autoimmune diseases were developed, accompanied by appearance of circulating autoantibodies in the recipient nu/nu mice that had been transplanted with cyclosporine A-treated donor thymic lobes of not only newborn but also adult mice (Fig. 7.2). At the time of sacrifice, the transplanted thymi from both neonatal and adult donors were histologically populated with massive lymphocytes, and the composition of thymocyte subsets was similar to that of a normal adult thymus. These results suggest the following: (1) normal thymus is continuously producing potential autoreactive T cells as well as Treg; (2) cyclosporine A can selectively abrogate the thymic production of Treg cells in mice at any age; (3) however, for autoreactive T cells to proliferate and differentiate into pathogenic effector T cells, active Treg must be absent in the periphery or have not yet migrated to the periphery. Thus, engrafting of the thymus from cyclosporine A-treated mice of any age into athymic nude mice or cyclosporine A administration to euthymic newborn mice can cause autoimmune disease, but its administration to euthymic adult mice does not.

7.2.3 EAO Induced by Whole-Body Irradiation

Total lymphoid irradiation is effective for treatment of lymphoid malignancies and autoimmune disease in humans and rodents. Furthermore, total lymphoid irradiation also establishes allograft tolerance when allogeneic bone marrow cells or solid organs are engrafted immediately after the irradiation. However, it was found that the irradiation can functionally alter the immune system and paradoxically break self-tolerance (Sakaguchi et al. 1994a). High dose (42.5 Gy), fractioned (2.5 Gy, 17 times) total lymphoid irradiation on mice caused various organ-localized autoimmune diseases involving EAO and autoimmune epididymitis (Fig. 7.1). The incidences of autoimmune gastritis, thyroiditis, sialadenitis, and EAO with epididymitis were approximately 75%, 4%, 7%, and 9%, respectively. Total lymphoid irradiation eliminated the majority of mature thymocytes and the peripheral T cells for 1 month, and inoculation of spleen cells, thymocytes, or bone marrow cells prepared from syngeneic non-irradiated mice within 2 weeks after total lymphoid irradiation effectively prevented the development of the autoimmune diseases. Depletion of $CD4^+$ T cells from the inoculated donor lymphocytes abrogated the disease preventive activity. $CD4^+$ T cells also appeared to mediate the autoimmune diseases because $CD4^+$ T cells from disease-bearing irradiated mice adoptively transferred the autoimmune lesions to syngeneic naïve mice (Fig. 7.3), indicating that autoimmune disease is caused by affecting the T cell immune system, rather than the target autoantigens, presumably by altering $CD4^+$ Treg-dependent control of autoreactive $CD4^+$ T cells. Furthermore, balb/c athymic nude mice spontaneously developed EAO with other autoimmune diseases when transplanted adult thymuses were irradiated before transplantation (Sakaguchi and Sakaguchi 1990) (Fig. 7.2). In this transplantation model, thymi were removed from donor mice 2 days after 9.0 Gy whole-body irradiation.

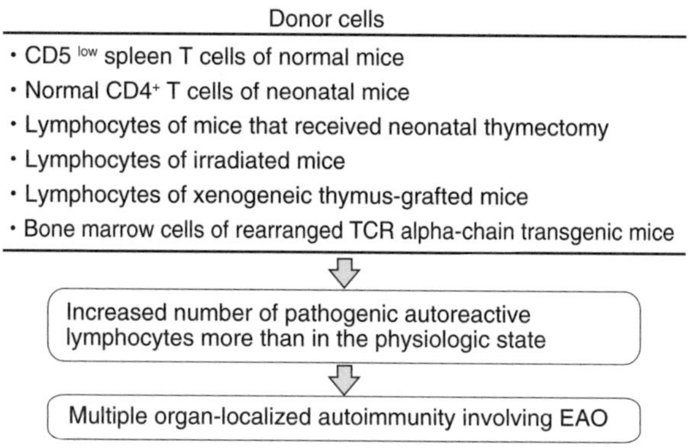

Fig. 7.3 EAO induced by adoptive cell transfer in mice

It must be also noted that irradiation alters not only the immune system but also the BTB. The BTB plays an important role in the intact spermatogenesis, and uncontrolled permeability of the BTB results in leakage of TGC autoantigens with the resultant anti-TGC autoimmune responses. A single local application of microwave electromagnetic pulse irradiation of non-thermal intensity to the testes (400 kV/m) resulted in decreased levels of mRNA and protein expressions of tight-junction-associated proteins (zonula occludens-1 and occludin) of the BTB, followed by the development of autoimmune process in the testes of mice and rabbits (Grigorev et al. 1981; Wang et al. 2010; Hou et al. 2012). The pathology was produced by both humoral and cellular immunity against testicular autoantigens and characterized by structural disturbance of the seminiferous tubular walls and the spermatogenic disturbance. Transforming growth factor-beta 3 is also a key molecule involved in the BTB permeability via regulation of tight junctions. In mice that had received electromagnetic radiation, transforming growth factor-beta 3 significantly decreased with increase of serum anti-sperm autoantibodies levels (Wang et al. 2010). On the contrary, increase of both mRNA and protein expressions of transforming growth factor-beta 3 with increase of the apoptotic TGC was also reported in electromagnetic pulse-exposed mice (Luo et al. 2013).

Exposure to ionizing radiation also induced male infertility, accompanied by increasing permeability of the BTB in mice (Son et al. 2015). The diameter and epithelial depth of the seminiferous tubules were significantly decreased in 1.7 Gy-irradiated mice, which showed significantly decreased levels of tight junction-associated proteins such as zonula occludens-1 and occludin-1 and increased serum anti-sperm autoantibodies compared with those of the non-irradiated animals. In 6.0 Gy-irradiated mice, serum anti-TGC autoantibody levels were also significantly elevated; however, lymphocytic infiltration was hardly seen in the testes in spite of exhibiting severe spermatogenic disturbance (Takahashi et al. 2017). It seems apparent that damage to the BTB integrity results in leakage of TGC autoantigens, leading to the induction of anti-TGC autoimmunity. Therefore, the ionizing irradiation should induce the spermatogenic disturbance by direct killing of TGC and also the BTB damage-induced defect of TGC differentiation. The following production of serum anti-TGC autoantibodies might infiltrate the seminiferous epithelium through the damaged BTB region and further damage the spermatogenic state.

Taken together, high-dose ionizing irradiation induces Treg depletion, TGC death, and the BTB disruption. However, it remains unknown how the systemic Treg depletion, TGC death, the BTB damage, and the following leakage of TGC autoantigens from the disrupted BTB cooperate with each other for EAO induction in irradiated mice. However, effects of irradiation on the testicular tissues should not be noted in EAO in non-irradiated mice that received $CD4^+$ T cells from disease-bearing irradiated mice and also in non-irradiated athymic nude mice engrafted with adult thymuses that had been irradiated before transplantation (Sakaguchi and Sakaguchi 1990) (Fig. 7.2).

7.2.4 EAO Induced by Transfer of Normal Lymphocytes

Transfer of adult CD5^{low} spleen T cells of normal mice to athymic nude mice, to mice without T cells, or to scid mice induces multiple organ-localized autoimmune diseases (Sugihara et al. 1988; Smith et al. 1992). The incidence of EAO was 40% (Sakaguchi et al. 1985) (Fig. 7.3). Therefore, the existence of pathogenic T cells in normal individuals, and their regulation by Treg, has been demonstrated on this EAO model. The CD4^{+}CD8^{-} subset represents mature thymocytes that have passed beyond the stage of T cell development in which the deletion of autoreactive T cells is expected. However, mature pathogenic autoreactive T cells are not deleted in normal thymus and can induce multiple organ-localized autoimmune diseases by their transfer to athymic nu/nu recipients. Transfer of unfractioned spleen T cells of normal adult donors did not evoke multiple organ-localized autoimmune diseases although transfer of fractioned CD4^{+} T cells that expresses a low level of cell surface CD5 molecules was able to do so. In this experimental system, splenic T cells of normal adult donors were treated with CD5 antibody and complement, and the residual T cells were then injected into recipients for induction of multiple organ-localized autoimmune diseases. Although 100% of T cells are known to be CD5^{+}, this treatment eliminated 95% of the CD4^{+} T cells, as demonstrable by flow cytometry. It is noted that the residual 5%, which expressed a low level of CD5 (CD4^{+} CD5^{low} T cells), were responsible for disease transfer (Smith et al. 1992).

EAO also develops in athymic syngeneic recipients of neonatal but not adult splenic CD4^{+} T cells (Fig. 7.3). This finding is consistent with the results of previous studies of V beta 11-positive T cells that are undeleted in neonatal thymus and are enriched in the neonatal spleen for recognition of the endogenous retroviral peptides and superantigens (Smith et al. 1989; Woodland et al. 1991; Dyson et al. 1991).

7.2.5 EAO Induced by Engraftment of Syngeneic Newborn Thymus

balb/c athymic nu/nu mice spontaneously developed EAO with other autoimmune diseases such as oophoritis gastritis, thyroiditis, arteritis, glomerulonephritis, and polyarteritis when transplanted with "newborn" (0 or 1 day old) balb/c thymus (Sakaguchi and Sakaguchi 1990) (Fig. 7.2). The incidences of EAO, oophoritis gastritis, thyroiditis, vasculitis, and glomerulonephritis were approximately 8%, 25%, 61%, 4%, 23%, and 10%, respectively. Transplantation of thymus from adult balb/c mice was far less effective in inducing histologically evident autoimmune disease in athymic nu/nu mice. Furthermore, multiple organ-localized autoimmune diseases were not induced in athymic nu/nu mice grafted with syngeneic "embryonic" thymus (Nishigaki-Maki et al. 1999; Morimoto et al. 2000). To determine whether spontaneous autoimmune disease after thymus engrafting is unique to nu/nu mice, balb/c newborn thymi were engrafted into T cell-depleted balb/c mice that had received thymectomy at 6 weeks of age, irradiation at 2 weeks later at 9.0 Gy, and transplantation of 5 × 10^6 syngeneic bone marrow cells treated with anti-Thy-1.2 plus rabbit complement. The results showed that similar autoimmune diseases were produced in "newborn" thymus-engrafted T cell-depleted recipient mice but not in the engrafted normal recipients. These results indicate that the balb/c mice have pathogenic autoreactive T cells in their thymi, and such autoreactive T cells spontaneously expand and cause autoimmune disease when released to the T cell-deficient/eliminated periphery. Various manipulations that deplete Treg ($CD4^+CD25^+$ T cells) potentially activate orchitogenic $CD4^+$ T cells and promote EAO induction, but the presence of normal T cells including "natural" Treg suppresses the disease induction.

7.2.6 EAO Induced by Engraftment of Xenogeneic Thymus

Attempts were made to reconstitute T cell functions of nu/nu athymic nude mice by transplantation of xenogeneic thymic rudiments obtained from embryonic rats, rabbits, hamsters, guinea pigs, swine, and cows (Taguchi et al. 1986; Nishigaki-Maki et al. 1999). The results showed that these grafted mice gained T cell-mediated immune function and accepted skin grafts from the donor strain. All of the grafted thyme grew and formed proper thymic structure with host $CD90^+$ cells. Those mice generally survived more than 1 year without any severe infectious diseases under a conventional environment. However, they developed severe multiple organ-localized autoimmune diseases showing features similar to autoimmunity observed in the mice after neonatal thymectomy. Approximately 30% of the transplanted mice developed EAO (Fig. 7.2). This autoimmunity is also caused by a dysfunction of Treg. It is also noted that multiple organ-localized autoimmune diseases were not induced in nude mice grafted with syngeneic or allogeneic thymi of adult donors (Nishigaki-Maki et al. 1999; Morimoto et al. 2000).

In these chimeric animals, TCR alpha-beta expression pattern of the lymphocytes in the grafted thymi was quite similar to that of normal mouse thymocytes. Autoimmune lesions were successfully transferred into naïve nude mice or scid mice by donor spleen cells from the xenogeneic thymus-grafted nude mice (Nishigaki-Maki et al. 1999; Ohno et al. 1999) (Fig. 7.3). Sufficient $CD4^+$ T cells were observed in the donor lymphoid organs of all grafted nude mice, and removal of $CD90^+$ or $CD4^+$, but not $CD8^+$ cells from their spleen cells, eliminated the disease transfer activity (Ohno et al. 1999). Furthermore, positively fractioned $CD4^+$ T cells from the xenogeneic thymus-grafted nude mice were capable of inducing autoimmune lesions without the appearance of organ-specific autoantibodies, but the grade of lesions was lower than that in recipient mice that received unfractioned spleen cells. Transfer of sera from the grafted nude mice to scid mice did not induce any pathogenic features in the target organs, although deposition of immunoglobulins in the corresponding target organs was observed. This indicates that pathogenic $CD4^+$ T cells can induce autoimmune disease without B cell's help but that cooperation with functional B cells induces more severe damage (Ohno et al. 1999).

7.2.7 EAO Induced by Administration of Anti-IL-2 Receptor Antibody

During development of whole organism, tissue-specific Treg involved in self-tolerance is activated extrathymically by autoantigen from mature organs. Since it is speculated that not only pathogenic CD4$^+$ effector T cells but also CD4$^+$ Treg express the IL-2 receptor (CD25) as an activated T cell population, an attempt was made to eliminate these Treg from the developing immune system of neonatally thymectomized (C57BL/6 × A/J)F_1 mice by in vivo injection of rat monoclonal antibodies (IgG1) against mouse IL-2-receptor alpha (Taguchi and Takahashi 1996). In this experimental system, neonatal thymectomy was performed on day 7 after birth. As described above, day 3 thymectomy is effective to induce multiple organ-localized autoimmune diseases, while day 7 thymectomy is hardly effective. However, day 7-thymectomized mice developed EAO and other autoimmune diseases after the anti-IL-2 receptor antibody-treatment (Fig. 7.1), and their incidence and severity became apparently higher than control mice that had received day 7 thymectomy alone.

In next experiments, anti-IL-2 receptor alpha monoclonal antibodies were injected intraperitoneally into 10-day-old intact mice every other day for 2 weeks (Taguchi and Takahashi 1996). It was found that EAO with autoimmune epididymitis were induced along with other autoimmune inflammation in the prostate, stomach, lacrimal gland, salivary gland, thyroid, and the retina (Fig. 7.1), like in day 7-thymectomized mice injected with anti-IL-2 receptor alpha monoclonal antibodies. The results indicate that CD4$^+$ T cells expressing IL-2 receptor alpha play a critical role as Treg in the periphery for maintenance of immune tolerance. This study also suggests the importance of IL-2 receptor alpha expression on Treg, rather than on pathogenic (effector) autoreactive T cells. Considering that tissue autoantigens extrathymically induce activation of tissue-specific Treg involved in self-tolerance, testis-specific Treg may be induced by leaked autoantigens from maturing testis to circulatory system under normal condition. Such activated Treg probably expresses IL-2 receptor alpha, and this population may be eliminated by administration of anti-IL-2 receptor alpha monoclonal antibodies in vivo at the age of developing immune system of mice, consequently leading to uncontrollable activation of tissue antigen-specific pathogenic T cells.

7.2.8 EAO Induced by Transfer of Rearranged TCR Alpha-Chain Gene

Germ line expression of rearranged TCR alpha-chain transgenes with the IgH chain enhancer reproducibly elicits T cell-mediated EAO in 8 of 16 SWR/J-backcrossed mice with other autoimmune diseases in the thyroid gland, gastric mucosa, Langerhans islets, salivary gland, and ovaries in selected strains of normal mice (Sakaguchi et al. 1994b) (Fig. 7.4). These diseases can be adoptively transferred to syngeneic normal mice by CD4$^+$ T cells expressing rearranged TCR alpha-chain

Fig. 7.4 EAO induced by genetical manipulation of the immune system in mice

Gene manipulation

- Rearranged TCR alpha-chain gene transfer
- HLA-B27 gene transfer
- TAM gene knockout
- Aire gene knockout
- p35 gene knockout

⇩

Systemic and local defects in the regulation of innate and adoptive immunity

⇩

EAO with or without multiple organ-localized autoimmunity

transgenes. Normal organs transplanted in the transgenic mice were also destroyed by inflammation in an antigen-specific manner when the mice developed autoimmune disease in the corresponding organs. This indicates that the autoimmune diseases are produced by genetic manipulation of the T cell lineage but not the target autoantigens. Furthermore, transfer of the transgenic bone marrow cells to MHC-compatible scid mice also produces the same autoimmune disease as in the donors (Fig. 7.3). Therefore, it appears that the transgene-induced autoreactive effector T cells are neither deleted in the thymus nor rendered anergic upon contact with the normal target autoantigens but can be controlled by a T cell-dependent mechanism. This indicates that abnormality of the environment of T cell differentiation/selection in the thymus is not responsible for triggering the autoimmune responses in mice with germ line expression of rearranged TCR alpha-chain transgenes. In contrast, the development of autoimmune diseases in the recipient scid mice is effectively prevented by co-transfer of syngeneic non-transgenic T cells. Expansion/activation of such autoreactive T cells appears to be controlled in the normal periphery by a subpopulation of normal T cells. The repertoire of T cells is solely determined in the thymus by the TCR gene rearrangement and by subsequent positive/negative selections, in which T cells bearing high-affinity TCR for autoantigen expressed in the thymus are clonally deleted. Since the TCR plays the key role in growth/differentiation and repertoire selection of T cells, germline alteration of the TCR gene expression may affect the ontogeny of autoreactive T cells or their control in the thymus or periphery. It is likely that transgene expression may lead to the production of more numerous or more pathogenic autoreactive T cells than in the physiologic state, thereby causing autoimmune diseases.

7.2.9 EAO Induced by Transfer of HLA-B27 Gene

Humans who have inherited the human class I MHC allele HLA-B27 have a markedly increased risk of developing the multiple organ-localized autoimmune diseases termed HLA-B27 syndromes. Clinical features in HLA-B27 syndromes include anterior uveitis, ankylosing spondylitis, reactive arthritis, psoriatic arthritis, and inflammatory bowel disease such as ulcerative colitis and Crohn's disease. Although autoimmune orchitis has not been reported in men with HLA-B27 syndromes, these patients showed reduced sperm motility, higher plasma luteinizing hormone and follicle-stimulating hormone and lower testosterone levels compared with control subjects (Villiger et al. 2010; Ramonda et al. 2014).

To investigate the role of HLA-B27, both HLA-B27 and human B2-microglobulin genes were introduced into rats (Hammer et al. 1990; Taurog et al. 2012). In the transgenic rat, EAO with autoimmune epididymitis and other inflammatory diseases involving the gastrointestinal tract, peripheral and vertebral joints, skin, nails, and heart were found (Hammer et al. 1990) (Fig. 7.4). Inflammation was first evident in the ductuli efferentes as early as age 30 days, the age when meiotic TGC first appear in the seminiferous tubules (Taurog et al. 2012). The inflammation was initially composed of neutrophils, later became granulomatous, but remained largely confined to the ductuli efferentes until almost 2 months later. The EAO was macroscopically manifested by a progressive enlargement of the testes followed by testicular atrophy, with resultant infertility. It took another 3 months for inflammation shifts from the ductuli efferentes to the testis with the spermatogenic disturbance. Anti-TGC antibodies and anti-sperm antibodies appeared in the rat serum after age 70 days. Histologically, the tunica albuginea was thickened by connective tissue, which contained active angioblasts and fibroblasts as well as large numbers of lymphocytes and plasma cells. The testes often contained numerous granulomas with necrotic centers surrounded by epithelioid macrophages and giant cells and peripherally by lymphocytes, plasma cells, and fibroblasts. Cells infiltrating the testes were predominantly $CD4^+$ T cells and $CD68^+$ or $CD163^+$ macrophages. The epididymis frequently contained granulomas similar to those found in the testis, along with dilated tubules containing necrotic cellular debris. The interstitium of the epididymis was expanded by lymphocytes, plasma cells, epithelioid macrophages, and moderate fibrosis. It is noted that, severe EAO occurs in the transgenic rats several months before the onset of joint disease.

The levels of IFN-gamma, IL-10, and IL-17 were elevated in the ductuli efferentes, epididymis, and testis. In addition, levels of IL-12A, IL-22, IL-23A, and IL-23 receptor were found to be elevated in the ductuli efferentes. With regard to the immune mechanisms driving EAO, it is not yet clear whether the inflammation in the ductuli efferentes is initially driven by a transgene-induced defect in the regulation of innate immunity or whether the rats have preexisting effector pathogenic T cells that induce inflammation upon contact with TGC autoantigens. The influx of neutrophils in the earliest lesions in the ductuli efferentes suggests that innate immune signals are involved in producing an IL-17 response.

7.2.10 EAO Induced by Knockout of TAM Receptor Tyrosine Kinases Triple Genes

Tyro-3, Axl and Mer (TAM) receptors belong to a subfamily of receptor tyrosine kinases. They are critical for engulfment and efficient clearance of apoptotic cells by macrophages (Scott et al. 2001). Under normal condition, rapid clearance of apoptotic cells is important to inhibit inflammation and autoimmune responses against intracellular autoantigens. Therefore, TAM receptors are negative regulators of TLR-initiated systemic innate immunity and play critical roles in regulating immune responses (Lu et al. 1999; Sun et al. 2010). Mutant mice that lack these receptors develop a severe lymphoproliferative disorder accompanied by broad-spectrum autoimmunity in the lung, liver, kidney, heart, pancreas, intestine, skeletal muscle, eye, brain, and spinal cord (Lu and Lemke 2001). These phenotypes result from a deficient in the clearance of apoptotic cells and a hyperactivation of antigen-presenting cells in which the three receptors are normally expressed.

TAM receptors are also abundantly expressed in Sertoli cells and Leydig cells under normal state and therefore regulate the tissue homeostasis in immune-privileged testis (Deng et al. 2016). They facilitate phagocytic clearance of apoptotic TGC by Sertoli cells (Xiong et al. 2008). The removal of apoptotic TGC by phagocytes facilitates the elimination of the autoantigens, which may reduce endogenous inflammation. Moreover, various TLRs are expressed and functional in Sertoli cells, and TAM receptors inhibit TLR-mediated inflammatory cytokine production by Sertoli cells. It was found that TAM receptor tyrosine kinases triple knockout (TAM$^{-/-}$) mice exhibit impaired spermatogenesis with resultant male infertility (Lu et al. 1999; Sun et al. 2010; Zhang et al. 2013), although mice lacking any single receptor do not exhibit apparent pathology during their lifetime. TAM triple knockout (TAM$^{-/-}$) mice exhibit an excessive activation of TLR in response to its ligand polyinosinic-polycytidylic acid, resulting in the upregulation of various inflammatory cytokines and show multiple severe defects of the spermatogenesis, systemic immune homeostasis, and clearance of apoptotic TGC (Fig. 7.4). After the onset of sexual maturity, TGC were progressively degenerated, and macrophages and lymphocytes infiltrated into the testis as TAM$^{-/-}$ mice aged. Moreover the integrity of BTB was impaired, and anti-TGC autoantibodies were produced. TNF-alpha, IL-6, and monocyte chemotactic protein-1 were upregulated in the testis of TAM$^{-/-}$ mice and predominantly located in Sertoli cells. Secretion of other cytokines, such as IL-1 beta, and interferons alpha and beta were also elevated (Sun et al. 2010). In vitro assays showed that TAM$^{-/-}$ Sertoli cells secrete significantly high levels of inflammatory cytokines compared with wild-type Sertoli cells after co-culture with apoptotic TGC.

7.2.11 EAO Induced by Knockout of the Autoimmune Regulator (Aire) Gene

Educational immune tolerance to self-antigens, composed of the negative selection of autoreactive T cells and the generation of Treg, is induced primarily in the thymus where tissue-restricted antigens are presented to T cells by the thymic stromal cells—a process known as central tolerance regulated by the Aire (Chan and Anderson 2015). The Aire is a promiscuous thymic transcription factor involved in controlling expression of tissue-restricted antigens for presentation during the establishment of central tolerance in the thymus (Pitkanen and Peterson 2003;

Eldershaw et al. 2011). The loss of this protein is responsible for the autoimmune polyendocrinopathy syndrome or autoimmune polyendocrinopathy-candidiasis-ectodermal dystrophy (APECED) because of a defect in thymic negative selection (Kisand and Peterson 2011; Taniguchi and Anderson 2011). In immune responses by challenging with exogenous antigens, the peripheral T cells of mice with a disrupted Aire gene have approximately fivefold increased proliferation (Ramsey et al. 2002). Although the Aire is expressed heavily in the thymic epithelial cells and is involved in maintaining self-tolerance, the testis is the most predominant extrathymic location of the Aire (Schaller et al. 2008; Radhakrishnan et al. 2016). In particular, spermatogonia and spermatocytes significantly express Aire. RT-PCR analyses also revealed the expression of Aire in mouse ovary, lung, kidney, and adrenal gland (Ruan et al. 1999). It is suggested that extrathymic Aire-expressing cells have an important role in the clonal deletion of autoreactive $CD8^+$ T cells (Taniguchi and Anderson 2011).

Mice with a targeted deletion of the Aire gene develop normally; however, the absence of the Aire protein influences ectopic expression of peripheral tissue antigens in thymic medullary epithelial cells, resulting in the development of an autoimmune disorder similar to APECED including multiple-organ lymphocytic infiltration and circulating autoantibodies (Ramsey et al. 2002; Villasenor et al. 2005). In the testis of Aire-deficient mice, the scheduled apoptotic wave of TGC, which is necessary for normal spermatogenesis, is decreased, and sporadic apoptosis in adults is increased. Moreover, they were infertile with anti-sperm autoantibody formation and frequent inflammatory cell infiltration in the epididymal interstitium (Hubert et al. 2009; Hedger 2011a, b). However, typical inflammatory lesion was not seen in the testis.

7.2.12 EAO Induced by Knockout of IL-12/IL-35 Common Subunit p35 Gene

The IL-6/IL-12 family cytokines involving IL-12 (p35/p40), IL-23 (p19/p40), IL-27 (p28/Epstein-Barr virus-induced gene 3 [EBI3]), and IL-35 (p35/EBI3) play critical roles in the regulation of various immune responses. This family of cytokines has unique characteristics: they are heterodimers comprising two different subunits, and one subunit of the cytokines receptor is sometimes shared with more than two cytokines. IL-35, a novel anti-inflammatory cytokine, that is, produced by Foxp3+ Treg, suppresses cell proliferation and downregulates Th17 cell development (Collison et al. 2007). In mice with congenital lack of EBI3, p35, and IL-12 receptor beta 2, mild but significant infiltration of lymphocytes into the testicular interstitium was found with increased IFN-gamma mRNA expression in the testes and autoantibody production against spermatids (Terayama et al. 2014). Spermatogenic disturbance was very focally but frequently observed in the seminiferous tubules surrounded by infiltrating lymphocytes. In particular, p35-deficient mice showed the most severe spermatogenic disturbance. It is noted that no significant phenotype of inflammatory lesion was found throughout the body except for the testis.

In wild-type mice, expression of EBI3 was markedly increased at both mRNA and protein levels in the testes of 10–12-week old mice as compared with levels in 2-week old mice, whereas the mRNA expression of p40 was markedly decreased and that of p35 was conserved between these two groups (Terayama et al. 2014). Immunohistochemical analyses revealed that capillary endothelial cells and peritubular myoid cells surrounding the seminiferous tubules were highly positive for p35, and CD163-positive resident macrophages were also positive for p35 and EBI3. Therefore, the developmental expression of p35/EBI3 may function for prevention of autoimmune reaction in the testis. The p35 may help in maintaining the testicular immune privilege, in part in an IL-35-dependent manner.

References

Chan AY, Anderson MS. Central tolerance to self revealed by the autoimmune regulator. Ann N Y Acad Sci. 2015;1356:80–9.

Collison LW, Workman CJ, Kuo TT, Boyd K, Wang Y, Vignali KM, Cross R, Sehy D, Blumberg RS, Vignali DA. The inhibitory cytokine IL-35 contributes to regulatory T-cell function. Nature. 2007;450:566–9.

Del Rio R, Sun Y, Alard P, Tung KS, Teuscher C. H2 control of natural T regulatory cell frequency in the lymph node correlates with susceptibility to day 3 thymectomy-induced autoimmune disease. J Immunol. 2011;186:382–9.

Deng T, Chen Q, Han D. The role of TAM receptor tyrosine kinases in the mammalian testis and immunoprivileged sites. Front Biosci. 2016;21:316–27.

Dyson PJ, Knight AM, Fairchild S, Simpson E, Tomonair K. Genes encoding ligands for deletion of V beta11 T cells cosegregate with mammary tumor virus genomes. Nature. 1991;349:431–532.

Eldershaw SA, Sansom DM, Narendran P. Expression and function of the autoimmune regulator (Aire) gene in non-thymic tissue. Clin Exp Immunol. 2011;163:296–308.

Filaci G, Fenoglio D, Indiveri F. $CD8^+$ T regulatory/suppressor cells and their relationships with autoreactivity and autoimmunity. Autoimmunity. 2011;44:51–7.

Grigorev VV, Ogurtsov RP, Zubzhitsi IN. Immunomorphologic changes in the testes upon exposure to a microwave electromagnetic field. Arkh Anat Gistol Embriol. 1981;80:69–75.

Hammer RE, Marika SD, Richardson JA, Tang JYP, Taurig JD. Transgenic rats expressing HLA-B27 and human b2 microglobulin with spontaneous inflammatory disease in multiple organ systems: an animal model of HLA-B27-associated disease. Cell. 1990;63:1099–112.

Hattori M, Brandon MR. Thymus and the endocrine system: ovarian dysgenesis in neonatally thymectomized rats. J Endocrinol. 1979;83:101–11.

Hedger MP. Toll-like receptors and signaling in spermatogenesis and testicular responses to inflammation-a perspective. J Reprod Immunol. 2011a;88:130–41.

Hedger MP. Immunophysiology and pathology of inflammation in the testis and epididymis. J Androl. 2011b;32:625–40.

Hiramine C, Hojo K, Matsumoto H, Koseto M, Itoh M. Differential effect of cyclosporine in vivo on the distribution of T cell subsets in the thymus, spleen, and lymph nodes. Transplantation. 1989a;47:499–503.

Hiramine C, Hojo K, Koseto M, Itoh M. The effect of cyclosporine on thymic epithelial cells-an immunohistochemical study. Thymus. 1989b;14:213–21.

Hou WG, Zhao J, Li Z, Li W, Li T, Xiong LZ, Zhang YQ. Effects of electromagnetic pulse irradiation on the mouse blood-testicle barrier. Urology. 2012;80(225):e1–6.

Hubert FX, Kinkel SA, Crewther PE, Cannon PZ, Webster KE, Link M, Uibo R, O'Bryan MK, Meager A, Forehan SP, Smyth GK, Mittaz L, Antonarakis SE, Peterson P, Health WR, Scott

HS. Aire-deficient C57BL/6 mice mimicking the common human 13-base pair deletion mutation present with only a mild autoimmune phenotype. J Immunol. 2009;182:3902–18.

Itoh M, Takahashi T, Sakaguchi N, Kuniyasu Y, Shimizu J, Otuka F, Sakaguchi S. Thymus and autoimmunity: production of $CD25^{+}CD4^{+}$ naturally anergic and suppressive T cells as a key function of the thymus in maintaining immunologic self-tolerance. J Immunol. 1999;162:5317–26.

Jones LA, Chin T, Merriam GR, Nelson LM, Kruisbeck AM. Failure of clonal deletion in neonatally thymectomized mice: tolerance is preserved through clonal anergy. J Exp Med. 1990;139:1277–85.

Kisand K, Peterson P. Autoimmune polyendocrinopathy candidiasis ectodermal dystrophy: known and novel aspects of the syndrome. Ann N Y Acad Sci. 2011;1246:77–91.

Kojima A, Spencer CA. Genetic susceptibility to testicular autoimmunity: comparison between postthymectomy and postvasectomy models in mice. Biol Reprod. 1983;29:195–205.

Kojima A, Prehn RT. Genetic susceptibility to post-thymectomy autoimmune diseases in mice. Immunogenetics. 1981;14:15–27.

Lipscomb HL, Gardner PJ, Sharp G. The effect of neonatal thymectomy on the induction of autoimmune orchitis in rats. J Reprod Immunol. 1979;1:209–17.

Luo Y, Wang X, Chen Y, Xu S, Ding G, Shi C. Effects of electromagnetic radiation on morphology and TGF-beta3 expression in mouse testicular tissue. Toxicology. 2013;310:8–14.

Lu Q, Gore M, Zhang Q, Camenisch T, Boast S, Casagrandra F, Lai C, Skinner MK, Klein R, Matsushima GK, Earp HS, Goff SP, Lemke G. Tyro-3 family receptors are essential of mammalian spermatogenesis. Nature. 1999;398:723–8.

Lu Q, Lemke G. Homeostatic regulation of the immune system by receptor tyrosine kinases of the Tyro 3 family. Science. 2001;293:306–11.

Miller JF. Analysis of the thymus influence in leukaemogenesis. Nature. 1961;191:248–9.

Morimoto T, Nishigaki-Maki K, Ohno K, Ikeda H, Takeuchi M, Ueda T, Takahashi T, Taguchi O. Transplantation of xenogeneic embryonic thymus to athymic nude mice induces acquisition of distorted immunity. Transplant Proc. 2000;32:956–7.

Nishigaki-Maki K, Takahashi T, Ohno K, Morimoto T, Ikeda H, Takeuchi M, Ueda M, Taguchi O. Autoimmune diseases developed in athymic nude mice grafted with embryonic thymus of xenogeneic origin. Eur J Immunol. 1999;29:3350–9.

Nishizuka Y, Sakakura T. Thymus and reproduction: sex linked dysgenesis of the gonad after neonatal thymectomy. Science. 1969;166:753–5.

Nishizuka Y. A novel experimental system of organ-localized autoimmune disease in the mouse. Acta Pathol Jpn. 1982;32:211–22.

Ohno K, Takahashi T, Maki K, Ueda M, Taguchi O. Successful transfer of localized autoimmunity with positively selected $CD4^{+}$ cells to scid mice lacking functional B cells. Autoimmunity. 1999;29:103–10.

Pitkanen J, Peterson P. Autoimmune regulator: from loss of function to autoimmunity. Genes Immun. 2003;4:12–21.

Radhakrishnan K, Bhagya KP, Kumar AT, Devi AN, Sengottaiyan J, Kumar PG. Autoimmune regulator (Aire) is expressed in spermatogenic cells, and it altered the expression of several nucleic-acid-biding and cytoskeletal proteins in germ cell 1 spermatogonial (GC1-spg) cells. Mol Cell Proteomics. 2016;15:2686–98.

Ramonda R, Foresta C, Ortolan A, Bertoldo A, Oliviero F, Lorenzin M, Pizzol D, Punzi L, Garolla A. Influence of tumor necrosis factor alpha inhibitors on testicular function and semen in spondyloarthritis patients. Fertil Steril. 2014;101:359–65.

Ramsey C, Winqvist O, Puhakka L, Halonen M, Moro A, Kampe O, Eskelin P, Pelto-Huikko M, Peltonen L. Aire deficient mice develop multiple features of APECED phenotype and show altered immune response. Hum Mol Genet. 2002;11:397–409.

Ruan QG, Wang CY, Shi JD, She JX. Expression and alternative splicing of the mouse autoimmune regulator gene (Aire). J Autoimmun. 1999;13:307–13.

Sakaguchi S, Fukuma K, Kuribayashi K, Masuda T. Organ-specific autoimmune diseases induced in mice by elimination of T cell subset. I. Evidence for the active participation of T cell in natu-

ral self-tolerance; deficit of a T cell subset as a possible cause of autoimmune disease. J Exp Med. 1985;161:72–87.
Sakaguchi S, Sakaguchi N. Thymus and autoimmunity. Transplantation of the thymus from cyclosporine A-treated mice causes organ-specific autoimmune disease in athymic nude mice. J Exp Med. 1988;167:1479–85.
Sakaguchi S, Sakaguchi N. Organ-specific autoimmune disease induced by elimination of T cell subsets. V. Neonatal administration of cyclosporine A causes autoimmune disease. J Immunol. 1989;142:471–80.
Sakaguchi S, Sakaguchi N. Thymus and autoimmunity: Capacity of the normal thymus to produce self-reactive T cells and conditions required for their induction of autoimmune disease. J Exp Med. 1990;172:537–45.
Sakaguchi N, Sakaguchi S. Causes and mechanism of autoimmune disease: cyclosporine A as a probe for the investigation. J Invest Dermatol. 1992;98:79S–6S.
Sakaguchi N, Miyai K, Sakaguchi S. Ionizing radiation and autoimmunity. Induction of autoimmune disease in mice by high dose fractionated total lymphoid irradiation and its prevention by inoculating normal T cells. J Immunol. 1994a;152:2586–95.
Sakaguchi S, Ermak TH, Toda M, Berg LJ, Ho W, de St Groth BF, Peterson PA, Sakaguchi N, Davis MM. Induciton of autoimmune disease in mice by germline alteration of the T cell receptor gene expression. J Immunol. 1994b;152:1471–84.
Sakaguchi S, Sakaguchi N, Asano M, Itoh M, Toda M. Immunologic self-tolerance maintained by activated T cells expressing IL-2 receptor alpha-chains (CD25). J Immunol. 1995;155:1151–64.
Scott RS, McMahon EJ, Pop SM, Reap EA, Caricchio R, Cohen PL, Earp HS, Matsushima GK. Phagocytosis and clearance of apoptotic cells is mediated by MER. Nature. 2001;411:207–11.
Schaller CE, Wang CL, Beck-Engeser G, Goss L, Scott HS, Anderson MS, Wabl M. Expression of Aire and the early wave of apoptosis in spermatogenesis. J Immunol. 2008;180:1338–43.
Smith H, Chen IM, Kubo R, Tung KSK. Neonatal thymectomy results in a repertoire enriched in T cells deleted in adult thymus. Science. 1989;245:749–52.
Smith H, Sakamoto Y, Kasai K, Tung KSK. Effector and regulatory cells in autoimmune oophoritis elicited by neonatal thymectomy. J Immunol. 1991;147:2928–33.
Smith H, Lou YH, Lacy P, Tung KSK. Tolerance mechanism in ovarian and gastric autoimmune disease. J Immunol. 1992;149:2212–8.
Smith TR, Kumar V. Revival of $CD8^+$ Treg-mediated suppression. Trends Immunol. 2008;29:337–42.
Son Y, Heo K, Bae MJ, Lee CG, Cho WS, Kim SD, Yang K, Shin IS, Lee MY, Kim JS. Injury to the blood-testis barrier after low-dose-rate chronic radiation exposure in mice. Radiat Prot Dosim. 2015;167:316–20.
Sugihara S, Izumi Y, Yoshioka T, Yagi H, Tsujimura T, Tarutani O, Kohno Y, Murakami S, Hamaoka T, Fujiwara H. Autoimmune thyroiditis induced in mice depleted of particular T cell subsets. I. Requirement of Lyt-1 dull L3T4 bright normal T cells for the induction of thyroiditis. J Immunol. 1988;141:105–13.
Sun B, Qi N, Shang T, Wu H, Deng T, Han D. Seroli cell-initiated testicular innate immune response through toll-like receptor-3 activation is negatively regulated by Tyro3, Axl, and Mer receptors. Endocrinology. 2010;151:2886–97.
Taguchi O, Nishizuka Y, Sakakura T, Kojima A. Autoimmune oophoritis in thymectomized mice: detection of circulating antibodies against oocytes. Clin Exp Immunol. 1980;40:540–3.
Taguchi O, Nishizuka Y. Experimental autoimmune orchitis after neonatal thymectomy in the mouse. Clin Exp Immunol. 1981;46:425–34.
Taguchi O, Takahashi T, Seto M, Namikawa R, Matsuyama M, Nishizuka Y. Development of multiple organ-localized autoimmune diseases in nude mice after reconstitution of T cell function by rat fetal thymus graft. J Exp Med. 1986;164:60–71.
Taguchi O, Nishizuka Y. Self-tolerance and localized autoimmunity: mouse models of autoimmune disease that suggest that tissue specific suppressor T cells are involved in tolerance. J Exp Med. 1987;165:146–56.

Taguchi O, Takahashi T, Nishizuka Y. Self-tolerance and localized autoimmunity. Curr Opin Immunol. 1990;2:576–81.

Taguchi O, Kotani K, Ikeda H, Kezuka T, Takeuchi M, Takahashi T. Tissue-specific suppressor T cells involved in self-tolerance are activated extrathymically by self-antigens. Immunology. 1994;82:365–9.

Taguchi O, Takahashi T. Administration of anti-interleukin-2 receptor antibody in vivo induced localized autoimmune disease. Eur J Immunol. 1996;26:1608–12.

Takahashi K, Nagahori K, Qu N, Kuramasu M, Hayashi S, Hirai S, Hatayama N, Miyaso H, Ogawa Y, Itoh M. Effect of Goshajinkigan on the recovery of spermatogenesis after irradiation treatment in mice. 2017 (in preparation).

Tang XL, Smith TR, Kumar V. Specific control of immunity by regulatory CD8 T cells. Cell Mol Immunol. 2005;2:11–9.

Taniguchi RT, Anderson MS. The role of Aire in clonal selection. Immunol Cell Biol. 2011;89:40–4.

Taurog JD, Rival C, van Duivenvoorde LM, Satumira N, Dorris ML, Sun M, Shelton JM, Richardson JA, Hamra FK, Hammer RE, Tung KSK. Autoimmune epididymoorchitis is essential to the pathogenesis of male-specific spondylarthritis in HLA-B27-transgenic rats. Arthritis Rheum. 2012;64:2518–28.

Terayama H, Yoshimoto T, Hirai S, Naito M, Qu N, Hatayama N, Hayashi S, Mitobe K, Furusawa J, Mizoguchi I, Kezuka T, Goto H, Suyama K, Sakabe K, Itoh M. Contribution of IL-12/IL-35 common subunit p35 to maintaining testicular immune privilege. PLoS One. 2014;9(e):96120.

Tung KS, Smith S, Teuscher C, Cook C, Anderson RE. Murine autoimmune oophoritis, epididymoorchitis, and gastritis induced by day 3 thymectomy. Immunopathology. Am J Pathol. 1987a;126:293–302.

Tung KS, Smith S, Matzner P, Kasai K, Oliver J, Feuchter F, Anderson RE. Murine autoimmune oophoritis, epididymoorchitis, and gastritis induced by day 3 thymectomy. Autoantibodies. Am J Pathol. 1987b;126:303–14.

Tung KS, Teuscher C. Mechanisms of autoimmune disease in the testis and ovary. Hum Reprod Update. 1995;1:35–50.

Villasenor J, Benoist C, Mathis D. AIRE and APECED: molecular insights into an autoimmune disease. Immunol Rev. 2005;204:156–64.

Villiger PM, Caliezi G, Cottin V, Forger F, Senn A, Ostensen M. Effects of TNF antagonists on sperm characteristics in patients with spondyloarthritis. Ann Rheum Dis. 2010;69:1842–4.

Vojtiskova M, Pokorna Z. Prevention of experimental allergic aspermatogenesis by thymectomy in adult mice. Lancet. 1964;1:644–5.

Wang XW, Ding GR, Shi CH, Zeng LH, Liu JY, Li J, Zhao T, Chen YB, Guo GZ. Mechanisms involved in the blood-testis barrier increased permeability induced by EMP. Toxicology. 2010;276:58–63.

Woodland DL, Happ MP, Gollob KJ, Palmer E. An endogenous retrovirus mediating deletion of beta T cells? Nature. 1991;349:529–30.

Xiong W, Chen Y, Wang H, Wang H, Wu H, Lu Q, Han D. Gas6 and the Tyro 3 receptor tyrosine kinase subfamily regulate the phagocytic function of Sertoli cells. Reproduction. 2008;135:77–87.

Zhang X, Li N, Chen Q, Yan K, Liu Z, Zhang X, Liu P, Chen Y, Han D. Breakdown of immune homeostasis in the testis of mice lacking Tyro3, Axl and Mer receptor tyrosine kinases. Immunol Cell Biol. 2013;91:416–26.

The Future Directions of Testicular Autoimmunity Investigation

8

8.1 Introduction

It is noted that experimental autoimmune orchitis (EAO) can be induced without the use of any adjuvants in both immune-competent and immune-deficient animals. This means that both healthy and immune-compromised men may be easily affected by testicular autoimmunity. Normally, the TGC autoantigens are protected by two independent mechanisms: (1) the confinement of most of the autoantigens by a strong but regionally incomplete BTB and (2) the systemic and local immunoregulatory mechanisms that prevent activation of TGC specific autoreactive lymphocytes. Therefore, the susceptibility to testicular autoimmunity may be influenced at the levels of target TGC, supporting tissue surrounding target TGC and immune system. In particular, it should be clarified whether or how the relevant autoantigens are presented to specific T cells for induction or prevention of testicular autoimmunity.

8.2 Various Issues for Testicular Autoimmunity in the Future

8.2.1 Precise Epidemiology of Testicular Autoimmunity in Men

Testicular biopsies from infertile men have been found to contain immunopathological evidence of orchitis and testicular immune complexes, which are also found in EAO. At present, respective epidemiological data are very scarce. Clinically, testicular biopsy specimens from men with spermatogenic disturbance of immunologic origin are supposed to represent the final stage of the pathological process (post-active inflammation stage) in which the infiltration of immune reactants has already ceased and only the spermatogenic disturbance remains. In the majority of patients, diagnosis is hampered by an asymptomatic course of the disease and unspecific clinical signs. Therefore, immunological factors may be more often involved in male infertility than has been suspected if the patients can receive the

M. Itoh, *Testicular Autoimmunity*, DOI 10.1007/978-4-431-54460-9_8

medical examination more early. Furthermore, examination sites in the testis may affect the incidence of inflammation. Many histopathological studies revealed the frequent involvement of inflammatory cell infiltration at the mediastinum (the tubuli recti and the rete testis) (Hatakeyama 1984; Tung et al. 1987; Itoh et al. 1995b). Actually, differing from the common biopsy cases of convoluted seminiferous tubules at the peripheral testis, the sampling of tissue from the tubuli recti and the rete testis is very difficult because of the danger that biopsy-induced tissue injury may block TGC transport to the ductuli efferentes. However, if biopsy tissue can be taken from the tubuli recti and the rete testis regions safely, the incidence of lymphocytic infiltration in the testes of infertile men should become higher than reported. It should be also kept in mind that testicular biopsy artificially breaks BTB with the resultant exposure of TGC autoantigens to the immune system. Therefore, development of noninvasive test for diagnosis of orchitis is needed. Several different imaging methods such as color Doppler sonography and magnetic resonance imaging have been tried (Moraes et al. 2010).

As another noninvasive test, identification of specific markers of testicular autoimmunity has been awaited. Even though only anti-sperm antibodies, which represent humoral immunity, have been taken into account by many urologists or andrologists when assessing immunologic male infertility (Shibahara et al. 2005; Shiraishi et al. 2009), many reports on EAO imply that DTH response, cellular immunity, is more critical for the disease induction than humoral immunity in spite of no use of DTH-inducing CFA (Sakamoto et al. 1985; Sakamoto and Nomoto 1986; Itoh et al. 1991a, b, c, 1992b; Itoh 2009). Considering that the DTH intensity against TGC well correlated with EAO development (Qu et al. 2014), in vivo assay of DTH response on injection of some specific TGC autoantigens or in vitro assay of cytokines secretion or cell proliferation of isolated lymphocytes stimulated with TGC autoantigens may be effective for screening and predicting methods to detect whether testicular autoimmunity is involved or not in infertile male patients. In immunologically infertile women, a precise and objective method for the diagnosis was developed and examined, based on a one-step agarose leukocyte migration inhibition factor assay (Dimitrov et al. 1992). The migration areas are evaluated by a computer-assisted image analysis system. The radial migration indexes and area migration indexes are computed and expressed as a migration index percentage for each patient and control. Therefore, development of a reliable, standardized testing protocol for diagnosis of autoimmune orchitis will contribute to grasp precise epidemiology of testicular autoimmunity in men.

Most recently, a new noninvasive biomarker for the diagnosis of testicular inflammation was reported (Fijak et al. 2014). In sera from infertile azoospermic patients with histologically confirmed testicular inflammation, significantly elevated titers of autoantibodies against disulfide isomerase family A, member 3 (ER-60), were found. Proteins in lysates of normal testicular tissue have 14 proteins that immunoreacted with a majority of sera of patients with testicular inflammation. Of these 14 proteins, ER-60, transferrin, and chaperonin containing T-complex protein 1, subunit 5, were considered as specific. Since ER-60 reacted with 92% of patient sera, an ER-60-autoantibody ELISA was developed. Therefore, measurement of ER-60 autoantibody titers in serum could be a novel noninvasive marker for the diagnosis of asymptomatic testicular inflammation causing male fertility disturbances.

Although many patients with idiopathic male infertility are asymptomatic, chronic genitourinary inflammation often results in leukocytospermia, an elevated number of leukocytes in semen. Hagen et al. (2015) evaluated expression of TLR-2, TLR-4, cyclooxygenase-2, and nuclear factor-like 2 in semen samples of age-matched infertile patients with and without leukocytospermia by the usage of specific Western blot evaluation, cytokine array, and immunofluorescence microscopy followed by computer-based analysis. Differential cytokine profiling of seminal plasma by antibody array revealed upregulation of the four pro-inflammatory chemokines in leukocytospermia. Therefore, TLR-2, TLR-4, cyclooxygenase-2, and nuclear factor-like 2 in semen can serve as novel biomarkers for idiopathic and asymptomatic male infertility patients.

8.2.2 Pathogenesis of the Onset of Autoimmune Inflammation in the Testis

Investigation of initial stage of testicular autoimmunity should lead to understanding of first contact between immune cells and testicular autoantigens in the testis. There are many EAO models nowadays, but there is still limited information of mode of EAO onset. Investigation of start of inflammatory cell infiltration in various EAO models may be useful for understanding its pathophysiology. Spermatids and spermatozoa are apparently foreign cells for females, prepubertal males, and neonatally castrated males. Therefore, transfer of lymphocytes obtained from syngeneic females, prepubertal males, or neonatally castrated males into adult male animals may be also valid to study the onset of contact between lymphocytes and TGC autoantigens in the testis.

In the testis, testis-specific effector $CD4^+$ T cells can recognize TGC autoantigens on antigen-presenting cells in the testis before EAO induction. Under normal condition, many TGC are degenerated in the seminiferous tubules, and their autoantigens should latently leaked, followed by endocytosis by various testicular somatic cells, such as Sertoli cells, peritubular myoid cells, testicular macrophages/dendritic cells, Leydig cells, and capillary endothelia. It is supposed that testicular macrophages/dendritic cells expressing MHC class II antigens surrounding the tubuli recti and rete testis are most important antigen-presenting cells for EAO induction; however, it remains unclear how TGC autoantigens leak outside the germ cell ducts and picked up by macrophages/dendritic cells in the testicular interstitium under physiological condition. It is also noted that mouse testicular cells express Fas ligand and have the potential to induce apoptotic death of activated T cells expressing Fas (CD95). To establish EAO, the orchitogenic T cells must escape the T cell killing mechanism by testicular cells. One possible mechanism is that the testis-specific effector T cells are resistant to the Fas-mediated cell death induced by the Fas ligand on testicular cells because Fas-mediated signaling does not always induce apoptosis. Alternatively, there is another possibility that EAO induction modulates expression of the Fas ligand on the testicular cells, which allow the testis-specific T cells to escape from apoptosis induction.

The role of humoral immunity in EAO induction still remains obscure. The histopathologic distribution of the initiation of inflammation differs between active and passive EAO (Tung et al. 1987; Itoh et al. 1991c, 1992b). Active EAO induced by testicular homogenate+CFA+BP immunization initially affects subcapsular seminiferous tubules far from the rete testis. In contrast, passive EAO by transfer of $CD4^+$ T cells obtained from testicular homogenate+CFA+BP-immunized donor mice preferentially induce inflammation in the tubuli recti adjacent to the rete testis. In TGC-induced EAO, active EAO is characterized by orchitis that preferentially affects the tubuli recti and the rete testis and by the absence of epididymo-vasitis; however, passive EAO is consistently accompanied by epididymo-vasitis. It is supposed that both cellular and humoral immune responses are induced in active EAO, while cellular rather than humoral immunity is critical for passive EAO. This indicates that EAO is generally $CD4^+$ T cell dependent, but B cells and plasma cells also affect the start of EAO.

Although Th1 cells were thought to be the main drivers of organ-specific autoimmunity, animals lacking the Th1 signature cytokines and molecules are not resistant, but more susceptible to multiple autoimmune diseases (Ferber et al. 1996; Jones et al. 1997; Matthys et al. 1999). In these animals, the generation of a unique $CD4^+$ T cell subset, named Th17 cells, is involved. Th17 cells produce the effector cytokine IL-17, which promote tissue inflammation and neutrophil recruitment for host defense and also are primarily associated with autoimmune inflammation (Korn et al. 2009). Actually, in testicular antigens+CFA+BP-induced EAO lesion, $CD4^+IL\text{-}17^+$ and $CD8^+IL17^+$ were immunohistochemically identified (Jacobo et al. 2011a, b). The addition of IL-17A to normal rat Sertoli cell cultures induced a significant decline in transepithelial electrical resistance and a reduction of occluding expression and redistribution of occludin and claudin-11, altering the Sertoli cell tight junction barrier (Perez et al. 2014). Also in vivo, intra-testicular injection of recombinant rat IL-17A in rats induced increased the BTB permeability and delocalization of occludin and claudin-11. Therefore, involvement of Th17 cells for the start of testicular inflammation will be studied in other EAO models.

8.2.3 Pathophysiologic Relation Between Chronic Inflammation in the Testis and Prolonged Spermatogenic Disturbance

The target finding by orchitogenic lymphocytes was antigen-specific, but the following tissue damage leading to spermatogenic disturbance may be produced by an antigen nonspecific fashion in EAO. Previously, the pathogenesis for TGC depletion in EAO lesion was often attributed to an influx of specific autoantibodies into the germ cell ducts with a leaky BTB; however, recently, much attention is being paid to the effect of cytokines on the function of Sertoli cells, Leydig cells, and the developing TGC (Itoh et al. 1992b, 1993). IL-1, IL-6, IL-17, IFN-gamma, TNF-alpha, and transforming growth factor-beta have been reported to affect Sertoli cells and the inter-Sertoli cell junctions as the BTB (Banks and Kastin 1992; Plotkin et al. 2000; Lui et al. 2003; Li et al. 2006; Sarkar et al. 2008; Wang and Lui 2009; Lie et al. 2011; Lydka et al. 2012; Perez et al. 2012, 2014; Zhang et al. 2014b). If this hypothesis is correct, the depletion of TGC should be induced without a direct contact of TGC with specific autoantibodies or specific $CD4^+$ T cells during EAO.

The vitro experiments on seminiferous tubule cultures showed that IFN-gamma and TNF-alpha induced apoptosis of TGC through the Fas/Fas ligand system (Riccioli et al. 2000). It is indicated that the Fas/Fas ligand system mediates apoptosis of TGC in the injured testis but not in the normal testis having spontaneous apoptosis (Koji 2001; Koji et al. 2001). It was also demonstrated that IL-6 induced apoptosis of TGC in isolated seminiferous tubules in rats (Rival et al. 2006). Clinically, the semen IL-6 level is increased in vasectomy reversal patients (Nandipati et al. 2005). Local injection of IFN-gamma into the testis in vivo induced a direct cytotoxic effect on TGC, indicating that IFN-gamma is also harmful to the seminiferous epithelium (Natwar et al. 1995). In addition, IFN-gamma was shown to increase the expression of Fas in Sertoli cells and makes these cells susceptible to Fas ligand-mediated cytotoxicity in the seminiferous epithelium (Riccioli et al. 2000). IFN-alpha is produced predominantly by leukocytes in man, and most cell types are able to produce IFN-alpha in the mouse. In transgenic mice using a plasmid containing IFN-alpha gene, aberrant expression of the introduced IFN-alpha gene occurs only in the testis, in which an ongoing degeneration of TGC leading to calcium deposits and atrophy of the seminiferous tubules were found (Hekman et al. 1988). Intra-testicular injection of recombinant rat IL-17A to rats induced focal inflammatory cell infiltration in the interstitium and germ cell sloughing in adjacent seminiferous tubules. $ED1^+$ macrophages were the main population infiltrating the interstitium following IL-17A injection (Perez et al. 2014). Therefore, IL-17A may facilitate the recruitment of immune cells to the testicular interstitium, resulting in the spermatogenic disturbance.

Coxsackievirus and adenovirus receptor is a junction molecule that is expressed on Sertoli cells and TGC. It mediates Sertoli cell-TGC adhesion and facilitates migration of preleptotene/leptotene spermatocytes across the BTB, suggesting that coxsackievirus and adenovirus receptor-based cell adhesion and migration are crucial for spermatogenesis (Gao and Lui 2014). Combined treatment with IFN-gamma+TNF-alpha exerts a synergistic effect by downregulating mRNA of coxsackievirus and adenovirus receptor and its protein levels. Therefore, downregulation of coxsackievirus and adenovirus receptor by IFN-gamma+TNF-alpha treatment may provide an explanation of how TGC are sloughing in the seminiferous epithelium during testicular inflammation.

It became evident that damaged TGC products induce expression of various inflammatory mediators, including TNF-alpha, IL-1-beta, IL-6, and monocyte chemotactic protein-1, in Sertoli cells. Notably, the damaged TGC products-induced inflammatory gene expression was significantly reduced by knockout of TLR-2 and TLR-4 (Zhang et al. 2013a). Monocyte chemotactic protein-1 secreted by Sertoli cells after stimulation with damaged TGC products promotes migration of macrophages around the seminiferous tubules. Accumulated macrophages might deteriorate the spermatogenic disturbance. Indeed, busulfan-induced spermatogenic disturbance in vivo upregulates TNF-alpha and monocyte chemotactic protein-1 expression in Sertoli cells and facilitates macrophage migration into the testis in wild-type mice. These phenomena were not observed in TRL2$^{-/-}$TLR4$^{-/-}$ mice. It indicates that damaged TGC products induce inflammatory gene expression in Sertoli cells via the activation of TLR-2 and TLR-4, which may initiate prolonged inflammatory responses in the testis. However, clinical reports of the detection of various cytokines in testis biopsy specimens from infertile men have been still limited. To elucidate the mechanisms underlying the spermatogenic disturbance during human immune orchitis, functional analyses of cytokines and establishment of cytokine therapies in various EAO models will be expected.

Additionally, factors of damage to the spermatogenesis other than cytokines must also be kept in mind. Testicular inflammation may elevate the organ temperature and also disturb microcirculation in the testis, resulting in heat and ischemic damage to the seminiferous epithelium. Preferential accumulation of lymphocytes around the tubuli recti in EAO may cause dysfunction of valve structure of modified Sertoli cells inside the tubuli recti and then increase intra-seminiferous tubular pressure. A recent study showed that an impaired removal of apoptotic TGC induce noninfectious testicular inflammation, thus favoring testicular autoimmunity (Schuppe and Meinhardt 2005; Schuppe et al. 2008; Pelletier et al. 2009). The meaning of phagocytic removal of apoptotic TGC by Sertoli cells should be also an interesting topic to be investigated in field for maintaining testicular immune microenvironment.

During EAO, the spermatogenic disturbance may involve both failure of TGC differentiation and facilitation of TGC death (Kuerban et al. 2012). It remains unclear whether TGC death is by necrosis, apoptosis, or cell death involving autophagy. Recently, autophagy has been focused in various cells (Enomoto et al. 2007; Yokoyama et al. 2008; Kawakita et al. 2009; Ohtomo et al. 2010; Kawaguchi et al. 2011; Komatsu et al. 2012). It may be that TGC leaked out of BTB receive necrosis; however, TGC death inside the BTB results from not only apoptosis and but also autophagy. Besides initiating apoptotic pathways, EAO also may induce autophagic pathways in TGC and/or Sertoli cells, including autophagosome formation (Bustamanter-Marin et al. 2012; Eid et al. 2012, 2015; Han et al. 2015).

8.2.4 Identification of Relevant Autoantigens for Autoimmune Orchitis

Testicular autoantigens expressed in haploid TGC appear after puberty when immunocompetence has been already established. A large number of testis-specific autoantigens are present not only on spermatids and spermatozoa but also on spermatogonia, spermatocytes, Sertoli cells, Leydig cells, and basement membrane of the tubular walls (Sato et al. 1981; Lustig et al. 1982, 1987; Ichinohasama et al. 1986; Yule et al. 1988). For a more complete understanding of the immune pathogenesis of EAO, molecular and biochemical approaches to

TGC autoantigens from mice at different weeks after birth are needed. However, the molecular structure of autoantigens relative to EAO has been little characterized. Considering that testicular homogenate+CFA+BP-induced EAO involves immune responses against various antigens, it may be difficult to clear which proteins are target antigens that are critical for EAO induction. To identify the target autoantigens effectively, its investigation using EAO models induced by no use of any chemical or bacterial agents such as active EAO induced by immunization with testicular antigens alone and spontaneous EAO after manipulation of immune system may be easy and useful.

Although EAO-inducing TGC are highly species-specific, there are also common testicular antigens among different species for eliciting anti-TGC DTH with or without involving EAO (Yoshida et al. 1979, 1981; Adekunle et al. 1987; Qu et al. 2017). Moreover, sporadic orchitis and spermatogenic disturbance were observed with immunization with non-testicular antigens such as brain, spinal cord, thyroid gland, kidney, adrenal gland, and ovary emulsified in CFA and concomitant intravenous injection with BP (Adekunle et al. 1987). Therefore, EAO-inducing T cells can be also activated by stimulation with non-testicular peptides that cross-react with testicular autoantigens at the level of the TCR. This molecular mimicry depends in part on the sharing between unrelated peptides of the few critical amino acids that are required for activation of pathogenic orchitogenic T cells. If the candidate purified autoantigen-specific $CD4^+$ T cell clone is established and shown to induce EAO by adoptive transfer to naïve recipients, we can identify the purified protein as the target autoantigen of EAO in the future.

8.2.5 Genetic Control of Autoimmune Orchitis

Identification of susceptible and resistant strains of inbred mice and the phenotyping of segregating populations derived from them allow an estimation of the number of genes involved. Previous studies have demonstrated that genetic predisposition is a major contributor to EAO susceptibility and resistance. It should be also determined whether immune responses to relevant testicular autoantigens are primarily regulatory or active in nature for each strain. Research based on molecular linkage analysis of inbred mice has been embarked upon for mapping genes that influence the susceptibility and resistance to EAO. In general, the MHC is the primary genetic determination of autoimmune disease susceptibility with multiple additional interacting loci required.

In regard to EAO, Balb/c strain ($H\text{-}2^d$) is susceptible to testicular antigen+CFA+BP immunization but resistant to TGC immunization or neonatal thymectomy. C3H/He ($H\text{-}2^d$) strain is susceptible to TGC immunization but resistant to testicular antigen+CFA+BP immunization or neonatal thymectomy. C57BL/6 ($H\text{-}2^b$) strain is susceptible to testicular antigen+CFA+BP immunization or neonatal thymectomy but resistant to TGC immunization. In contrast, A/J strain ($H\text{-}2^a$) is susceptible to the all three EAO models. Therefore, genetic susceptibility to EAO differs among the three disease models (Itoh et al. 1991a; Tokunaga et al. 1993a, b; Kojima and

Prehn 1981; Kojima and Spencer 1983; Teuscher et al. 1985a, b). Identification of susceptible and resistant strains of inbred mice and the phenotyping of segregating populations derived from them allow an establishment of the number of genes involved in each EAO model. Genetic analysis of inbred mouse strains until now indicates that susceptibility or resistance to EAO is polygenic and strongly influenced by both H-2-linked and non-H2-linked genes (Person et al. 1992). However, the identification and characterization of non-MHC genes have been problematic, since most autoimmune diseases are polygenic with the individual genes exhibiting only partial or minimal penetrance.

There are also some EAO models developed by gene manipulations such as rearranged TCR alpha-chain gene transfer, HLA-B27 gene transfer, TAM gene knockout, Aire gene knockout, and p35 gene knockout (Hammer et al. 1990; Sakaguchi et al. 1994; Lu et al. 1999; Hubert et al. 2009; Sun et al. 2010; Taurog et al. 2012; Zhang et al. 2013b; Terayama et al. 2014). Trials of these gene manipulations on various murine inbred strains may also contribute to the understanding of genetic control of EAO.

8.2.6 Therapeutic Control of Autoimmune Orchitis by Treg

The effective treatment of organ-specific inflammatory disorders of putative autoimmune origin is an ongoing goal in clinical medicine. Because the lymphocytic infiltration of the testis, the disturbance of spermatogenesis and the occurrence of DTH responses against testicular antigens can be observed in cases of human immunologic infertility (Anderson and Hill 1998); EAO should be used as in vivo tool for studying immuno-inflammatory pathways and immunotherapeutic approaches for the treatment of the human orchitis.

Cyclosporine A and deoxyspergualin have been used for the EAO treatment (Hojo and Hiramine 1985; Ablake et al. 2002). For specific inhibition of disease, adoptive transfer of tissue antigen-specific Treg may offer one of the effective treatments. In the normal state, there may be pathogenic clones reactive to autoantigens of TGC and clones to regulate such autoreactive cells, but these clones may keep silent in the appropriate balance between the clones. Strong proliferation of TGC-specific effector clones may occur after two or three injections with TGC, but the predominance of TGC-specific Treg clones may be generated in the course of more repeated immunization (Itoh et al. 1992a, b). Antigen-specific regulation of EAO has been also demonstrated following repeated intravenous injection of deaggregated, soluble testis antigens (Mukasa et al. 1992). Mice treated in this manner developed long-lasting resistance to the induction of EAO from subsequent challenge with TGC. In EAO developed in mice that received various immune-manipulations by neonatal thymectomy, irradiation, or drugs, specific deletion or dysfunction of T cell population, both naturally occurring Treg and inducible Treg, should illustrate the complex nature and balance of immunoregulation. Therefore, multiple Treg populations may be present and participate for EAO regulation.

8.2.7 Effects of Environmental Toxicants on Autoimmune Orchitis

Although the mechanisms for the development of autoimmune diseases remains obscure, accumulating evidence suggests that these increasingly recognized disorders result from environmental or occupational exposures of noninfectious agents in genetically susceptible individuals (Miller 2014). Impaired health status such as malnutrition, obesity, alcohol, tobacco, or illicit drug use may affect spermatogenesis (Eid et al. 2012, 2015). Nowadays, we can take various medicines and are daily exposed to various environmental toxicants of low doses (Ishihara et al. 2000; Gu et al. 2003; Ablake et al. 2004; Miyaso et al. 2010, 2014a, b; Kitaoka et al. 2013; Ogawa et al. 2013; Hirai et al. 2015). Some of them have ability to affect testicular function or immune function. To investigate whether various chemicals such as cadmium, uranium, phthalic acid esters, tamoxifen, diethylstilbestrol, bisphenol A, decabromodiphenyl ether, flutamide, alcohol, and cigarette smoking affect the incidence and severity of testicular autoimmunity is also valid (Fig. 8.1). The increased output of these chemicals has drawn a large number of people into contact with these elements. Malenchenko et al. (1978) were the first to investigate the effect of an environment chemical on the EAO induction by the use of uranium. Recently, it has appeared that low dose exposure of cadmium or phthalic acid significantly increased susceptibility of EAO (Ogawa et al. 2013; Hirai et al. 2015). Neonatal treatment with estrogen developed severe epididymo-vasitis later (Naito et al. 2014). It was also found that neonatal exposure to diethylstilbestrol, artificial estrogenic compound, induced epididymitis in all treated mice after 5 weeks of age and also evoked orchitis in some mice after 12 weeks of age (Miyaso et al. 2014a, b). These inflammatory lesions may be of "autoimmune/autoinflammatory syndrome induced by adjuvants (ASIA)," in which estrogen acts as an adjuvant in male mice. A study of the effect of di-(2-ethylhexyl) phthalate on the testicular immune microenvironment revealed that lymphocytes and F4/80- and MHC class II antigen-positive cells were significantly increased with the elevation of IL-10 and IFN-gamma mRNA expressions in the testes (Kitaoka et al. 2013). Histochemical

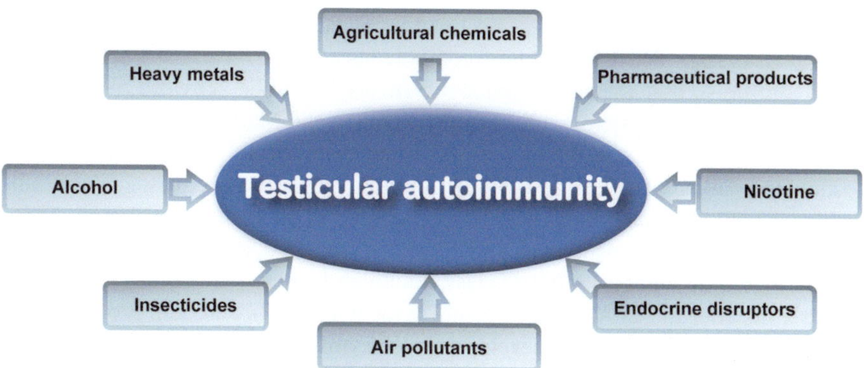

Fig. 8.1 Various environmental toxicants for possible modulation of the testicular autoimmunity

analyses involving horseradish peroxidase as a tracer showed that a little blood-borne horseradish peroxidase had infiltrated into the lumen of a few seminiferous tubules beyond the BTB. Age- and species-dependent infiltration of macrophages into the testes of rats and mice exposed to phthalate was also demonstrated (Murphy et al. 2014). In that study, a significant increase in monocyte chemoattractant protein-1 by peritubular myoid cells occurred 12 h after phthalate exposure.

In regard to the effect of other environmental factors on testicular autoimmunity, it may be also valuable whether exposure to an electromagnetic wave and field could affect EAO (Grigorev et al. 1981; Naito et al. 2012; Hanci et al. 2013). Exposure to a 900-MHz electromagnetic field in the prenatal term on the 21-old-day rat induced irregularities in seminiferous epithelium and tubular basal membrane accompanied by decreased diameter of the seminiferous tubules. Apoptotic index, lipid peroxidation, and DNA oxidation were higher than controls (Hanci et al. 2013). The increased TGC apoptosis may give specific lymphocytes a chance to react with TGC autoantigens more easily.

8.2.8 Immunopathology of the Male Reproductive Organs During Prolonged Sensitization with Xenoantigens

In the "autoimmune/autoinflammatory syndrome induced by adjuvants" (ASIA), different conditions induced by various adjuvants such as infectious fragments, hormones, aluminum, silicone, and metal are included, and the syndrome is characterized by common signs and symptoms, resulting in boosting the immune response and triggering the development of autoinflammatory phenomena (Loyo et al. 2012; Cruz-Tapias et al. 2013; Lujan et al. 2013; Colafrancesco et al. 2014).

CFA and BP have been used as adjuvants for EAO induction. Treatment with CFA and BP releases various pro-inflammatory cytokines involving IL-1-beta, IL-6, IL-12 TNF-alpha, and IFN-gamma in vivo (Mielcarek et al. 2001; Tonon et al. 2002; Raghavendra et al. 2004). In mice that were intravenously injected with BP alone, systemic inflammation involving hepatosplenomegaly and lymphadenopathy was induced, and the ductuli efferentes, the epididymis, the vas deferens, and the accessory sex glands in BP-injected mice received inflammatory cell infiltration (Itoh et al. 1995a). The mycobacterial components within CFA signal T cells assume a Th1 profile so that various lymphocytic clones should be activated, resulting in enhancement of the systemic inflammation (Billiau and Matthys 2001). Indeed, the employment of CFA and BP has proved to be instrumental in the breakdown of testicular immune privilege and microcircumstance for the spermatogenesis indirectly, as well as in augmenting of DTH (Pelletier et al. 1981; Sewell et al. 1986; Adekunle et al. 1987; Lustig et al. 1987; Mealy et al. 1990; Perez et al. 2011, 2012). Furthermore, the number of MHC class II antigen-bearing macrophages increased in the testis after the CFA+BP treatment (Tung et al. 1987), and both production of anti-TGC autoantibodies and development of cytolytic activity of T cells against TGC are inducible without the use of testicular antigens for sensitization (Ben et al.

1986; Musha et al. 2013). Therefore, CFA+BP treatment also may induce ASIA-like condition. Therefore, there is a possibility that EAO may be inducible with CFA+BP treatment alone if some optimal conditions such as more prolonged, chronic, and repeated sensitization with the adjuvants or other xenogeneic antigens are devised.

It is of considerable interest to know what happens in the host associated with the failure in the elaborate systemic immune system. Presumably such a critical situation could be created experimentally in animals by enforced overwork of the immune system, e.g., by repeated immunizations with an appreciable but not tolerogenic amount of xenoantigens over an extended period. Historically, Okabayashi and his colleagues (1980) had innovatively investigated prolonged sensitization with xenoantigens such as ovalbumin, hemolytic streptococci, *Escherichia coli*, bovine serum albumin, and horse serum over a year (Fig. 8.2). They had carried out a series of experiments in the experimental animals to clarify the overall sequence of events taking place in the immune system of the host by means of chronic and prolonged antigenic stimulation by using foreign proteins or bacterial antigens (Okabayashi 1964, 1967a, b, 1972, 1973, 1979). With such repeated immunization, the animals showed an enhanced immune cell proliferation in the lymphoid organs, together with accelerated hematopoiesis in the bone marrow. However, the reactivity of the immune system may not be permanent. Following continued antigen administration, the systemic immune reaction developed to the highest level during the middle stage but gradually became less reactive. A wasting in the systemic immune reaction thus ensued in the terminal stage as evidenced by progressive exhaustion of lymphoid responses. The bone marrow likewise showed prominent hypoplasia with or without fibrosis, and a variety of diseases of the blood, organs, and tissues such as mucoid, fibrinoid, hyaline, and amyloid degeneration occurred in sequence. Okabayashi had emphasized that before entering into the overt anergic or exhausted terminal phase, certain immunologic disorders develop in the later stage of prolonged antigenic stimulation which are significantly different from those observed during the early stages. Alterations of the organs and tissues gradually became degenerative in nature; however, under conditions of the imbalance in the wasting immune system, there appeared not only the degenerative conversion of the inflammatory process but also the development of "autoimmunization." The resulting dysplasia of lymphoid tissues and imbalance of the immune cell population, which could be interpreted in terms of the disturbance in immunological regulation, may induce "autoimmune diseases in the wasting immunity." Therefore, the chronically sensitized host is affected by systemic immune reaction for a long period, and prolonged antigenic sensitization induces all four immunopathies composed of immunoproliferative diseases, allergic and hypersensitivity diseases, immunodeficiency diseases, and autoimmune diseases (Fig. 8.3). Although the heart, kidneys, and various lymphoid organs have been well investigated (Okabayashi et al. 1980), it should be of interest to investigate whether and how the testis and other male reproductive organs are immunopathologically affected during prolonged sensitization with xenoantigens.

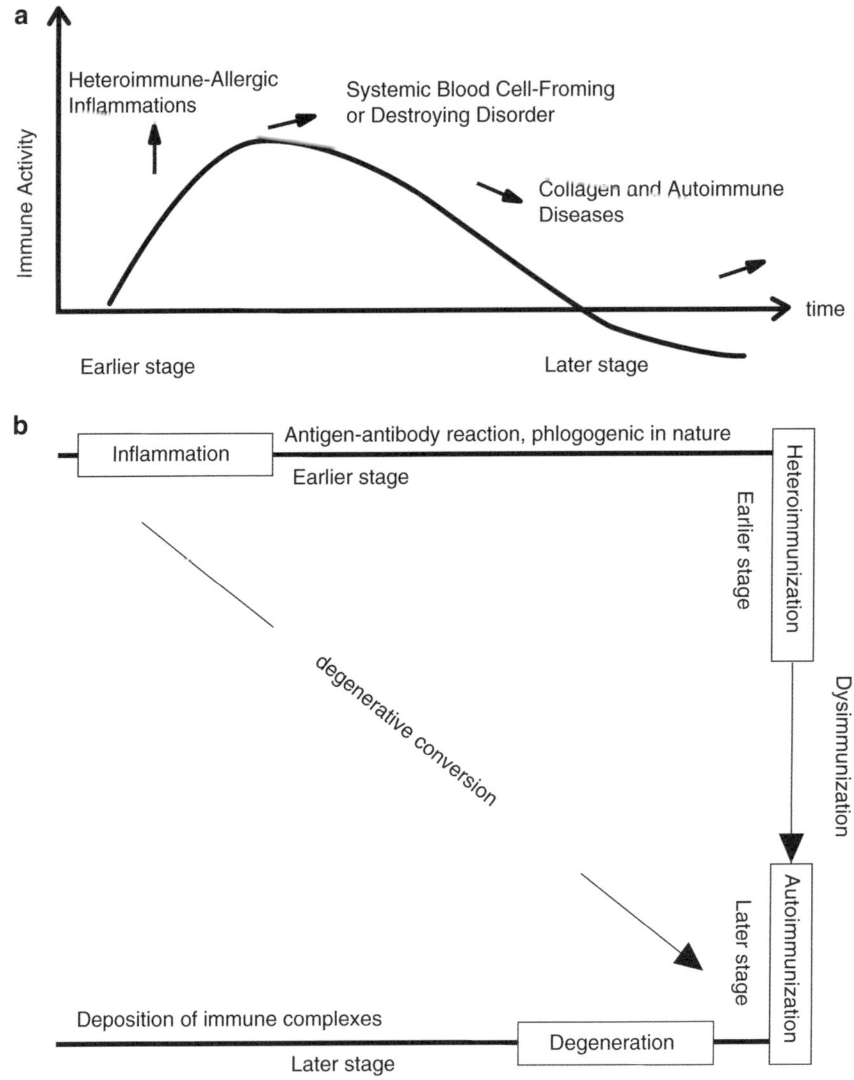

Fig. 8.2 Prolonged antigenic sensitization. (**a**) Chronology and deployment of the systemic immune reaction and its disorders. (**b**) Prominence of degenerative conversion and dysimmunization resulting in autoimmune diseases (autoimmunization) in the later stage (Okabayashi et al. 1980. Partly modified)

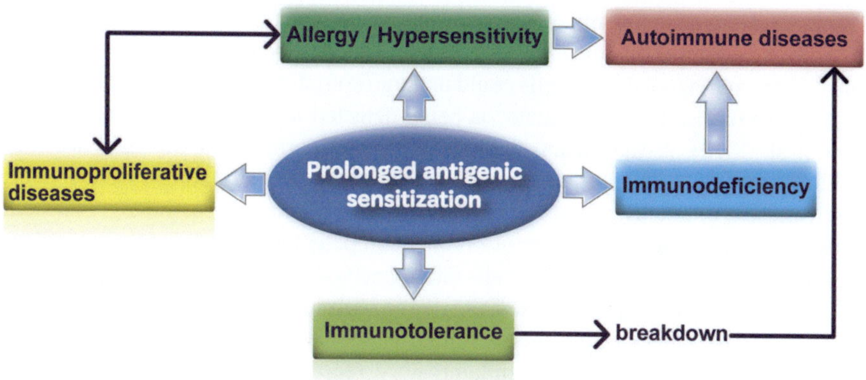

Fig. 8.3 The effects of prolonged antigenic sensitization on the immune system

8.2.9 Transplant Immunology of the Testis at Cellular, Tissue, and Organ Levels

In animals that received allogeneic or xenogeneic cells, tissues, or organs, "graft-versus-host reaction" or "transplant rejection" occurs if some immunosuppressive treatments are not given. In testicular immunology, four transplantation models described below may help the investigation on physiology of testicular immune privilege.

8.2.9.1 Transplantation of Spermatogonial Stem Cells into the Seminiferous Tubules

Spermatogonial stem cells are foundation of spermatogenesis and are characterized by their ability to self-renew and to produce differentiated progeny that forms spermatozoa. It has been known that rat spermatogenesis can occur in the seminiferous tubules of immune-depressed recipient mice after transplantation of rat spermatogonical stem cells. This transplant model should be useful for further study of testicular immune privilege. In previous studies on xenogeneic spermatogonial stem cells transplantation, to avoid immunologic rejection, inherently immunodeficient or experimentally immunosuppressed adult mice were used as the recipients. In another study, hamster spermatogenesis could be induced within the seminiferous tubules of rats when the hamster spermatogonial stem cells were transplanted to the testes of infant rats that have immaturity in both the immune system and the seminiferous epithelium (Tanaka et al. 1997). Before the xenogeneic spermatogonial stem cells, recipients are conventionally pretreated with busulfan for depletion of endogenous TGC (Clouthier et al. 1996). However, high-dose busulfan has a detrimental effect on the Sertoli cell secretory function and subsequently impaired the recipient Sertoli cell capacity to support donor spermatogonial stem cell differentiation or sometimes results in death of recipients. Later, transplantation of rat spermatogonial stem cells into immunocompetent mice was examined. The results showed that some transplanted spermatogonial stem cells could undergo complete spermatogenesis in recipient mouse testes, the rat spermatozoa being detected in the recipient epididymides (Qu et al. 2012). A significant increase in mouse spermatozoa was also noted in epididymides of recipient mice regardless of whether rat spermatozoa were concurrently present or not. These results suggest that transplanted rat spermatogonial stem cells can be tolerated in the testes of immunocompetent mice and that the transplantation of rat spermatogonial stem cells simultaneously stimulated endogenous spermatogenesis in the recipient mice. Despite the high immunogenicity of xenogeneic TGC, they can remain within the seminiferous tubules, epididymal ducts, and vasa deferentia without eliciting any inflammatory reactions. Although busulfan suppresses bone marrow function, it appeared that immune functions in busulfan-treated mice recovered to normal level when spermagonial stem cells were transplanted (Hirayanagi et al. 2015). The analysis of the experimental model will be followed with interest.

Transplantation of spermatogonial cells to or from mutant mice was also examined. Claudin-5 is expressed in Sertoli cells, spermatogonia, and preleptotene spermatocytes. It contributes to the formation of the BTB and regulated by the transcription factor Ets variant gene-5 (Etv5) (Morrow et al. 2009). The transcription factor Etv5 is essential for spermatogonial stem cell self-renewal, as the targeted deletion of the Etv5 gene in mice (Etv5$^{-/-}$) results in only the first wave of spermatogenesis, and all spermatogonial stem cells are lost during this time, causing a Sertoli cell-only phenotype (Schlesser et al. 2008; Tyagi et al. 2009). Reciprocal transplants of neonatal germ cells from wild-type and Etv5$^{-/-}$ testes were performed to determine the role of Etv5 in Sertoli cells and germ cells. Etv5 appears to be needed in both cell types for normal spermatogenesis. It is noted that Etv5$^{-/-}$ recipients displayed EAO-like lesions composed of deficient formation of the BTB, increased interstitial inflammation, and involution of the seminiferous tubules after transplantation of wild-type spermatogonial stem cells (Morrow et al. 2007). Preliminary studies suggest that the BTB is abnormal in the Etv5$^{-/-}$ mouse. The tight junctional protein claudin-5 was decreased in testes of neonatal Etv5$^{-/-}$ mice. Immunobiological analyses between transplanted stem cells and host somatic testicular cells should be significant for further study of testicular immune circumstance.

8.2.9.2 Transplantation of Testicular Somatic Cells into the Testis

For treatment for male infertility, Malolina et al. (2014) determined whether testicular cell transplantation is effective at repairing testicular injury induced by herpes simplex virus orchitis. ROSA26 mice were used as donors, and the recipients were C57BL/6 mice after herpes simplex virus testicular inoculation. In recipient testes, donor Sertoli cells formed new seminiferous tubules. At day 150, the seminiferous epithelium was completely recovered in some recipient tubules, and elongated spermatids were observed, indicating the effectiveness of allogeneic testicular somatic cell transplantation for restoration of spermatogenesis damaged by viral infections.

It is well known that cadmium exhibits severe gonadotoxicity inducing irreversible damage to the seminiferous epithelium (Ogawa et al. 2013). When Sertoli cells recovered and dissociated from donor testes were microinjected into recipient testes treated with cadmium in mice, they formed mature seminiferous tubule structures and supported spermatogenesis (Shinohara et al. 2003). Furthermore, transplantation of wild-type Sertoli cells into infertile Steel/Steel (dickie) testes created a permissive testicular microenvironment for generating spermatogenesis.

Seminiferous tubular cells were transplanted from normal immature transgenic donor rats into the testis of irradiated recipient rats. In many seminiferous tubules, the donor Sertoli cells formed abnormal spherical structures in the lumen, but in some tubules they formed a normal-appearing epithelium with only isolated spermatogonia, on the basement membrane (Zhang et al. 2009). When the donor tubular cells were injected into the interstitial region of the testis, they formed tubule-like structures containing Sertoli cells and isolated spermatogonia, both of donor origin. Especially, in host tubules adjacent to these newly formed donor-cell tubules or adjacent to the endogenous tubules with abnormal donor Sertoli cell structures, endogenous spermatogonia differentiated to the spermatocytes or even to spermatid stages. In the testicular interstitium around these newly donor cell-formed tubules and the host tubules with abnormal donor Sertoli cell structures, EAO-like lesions involving many circulating and resident macrophages accumulated in the interstitium were present. Therefore, the donor Sertoli cells that colonized the seminiferous tubules did not directly support recovery of spermatogenesis. Instead, the colonizing Sertoli cells acted indirectly on the interstitium to stimulate localized differentiation of endogenous spermatogonia. The further analyses of Sertoli cell transplantation should light on immunobiological milieu of supporting tissue for TGC. Transplantation of Leydig cells, testicular macrophages, and peritubular myoid cells may be also valid for study of recovery of spermatogenesis and local immune circumstance.

8.2.9.3 Transplantation of Whole Testis

The testis is regarded as an immune-privileged organ in that allogeneic tissue can be successfully transplanted into the testicular interstitium or transplanted allogeneic testicular tissue is resistant to the rejection. However, to investigate its immune privilege more clearly, transplantation of whole donor testis should be tried by surgical anastomosis with recipient's blood vessels. Transplantation of a set of testis with testicular artery and vein, ductuli efferentes, epididymides and a part of vas deferens into syngeneic males, allogeneic males, xenogeneic males, syngeneic male that were castrated at various ages, or syngeneic females may be helpful for studying testicular immunology. If the immune privilege status in the transplanted organs is broken down in recipients, EAO-like lesions may be induced in the transplanted organ. Lee et al. (1971) are the first to transplant allogeneic testis in the rat. In the allogeneic testis, perivascular mononuclear cellular infiltrates first appeared at 18 h after testicular transplantation. On day 3, lymphocytes and macrophages were confined to the perivascular region, and none entered the seminiferous tubules. Necrosis of seminiferous epithelium first appeared on day 3 and became progressive thereafter.

Perivascular mononuclear cell infiltrates were also found in the epididymis during the first 7 days. The epididymal changes included infiltration of mononuclear cells in the epididymal tubular walls, infiltration of polymorphonuclear neutrophils, and formation of abscesses, followed by fibrosis and granuloma formation. However, technical difficulty for testis transplantation has disturbed its further study for long years. Most recently, a different and more convenient technique for the testis transplantation has been developed, and transplant immunology of the testis is now in progress in the rat (Yi et al. submitted).

8.2.9.4 Transplantation of Bone Marrow Cells

Clinically, gonadal function is a key to quality of life following bone marrow transplantation for patients with malignancy. In patients who underwent bone marrow transplantation for a variety of hematological malignancies, the patients sustained severe gonadal damage to both their seminiferous epithelium as well as the Leydig cell compartment (Chatterjee et al. 2001). This deficit has been mainly attributed to pre-transplantation conditioning, but lower sperm counts in human also appear to be associated with GVHD following allogeneic bone marrow transplantation. Indeed, recipients of allogeneic transplantation experienced significantly more severe damage to TGC compartment compared to those who received an autologous transplant (Kyriacou et al. 2003).

Earlier studies of transplantation outcomes have shown that male recipients of female HLA-identical hematopoietic stem cell transplants experience increased GVHD. Male recipients of transplants from female hematopoietic stem cell donors represent a special group in which donor T cells that are specific for minor histocompatibility antigens encoded by Y-chromosome gens may contribute to a GVHD (Randolph et al. 2004). In mice that had received allogeneic bone marrow transplantation, the intra-testicular infiltration of donor alloreactive T cells followed by injury to testicular cells occurred during an acute GVHD (Wagner et al. 2005). The nadir of Leydig cell volume density coincided with the peak of intra-testicular infiltration by donor T cells. Injury to Leydig cells correlated with an intra-testicular inflammatory response characterized by INF-gamma and TNF-alpha production. It is now in progress whether some histopathological changes are induced or not in testes of mice that received transplantation of bone marrow cells from syngeneic males, allogeneic males, syngeneic females, allogeneic females, and syngeneic male that had been castrated at various ages in our laboratory. The analysis of this experimental model should be obviously a topic of considerable ongoing interest.

In other studies, differentiation of bone marrow stem cells into male germ cell lineage has been tried (Ghasemzadeh-Hasankolaei et al. 2014; Zhang et al. 2014a). Allogeneic bone marrow mesenchymal stem cells were co-cultured in conditioned media derived from cultured Sertoli cells in vitro, and then induced stem cells were transplanted into the seminiferous tubules of a busulfan-induced rat model. The in vitro induced cells exhibited specific TGC gene and protein markers, and after implantation the donor cells survived and located at the basement membranes of the recipient seminiferous tubules. No tumor mass, immune response, or inflammatory reaction developed.

It is known that bone marrow also contains mesenchymal stem cells. In mice receiving testis rupture, single dose of 5×10^5 bone marrow-derived mesenchymal stem cells was delivered intravenously (Aghamir et al. 2014). In this model, bone marrow-derived mesenchymal stem cells transfusion showed immunosuppressive effects on anti-sperm antibody production. Transplantation of mesenchymal bone marrow stem cells into the seminiferous tubules of recipient animals has been also noted (Lassalle et al. 2008; Horn et al. 2008; Zhang et al. 2014a). In recipient mice, the donor cells survived and located at the basement membranes of the seminiferous epithelium, and cellular organization of the seminiferous epithelium was found, but the improvement in spermatogenesis was quite incomplete, and no inflammatory reactions developed. On the other hand, recovery of spermatogenesis in busulfan-treated rats after local transfer of adipose tissue-derived mesenchymal stem cells was reported (Cakici et al. 2013). Therefore, transplanted bone marrow cells have a capability to induce GVHD or immunosuppression and also differentiation to male germ cell lineage. Immunobiological analyses on between transplanted stem cells and host somatic testicular cells should be significant for further study of testicular immune circumstance.

8.2.10 Biology of Relation Between Innate and Adaptive Immunity for Autoimmune Orchitis

TGC and immune cells are cores for life, but the own immune cells sometimes attack TGC auto-immunologically. In particular, testicular autoantigens, expressed on haploid TGC, appear after puberty and are not available to interact with lymphocytes early in life. The mechanisms underlying the testicular immune privilege have been investigated for several decades. Considering that central tolerance might require the interaction between developing TGC and developing lymphocytes before puberty, it has been assumed that regulatory mechanisms other than the central tolerance, such as innate immunity and peripheral tolerance, might prevent testicular autoimmunity and inflammation.

Before evolution and development of adoptive immunity, the testis mounts appropriate local innate immunity against invading pathogens. During infections, activation of inflammation is triggered by recognition of specific motifs, or pathogen-associated molecular patterns, found on bacterial, viral, fungal, and protozoan pathogens, medicated by specific pattern recognition receptors. The best characterization of these receptors is the TLR, which recognize bacterial and viral nucleic acids and other molecules unique to pathogens, including lipopolysaccharide, bacterial lipopeptides, and peptidoglycans (Kawai and Akira 2010). TLR recognize pathogen-associated molecular patterns and elicit antimicrobial immune responses. The innate defense system in the testis is also being revealed based on the identification of pattern recognition receptor-initiated immune responses (Chen et al. 2016). Therefore, TLR in Sertoli cells and testicular macrophages may play important roles in initiating testicular innate immune response. If adaptive immunity is normally modulated within the testis to minimize responses against TGC, innate immunity becomes more important for protecting the testis against infection and tumors. However, innate immunity against live *Escherichia coli* inside the seminiferous tubules leads to local inflammation with the resultant long-term damage to the seminiferous epithelium (Demir et al. 2007). It was demonstrated that damaged TGC products in the seminiferous tubules induce expression of various inflammatory mediators, including TNF-alpha, IL-1-beta, IL-6, and macrophage chemotactic protein 1, in Sertoli cells (Zhang et al. 2013a). Notably, damaged TGC-induced inflammatory gene expression was significantly reduced by knockout TLR-2 or TRL-4 and abolished by double knockout TLR-2 and TLR-4 (TLR-$2^{-/-}$TLR-$4^{-/-}$). This indicates that damaged TGC induce inflammatory gene expression in Sertoli cells via the activation of TLR-2 and TLR-4, which may initiate noninfectious inflammatory responses in the testis. Tyro-3, Axl, and Mer (TAM) receptors belong to a subfamily of receptor tyrosine kinases and are negative regulators of TLR-initiated systemic innate immunity and play critical roles in regulating immune responses (Lu et al. 1999; Sun et al. 2010). Mutant mice that lack these receptors develop the upregulation of various inflammatory cytokines, resulting in a severe lymphoproliferative disorder accompanied by broad-spectrum autoimmunity in the lung, liver, kidney, heart, pancreas, intestine, skeletal muscle, eye, brain, and spinal cord (Lu and Lemke 2001), and they also exhibit severe defects of the spermatogenesis and clearance of apoptotic TGC (Lu et al. 1999; Sun et al. 2010; Zhang et al. 2013a, b). TGC were progressively degenerated, and macrophages and lymphocytes infiltrated into the testis as $TAM^{-/-}$ mice aged. Moreover, the integrity of BTB was impaired, and anti-TGC autoantibodies were produced. TNF-alpha, IL-6, and monocyte chemotactic protein-1 were upregulated in the testis of $TAM^{-/-}$ mice and predominantly located in Sertoli cells. Secretion of other cytokines such as IL-1-beta and interferons alpha and beta were also elevated (Sun et al. 2010). Therefore, innate immunity in the testis may be involved for a first defense against testicular infection but also the start of testicular autoimmunity. Fine balance between the modulation of ability to resist infection or neoplasms and the attempt to minimize intra-testicular inflammation is important for ongoing spermatogenesis.

In addition to TLR, the cytosolic double-stranded RNA sensors, termed retinoic acid-inducible gene I-like receptors, NOD-like receptor members, and intracellular DNA sensors, have been also emerged as pattern recognition receptors that recognize a broad spectrum of pathogen-associated molecules patterns and damage-associated molecular patterns. The functions of the inflammasomes, an inflammation-promoting multiprotein oligomer consisting of caspase 1, apoptosis-associated speck-like protein, NOD-like receptor, and caspase 5, in the testis remain to be clarified (Zhao et al. 2014). The term "autoinflammatory syndrome" is caused by excessive inflammasome activation and characterized by unexplained episodes of fever and severe localized inflammation. The original definition was "seemingly unprovoked inflammation without high-titer autoantibodies or antigen-specific T cells" (McDermott et al. 1999). There is a well-confirmed evidence for "autoimmune/autoinflammatory syndrome induced by adjuvants (ASIA)" including the adjuvant arthritis model induced by injection of CFA in experimental animals (Shoenfeld and Agmon-Levin 2011; Colafrancesco et al. 2014). CFA-induced peripheral inflammation evokes pro-inflammatory cytokines such as IL-1-beta, IL-6 TNF-alpha, and IFN-gamma (Lapchak et al. 1992; Chuang et al. 1997; Raghavendra et al. 2004). In vivo intoxication with BP elicits a variety of physiological responses including a marked leukocytosis, disruption of glucose regulation, adjuvant activity, alterations in vascular function, hypersensitivity to vasoactive agents, and upregulation of MHC class II molecules (Tonon et al. 2002; Gao et al. 2003). BP-induced lymphocytosis is associated with alteration in thymocyte subpopulations (Person et al. 1992). BP primarily affects and depletes thymic T cells with an immature phenotype. However, in the periphery of BP-treated mice, the relative increase in the number of $CD4^+$ T cells is more than that of $CD8^+$ T cells. In regard to pro-inflammatory cytokines, BP treatment induced the release of IL-6, IL-12, and TNF-alpha (Mielcarek et al. 2001; Tonon et al. 2002). In regard to the testis, CFA+BP treatment evoked testicular dysfunction and also induced both cellular and humoral autoimmune responses against testicular autoantigens (Musha et al. 2013). Therefore, it may be possible that EAO is triggered by innate immunity following some optimal treatment with adjuvants alone. Moreover, there remains a possibility that tuberculosis, whooping cough, and vaccination for these two diseases affect testicular autoimmunity clinically.

From the point of view of immune evolution, it may be interesting to try experimental testicular inflammation of autoimmune and non-autoimmune origins in primitive mammals such as *Suncus murinus* and nonmammals such as reptiles, birds, amphibians, fishes, and primitive animals. If male reproductive immunology in mammals is compared with that of other species, we may be able to derive some unknown findings about relation between TGC and immune cells. In regard to the fish, EAO has been demonstrated in Atlantic salmon and rainbow trout following intramuscularly immunization with the testicular homogenate+CFA (Laird et al. 1980; Secombes et al. 1985a, b). Although granulomatous EAO could completely fill the seminiferous tubules and sperm duct, the lesion had no inhibitory effect on spermatogenesis during a subsequent maturation in the fishes. Immunization with testicular homogenate containing haploid TGC+CFA developed EAO, but immunization with testicular homogenate containing only premeiotic TGC+CFA did not induce EAO in the fishes (Secombes et al. 1985b). In testicular homogenate+CFA-induced EAO of the Nile tilapia, inflammatory cells were composed of lymphocytes, macrophages, eosinophils and plasma cells (Mochida et al. 1995). In regard to the bird, Wentworth and Mellen (1964) first succeeded in EAO induction in quails by immunization with testis in CFA. Later, the expression profiles of TLR were determined in the testis of roosters (Zhang et al. 2012). In roosters that were intravenously injected with lipopolysaccharide, expression of TLR4 was significantly upregulated in the tesits but not in the epididymis. Furthermore, expression of IL-1-beta, IL-6, and other chemokines was also upregulated by lipopolysaccharide injection (Zhang et al. 2012). The avian beta-defensins (avBD) are antimicrobial peptides and attack various microorganisms and may have efficacy to protect tissues from infection. In a study of the mRNA expressions of TLR and avBD of chicken spermatozoa incubated with lipopolysaccharide in vitro, TLR-2 to TRL-5, TRL-7, TLR-15, and TLR-21 were identified, and avBD-1, avBD-3, avBD-5, and avBD-7 to avBD-12 were also expressed by the incubated spermatozoa (Das et al. 2011). In the future, development of nonmammal EAO models with the lipopolysaccharide treatment or without depending on any bacterial component has been eagerly awaited.

In conclusion, the function of pattern recognition receptors and their role in negatively regulating systemic tolerance to testicular autoantigens are areas for future research. The coordination between immune privilege and local innate immune responses is critical in the maintenance of testicular immune homeostasis. Notably, the innate immune response is a double-edged sword in that defense against microbial pathogens is critical for hosts to recover from infectious diseases, while the inflammatory milieu may cause damage to the host. Dissection of its regulatory mechanisms in the testis could aid the establishment of preventive and therapeutic approaches for testicular autoimmunity.

8.2.11 Physiology of Natural Autoimmunity Against Testicular Antigens

The spermatogenesis starts at puberty when tolerance to various autoantigens was already established long ago. For humans, the entire process of spermatogenesis is estimated as taking more than 70 days (Heller and Clermont 1964; Amann 2008). Including the transport on germ cell duct system, it takes approximately 3 months. The testis produces 200–300 million spermatids and spermatozoa daily; however, only half or approximately 100 million of these become viable spermatozoa, and the rest of them die in the germ cell ducts (Johnson et al. 1983). Therefore, new differentiation autoimmunogenic antigens derived from many dying spermatozoa should be highly and continuously exposed to the immune system beyond the BTB. Therefore, effective clearance of dying TGC is required for homeostasis of male reproductive system. Obviously, the homeostatic importance of autoclearance of TGC debris increases dramatically for prevention of testicular inflammation.

In general, "autoimmune disease" is a pathological state arising from abnormal immune responses against autoantigens. On the other hand, "autoimmunity" is the presence of self-reactive immune response involving autoantibodies and autoreactive T cells, with or without damage resulting from it. Recently, it has been accepted that harmless autoimmune responses termed "natural autoimmunity" or "physiologic autoimmunity" are an integral part of vertebrate immune systems, which do not reflect the potentially self-destructive activity of the immune system (Doria et al. 2012; Poletaev et al. 2012; Poletaev 2014). The desired, nondestructive level of physiologic autoimmunity is ensured by mechanisms of combined negative/positive selection during immune maturation. Actually, anti-sperm autoantibodies and anti-TGC autoantibodies are detectable in normal males, indicating the presence of the natural autoimmunity against testicular antigens (Itoh et al. 1989; Hirai et al. 2013; Musha et al. 2013). Therefore, in testicular autoimmunity, an intense autoimmunity induces autoimmune orchitis; however, a mild or faint autoimmunity may be beneficial and plays a role of one of the self-defense mechanisms of mammal system to survive (Fig. 8.2). Although it remains unclear how the natural autoimmunity works, an autoclearance function of the immune system may be mediated by natural anti-sperm autoantibodies. Indeed, multitudes of natural autoantibodies of Ig G and Ig M classes have been permanently synthesized, secreted, and presented in the blood serum of all healthy persons during life span (Lacroix-Desmazes et al. 1998), and large proportions of natural autoantibodies specifically bind to oxidation-associated neo-antigens that become exposed on dying cells (Chou et al. 2009). In the testis, many TGC die every day by physiological apoptosis and are replaced by new ones under normal condition. It is supposed that some TGC and epididymal spermatozoa autoantigens leaking to blood circulation are normally cleared by reaction with natural anti-TGC autoantibodies. Therefore, natural autoimmunity may be a ground for autoclearance of cell debris of strongly autoimmunogenic TGC.

While a high level of autoimmunity is unhealthy, a low level of autoimmunity may be healthy and beneficial to survive (Fig. 8.4). The autoimmune attack on cells may be the consequence of cycling metabolic processes necessary for the blood homeostasis. Furthermore, it may involve "idiotype-antiidiotypic mechanisms," proposed by Jerne (1974), wherein a network of antibodies capable of neutralizing self-reactive autoantibodies exists naturally within the body. Therefore, natural autoimmunity is involved in self-maintenance, self-reparation, and self-optimization and may provide a harmonious state under the constant pressure of the environment by autoreactive entity based on a complicated and interconnected network of natural autoantibodies and autoreactive lymphocytes (Poletaev 2014). In normal males, a physiological feedback mechanism involving various immune networks with anti-TGC autoantibodies and TGC-specific autoreactive lymphocytes may operate for prevention of the pathogenic autoimmunity.

It is known that "allergy" is an immune response bringing harm rather than defense in the body. Therefore, the physiological autoimmune processes are preferably in relation to the term "(natural) autoimmunity," while the pathogenic autoimmune ones

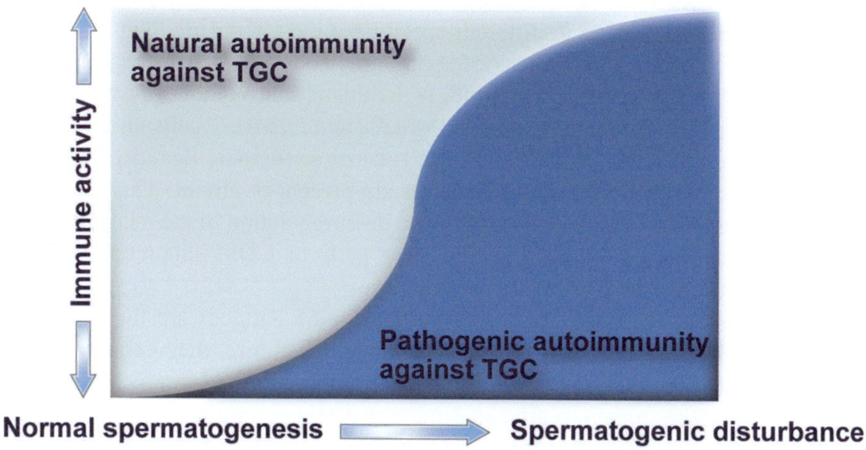

Fig. 8.4 Natural and pathogenic autoimmunity against TGC (testicular germ cells). Normal spermatogenesis is achieved under physiological condition of the natural autoimmunity

may be appropriately expressed as the term "auto-allergy" (Poletaev 2014). In general, as an intrinsic feature of the immune system, autoantibodies and autoreactive lymphocytes are permanently present throughout the organism life and form the interconnected system of self-recognition, and their functions are directed rather "inward" but not "outward" and are based on the intrinsic recognizing components of the "self." In other words, production of particular autoantibodies and autoreactive lymphocytes should not be considered a side effect but rather a physiological reflection of the immune system. In the future, differential and critical points between the natural (beneficial) autoimmune reactions and the pathogenic (harmful) ones against testicular antigens will be more investigated.

8.3 Concluding Remarks

Spermatogenesis is the process in which spermatozoa are produced from spermatogonial stem cells by way of mitosis and meiosis, and it starts at puberty and usually continues uninterrupted until death. In general, immunological competence is acquired during the perinatal period and consists of the ability to recognize all antigens present at that time as self. Thereafter, new antigen appearing within the organism is considered "nonself" or "neo-self" and, as immunological response, is raised against that antigen. Therefore, spermatids and spermatozoa appearing after puberty should be rich in antigens considered as "nonself" or "neo-self." One of the most intriguing aspects of testis is the ability to generate haploid TGC, which are "foreign" or "new" to the host without triggering immune activation. However, increasing evidence indicates that self-tolerance is a far more complex phenomenon, which involves clonal deletion, clonal anergy, idiotype network, clonal ignorance, and Treg. Indeed, experimental conditions in which lymphocytes recognizing testicular autoantigens are present without leading to testicular autoimmunity have been demonstrated. Central tolerance is established before birth or during the perinatal period in different species but clearly occurs long before the appearance of developing antigens of spermatids and spermatozoa in mammals. Peripheral tolerance, on the other hand, is maintained throughout life by interactions between TGC autoantigen-presenting cells and relative T cells under tolerizing conditions, in which some immunoregulatory cytokines, ligands, leukocyte subsets, or a combination of these elements are present or absent. This tolerizing interaction results in responses ranging from downregulation of the autoreactive T cells to the generation of $CD4^{+}CD25^{+}$ Treg cells or $CD8^{+}$ suppressor T cells (Mueller 2010; Hedger 2011).

Spermatids and spermatozoa with new developing antigens are the last to be developed in various cells of individual mammal. Therefore, they exhibit a quite high autoimmunogenicity, by which testicular autoimmunity is induced. Indeed, differing from other organ-specific autoimmune diseases, various EAO models can be easily produced without usage of any adjuvants in both immunocompetent and immunodeficient animals. Clinically, the chronic rather than acute inflammation in the testis of autoimmune or non-autoimmune origin can affect spermatogenesis, resulting in partial or complete male infertility. However, under normal condition, the local immunoregulatory environment, provided by the BTB, various testicular somatic cells, various intra-testicular cytokines and ligands, and intra-testicular innate and adoptive immunity systems, impedes testicular autoimmunity. Moreover, systemic immunoregulatory mechanisms acting on the autoreactive T cells play a critical protective role in testicular autoimmunity. While the testis is considered to be a remarkable immune-privileged site, the organ may easily receive acute or chronic autoimmune inflammation under some pathological milieu. It is suggested that continuous release of autoantigens of TGC and epididymal spermatozoa from the germ cell ducts to the circulation under normal and pathological conditions is responsible for maintaining peripheral tolerance to the autoantigens and also for evoking autoimmune responses to the autoantigens. Maintenance of normal spermatogenesis appears to depend on both the sequestered environment of TGC and the existence of a balance between immunological responsiveness and circulating TGC antigens in "natural autoimmunity." Further studies to know how the immunological and non-immunological circumstances protect the testis from the autoimmune attack will provide us important insights into interventions for male infertility. To grasp the circumstances, not only EAO models but also other various inflammation and transplantation models of the testis may be useful.

References

Ablake M, Itoh M, Kaneko T, Iimura A, Nakamura Y, Meroni P, Nicoletti F. Short-term prophylaxis with deoxyspergualin prevents testicular autoimmunity in mice. Eur J Parmacol. 2002;450:209–12.

Ablake M, Itoh M, Terayama H, Hayashi S, Shoji S, Naito M, Takahashi K, Suna S, Jitsunari F. Di-(2-ethlhexyl) phthalate induces severe aspermatogenesis in mice, however, subsequent antioxidant vitamins supplementation accelerates regeneration of the seminiferous epithelium. Int J Androl. 2004;27:274–81.

Adekunle AO, Hickey WF, Smith SM, Tung KSK, Teuscher C. Experimental allergic orchitis in mice IV. Preliminary characterization of the major murine testis specific aspermatogenic autoantigen(s). J Reprod Immunol. 1987;12:49–62.

Aghamir SM, Salavati A, Yousefie R, Tootian Z, Ghazaleh N, Jamali M, Azimi P. Does bone marrow-derived mesenchymal stem cell transfusion prevent antisperm antibody production after traumatic testis rupture? Urology. 2014;84:82–6.

Amann RP. The cycle of the seminiferous epithelium in humans: a need to revisit? J Androl. 2008;29:469–87.

Anderson DJ, Hill JA. Cell-mediated immunity in infertility. Am J Reprod Immunol Microbiol. 1998;17:22–30.

Banks WA, Kastin AJ. Human interleukin-1 alpha crosses the blood-testis barrier of the mouse. J Androl. 1992;13:254–9.

Ben K, Alexander NJ, Huso N. In vitro cell-mediated and complement-mediated cytotoxicity to murine testicular cells. Am J Reprod Immunol. 1986;12:33–7.

Billiau A, Matthys P. Models of action of Freund's adjuvants in experimental models of autoimmune disease. J Leukoc Biol. 2001;70:849–60.

Bustamanter-Marin X, Quiroga C, Lavandero S, Reyes JG, Moreno RD. Apoptosis, necrosis and autophagy are influenced by metabolic energy sources in cultured rat spermatocytes. Apoptosis. 2012;17:539–50. doi:10.1007/s 10495-012-0709-2.

Cakici C, Buyrukcu B, Duruksu G, Haliloglu AH, Aksoy A, Isik A, Uludag O, Ustun H, Subasi C, Karaoz E. Recovery of fertility in azoospermi rats after injection of adipose-tissue-derived mesenchymal stem cells: the sperm generation. Biomed Res Int. 2013; doi:10.1155/2013/529589.
Chatterjee R, Kottaridis PD, McGarrigle HH, Eliahoo J, McKeag N, Mackinnon S, Goldstone AH. Patterns of Leydig cell insufficiency in adult males following bone marrow transplantation for hematological malignancies. Bone Marrow Transplant. 2001;28:497–502.
Chen Q, Deng T, Han D. Testicular immunoregulation and spermatogenesis. Semin Cell Dev Biol. 2016.; pii: S1084-9521(16)30019-2
Chou MY, Fogelstrand L, Hartvigsen K, Hansen LF, Woelkers D, Shaw PX. Oxidation-specific epitopes are dominant targets of innate natural antibodies in mice and humans. J Clin Invest. 2009;119:1335–49.
Chuang YH, Chiang BL, Chou CC, Hsieh KH. Immune effector cells induced by complete Freund's adjuvant exert an inhibitory effect on antigen-specific type 2 T helper responses. Clin Exp Allergy. 1997;27:315–24.
Clouthier D, Avarbock M, Maika S, Hammer RE, Brinster RL. Rat spermatogenesis in mouse testis. Nature. 1996;381:418–21.
Colafrancesco S, Perricone C, Priori R, Valesini G, Shoenfeld Y. Sjogren's syndrome: another facet of the autoimmune/inflammatory syndrome induced by adjuvants (ASIA). J Autoimmun. 2014;51:10–6.
Cruz-Tapias P, Agmon-Levin N, Israeli E, Anaya JM, Shoenfeld Y. Autoimmune (auto-inflammatory) syndrome induced by adjuvants (ASIA)—animal models as a proof of concept. Curr Med Chem. 2013;20:4030–6.
Das SC, Isobe N, Yoshimura Y. Expression of Toll-like receptors and avian beta-defensins and their changes in response to bacterial components in chicken sperm. Poult Sci. 2011;90:417–25.
Demir A, Turker P, Onol FF, Sirvanci S, Findik A, Tarcan T. Effect of experimentally induced Escherichia coli epididymo-orchitis and ciprofloxacin treatment on rat spermatogenesis. Int J Urol. 2007;14:268–72.
Dimitrov DG, Sedlak R, Nouza K, Kinsky R. A quantitative objective method for the evaluation of anti-sperm cell-mediated immunity in humans. J Immunol Methods. 1992;154:147–53.
Doria A, Zen M, Bettio S, Gatto M, Bassi N, Nalotto L, Ghirardello A, Iaccarino L, Punzi L. Autoinflammation and autoimmunity: bridging the divide. Autoimmun Rev. 2012;12:22–30.
Eid N, Ito Y, Otsuki Y. Enhanced mitophagy in Sertoli cells of ethanol-treated rats: morphological evidence and clinical relevance. J Mol Histol. 2012;43:71–80.
Eid N, Ito Y, Otsuki Y. Ethanol-induced damage in the rat testis: oxidative stress-mediated germ cell apoptosis and vacuolization in Sertoli cells. Andrologia. 2015;47:3. doi:10.1111/and.12385.
Enomoto M, Tsuchida A, Miyazawa K, Yokoyama T, Kawakita H, Tokita H, Naito M, Itoh M, Ohyashiki K, Aoki T. Vitamine K2-induced cell growth inhibition via autophagy formation in cholangiocellular carcinoma cell lines. Int J Mol Med. 2007;20:801–8.
Ferber IA, Brocke S, Taylor-Edwards C, Ridgway W, Dinisco C, Steinman L, Dalton D, Fathman CG. Mice with a disrupted IFN-gamma gene are susceptible to the induction of experimental autoimmune encephalomyelitis (EAE). J Immunol. 1996;156:5–7.
Fijak M, Zeller T, Huys T, Klug J, Wahle E, Linder M, Haidl G, Allam JP, Pilatz A, Weidner W, Schuppe HC, Meinhardt A. Autoantibodies against protein disulfide isomerase ER-60 are a diagnostic marker for low-grade testicular inflammation. Hum Reprod. 2014;29:2382–92.
Gao JF, Call SB, Fillmore PD, Watanabe T, Meeker ND, Teuscher C. Analysis of the role of Bphs/Hrh1 in the genetic control of responsiveness to pertussis toxin. Infect Immun. 2003;71:1281–7.
Gao Y, Lui WY. Synergistic effect of interferon-gamma and tumor necrosis factor-alpha on coxsackievirus and adenovirus receptor expression: an explanation of cell sloughing during testicular inflammation in mice. Biol Reprod. 2014;90:59. doi:10.1095/biolreprod.113.113407.
Ghasemzadeh-Hasankolaei M, Sedighi-Gilani MA, Eslaminejad MB. Induction of ram bone marrow mesenchymal stem cells into germ cell lineage using transforming growth factor-beta superfamily growth factors. Reprod Domest Anim. 2014;49:588–98.
Grigorev VV, Ogurtsov RP, Zubzhitsi IN. Immunomorphologic changes in the testes upon exposure to a microwave electromagnetic field. Arkh Anat Gistol Embriol. 1981;80:69–75.

Gu H, Itoh M, Matsuyama N, Hayashi S, Iimura A, Nakamura Y, Miki T, Takeuchi Y. Toluene diisocyanate exposure induces laryngo-tracheal eosinophilia, which can be ameliorated by supplementation with antioxidant vitamins in guinea pigs. Acta Otolaryngol. 2003;123:965–71.

Hammer RE, Marika SD, Richardson JA, Tang JYP, Taurig JD. Transgenic rats expressing HLA-B27 and human b2 microglobulin with spontaneous inflammatory disease in multiple organ systems: an animal model of HLA-B27-associated disease. Cell. 1990;63:1099–112.

Hagen S, Khurana N, Chandra S, Abdel-Mageed AB, Mondal D, Hellstrom WJ, Sikka SC. Differential expression of novel biomarkers (TLR-2, TLR-4, COX-2, and Nrf-2) of inflammation and oxidative stress in semen of leukocytospermia patients. Andrology. 2015;3:848–55. doi:10.1111/andr. 12074.

Han SP, Zhou DX, Lin P, Qin Z, AN L, Zheng LR, Lei L. Formaldehyde exposure induces autophagy is testicular tissues of adult male rats. Environ Toxicol. 2015;30:323–31.

Hanci H, Odaci E, Kaya H, Aliyazicioglu Y, Turan I, Demir S, Colakoglu S. The effect of prenatal exposure to 900-MHz electromagnetic field on the 21-old-day rat testicle. Reprod Toxicol. 2013;42:203–9.

Hatakeyama S. Pathology of human testicular atrophy. J Jpn Soc Pathol. 1984;73:3–29.

Hedger MP. Immunophysiology and pathology of inflammation in the testis and epididymis. J Androl. 2011;32:625–40.

Hekman ACP, Trapman J, Mulder AH, van Gaalen JLM, Zwarthoff EC. Interferon expression in the testes of transgenic mice leads to sterility. J Biol Chem. 1988;263:12151–5.

Heller CG, Clermont Y. Kinetics of the germinal epithelium in man. Recent Prog Horm Res. 1964;20:545–71.

Hirai S, Naito M, Terayama H, Hatayama N, Qu N, Musha M, Itoh M. Serum autoantibodies in mice immunized with syngeneic testicular germ cells alone. Am J Reprod Immunol. 2013;70:509–17.

Hirai S, Naito M, Kuramasu M, Ogawa Y, Qu N, Terayama H, Hatayama N, Itoh M. Low-dose di(2-ethylhexyl) phthalate (DEHP) exposure increases susceptibility to testicular autoimmunity in mice. J Reprod Immunol. 2015;15:163–71.

Hirayanagi Y, Qu N, Hirai S, Naito M, Terayama H, Hayashi S, Hatakeyama N, Kuramasu M, Ogawa Y, Itoh M. Busulfan pretreatment for transplantation of rat spermatogonia differentially affects immune and reproductive systems in male recipient mice. Anat Sci Int. 2015;90:264–74.

Hojo K, Hiramine C. In vivo effects of cyclosporine A: abrogation of the induction of experimental allergic orchitis and sparing of the generation of suppressor cells. Int Arch Allergy Appl Immunol. 1985;78:63–70.

Horn MM, Paz AH, Duarte ME, Baldo G, Belardinelli MC, Matte U, Cirne-Lima EO, Passos EP. Germinative testicular cells and bone marrow mononuclear cells transplanted to a rat model of testicular degeneration. Cloning Stem Cell. 2008;10:543–6.

Hubert FX, Kinkel SA, Crewther PE, Cannon PZ, Webster KE, Link M, Uibo R, O'Bryan MK, Meager A, Forehan SP, Smyth GK, Mittaz L, Antonarakis SE, Peterson P, Health WR, Scott HS. Aire-deficient C57BL/6 mice mimicking the common human 13-base pair deletion mutation present with only a mild autoimmune phenotype. J Immunol. 2009;182:3902–18.

Ichinohasama R, Hirokawa K, Hatakeyama S. Spermatogenic disturbance induced in mice by combined local injection of monoclonal antibodies to Sertoli cell and to basal lamina of seminiferous tubules. Am J Reprod Immunol Microbiol. 1986;10:158–65.

Ishihara M, Itoh M, Miyamoto K, Suna S, Takeuchi Y, Takenaka I, Jitsunari F. Spermatogenic disturbance induced by di-(2-ethylhexyl) phthalate is significantly prevented by treatment with antioxidant vitamins in the rat. Int J Androl. 2000;23:85–94.

Itoh M, Chen XA, Takeuchi Y, Miki T. Morphological demonstration of the immune privilege in the testis using adjuvants: Tissue responses of male reproductive organs in mice injected with Bordetella pertussigens. Arch Histol Cytol. 1995a;58:575–9.

Itoh M, Hiramine C, Koseto M, Hojo K. Enzyme-linked immunosorbent assay (ELISA) for detecting antisperm antibodies in mice with testicular autoimmunity. Am J Reprod Immunol. 1989;21:9–15.

Itoh M, Hiramine C, Hojo K. A new murine model of autoimmune orchitis induced by immunization with viable syngeneic testicular germ cells alone. I. Immunological and histological studies. Clin Exp Immunol. 1991a;83:137–42.

Itoh M, Hiramine C, Tokunaga Y, Mukasa A, Hojo K. A new murine model of autoimmune orchitis induced by immunization with viable syngeneic testicular germ cells alone. II. Immunohistochemical findings of fully-developed lesion. Autoimmunity. 1991b;10:89–97.

Itoh M, Mukasa A, Tokunaga Y, Hiramine C, Hojo K. New experimental model for adoptive transfer of murine autoimmune orchitis. Andrologia. 1991c;23:415–20.

Itoh M, Mukasa A, Tokunaga Y, Hiramine C, Hojo K. Suppression of efferent limb of testicular autoimmune response by a regulatory CD4+ T cell line in mice. Clin Exp Immunol. 1992a;87:455–60.

Itoh M, Hiramine C, Mukasa A, Tokunaga Y, Fukui Y, Takeuchi Y, Hojo K. Establishment of an experimental model of autoimmune epididymo-orchitis mediated by T cell line in mice. Int J Androl. 1992b;15:170–81.

Itoh M, Hiramine C, Mukasa A, Tokunaga Y, Fukui Y, Takeuchi Y, Hojo K. Antigen non-specific tissue damage in T cell-mediated experimental autoimmune orchitis: preliminary characterization of a testis-specific T-cell line by using dermal tissue and cells. Andrologia. 1993;25:89–92.

Itoh M, de-Rooij DG, Takeuchi Y. Mode of inflammatory cell infiltration in testes of mice injected with syngeneic testicular germ cells without adjuvant. J Anat. 1995b;187:671–9.

Itoh M. Developmental relation between the gonads and the lymphoid organs. Reprod Immunol Biol. 2009;24:63–9.

Jacobo PV, Perez CV, Theas MS, Guazzone VA, Lustig L. CD4+ and CD8+ T cells producing Th1 and Th17 cytokines are involved in the pathogenesis of autoimmune orchitis. Reproduction. 2011a;141:249–58.

Jacobo P, Guazzone VA, Theas MS, Lestig L. Testicular autoimmunity. Autoimmun Rev. 2011b;10:201–4.

Jerne N. Towards a network theory of the immune system. Ann Immunol (Paris). 1974;125C:373–89.

Johnson L, Petty CS, Neaves WB. Further quantification of human spermatogenesis: germ cell loss during postprophase of meiosis and its relationship to daily sperm production. Biol Reprod. 1983;29:207–15.

Jones LS, Rizzo LV, Agarwal RK, Tarrant TK, Chan CC, Wiggert B, Caspi RR. IFN-gamma-deficient mice develop experimental autoimmune uveitis in the context of a deviant effector response. J Immunol. 1997;158:5997–6005.

Kawaguchi T, Miyazawa K, Moriya S, Ohtomo T, Che XF, Naito M, Itoh M, Tomoda A. Combined treatment with bortezomib plus bafilomycin A1 enhances the cytocidal effect and induces endoplasmic reticulum stress in U266 myeloma cells: crosstalk among proteasome, autophagy-lysosome and ER stress. Int J Oncol. 2011;38:643–54.

Kawai T, Akira S. The role of pattern-recognition receptors in innate immunity: update on Toll-like receptors. Nat Immunol. 2010;11:373–84.

Kawakita H, Tsuchida A, Miyazawa K, Naito M, Shigoka M, Kyo B, Enomoto M, Wada Y, Katsumata K, Ohyyashiki K, Itoh M, Tomoda A, Aoki T. Growth inhibitory effects of vitamin K2 on colon cancer cell lines via different types of cell death including autophagy and apoptosis. Int J Mol Med. 2009;23:709–16.

Kitaoka M, Hirai S, Terayama H, Naito M, Qu N, Hatayama N, Miyaso H, Matsuno Y, Komiyama M, Itoh M, Mori C. Effects on the local immunity in the testis by exposure to di-(2-ethylhexyl) phthalate (DEHP) in mice. J Reprod Dev. 2013;59:485–90.

Koji T, Hishikawa Y, Ando H, Nakanishi Y, Kobayashi N. Expression of Fas and Fas ligand in normal and ischemia-reperfusion testes: Involvement of the Fas system in the induction of germ cell apoptosis in the damaged mouse testis. Biol Reprod. 2001;64:946–54.

Koji T. Male germ cell death in mouse testes: possible involvement of Fas and Fas ligand. Med Electron Microsc. 2001;34:213–22.

Kojima A, Prehn RT. Genetic susceptibility to post-thymectomy autoimmune diseases in mice. Immunogenetics. 1981;14:15–27.

Kojima A, Spencer CA. Genetic susceptibility to testicular autoimmunity: comparison between postthymectomy and postvasectomy models in mice. Biol Reprod. 1983;29:195–205.

Komatsu S, Miyazawa K, Moriya S, Takase A, Naito M, Inazu M, Kohno N, Itoh M, Tomoda A. Clarithromycin enhances bortezomib-induced cytotoxicity via endoplasmic reticulum stress-mediated CHOP (GADD153) induction and autophagy in breast cancer cells. Int J Oncol. 2012;40:1029–39.

Korn T, Bettelli E, Oukka M, Kuchroo VK. IL-17 and Th17 cells. Ann Rev Immunol. 2009;27:485–517.

Kuerban M, Naito M, Hirai S, Terayama H, Qu N, Ikeda A, Musha M, Koji T, Itoh M. Involvement of Fas/Fas-L and Bax/Bcl-2 systems in germ cell death following immunization with syngeneic testicular germ cells in mice. J Androl. 2012;33:824–31.

Kyriacou C, Kottaridis PD, Eliahoo J, Mckeag N, Bomford J, McGarrigle HH, Linch DC, Mackinnon S, Chatterjee R. Germ cell damage and Leydig cell insufficiency in recipients of nonmyeloablative transplantation for haematological malignancies. Bone Marrow Transplant. 2003;31:45–50.

Lacroix-Desmazes S, Kaveri SV, Mouthon L, Ayouba A, Malanchere E, Coutinho A. Self-reactive antibodies (natural autoantibodies) in healthy individuals. J Immunol Methods. 1998;216:117–37.

Laird PLM, Wilson AR, Holliday FGT. Field trials of a method of induction of autoimmune gonad rejection in Atlantic salmon (Salmon salar L.). Reprod Nutr Dev. 1980;20:1781–8.

Lapchak PH, Guilbert LJ, Rabinovitch A. Tumor necrosis factor production is deficient in diabetes-prone BB rats and can be corrected by complete Freund's adjuvant: a possible immunoregulatory role of tumor necrosis factor in the prevention of diabetes. Clin Immunol Immunolathol. 1992;65:129–34.

Lassalle B, Mouthon MA, Riou L, Barroca V, Coureuil M, Boussin F, Testart J, Allemand I, Fouchet P. Bone marrow-derived stem cells do not reconstitute spermatogenesis in vivo. Stem Cells. 2008;26:1385–6.

Lee S, Tung KS, Orloff MJ. Testicular transplantation in the rat. Transplant Proc. 1971;3:586–90.

Li MW, Xia W, Mruk DD, Wang CD, Yan HH, Siu MK, Lei WY, Lee WM, Cheng CY. Tumor necrosis factor-alpha reversibly disrupts the blood-testis barrier and impairs Sertoli-germ cell adhesion in the seminiferous epithelium of adult rat testes. J Endocrinol. 2006;190:313–29.

Lie PP, Cheng CY, Mruk DD. Interleukin-1 alpha is a regulator of the blood-testis barrier. FASEB J. 2011;25:1244–53.

Loyo E, Jara LJ, Lopez PD, Puig AC. Autoimmunity in connection with a metal implant: a case of autoimmune/autoinflammatory syndrome induced by adjuvants. Auto Immun Highlights. 2012;4:33–8.

Lu Q, Gore M, Zhang Q, Camenisch T, Boast S, Casagrandra F, Lai C, Skinner MK, Klein R, Matsushima GK, Earp HS, Goff SP, Lemke G. Tyro-3 family receptors are essential of mammalian spermatogenesis. Nature. 1999;398:723–8.

Lu Q, Lemke G. Homeostatic regulation of the immune system by receptor tyrosine kinases of the Tyro 3 family. Science. 2001;293:306–11.

Lui WY, Lee WM, Cheng CY. TGF-betas: their role in testicular function and Sertoli cell tight junction dynamics. Int J Androl. 2003;26:147–60.

Lujan L, Perez M, Salazar E, Alvarez N, GImeno M, Pincrowski P, Irusta S, Santamaria J, Insausti N, Cortes Y, Figueras L, Cuartielles I, Vila M, Fantova E, Chapulle JL. Autoimmune/autoinflammatory syndrome induced by adjuvants (ASIA syndrome) in commercial sheep. Immunol Res. 2013;56:317–24.

Lustig L, Satz ML, Sztein MB, Denduchis B. Antigens of the basement membrane of the seminiferous tubules induce autoimmunity in Wistar rats. J Reprod Immunol. 1982;4:79–90.

Lustig L, Doncel GF, Berensztein-Denduchis B. Testis lesions and cellular and humoral immune responses induced in rats by immunization with laminin. Am J Reprod Immunol. 1987;14:123–8.

Lydka M, Bilinska B, Cheng CY, Mruk DD. Tumor necrosis factor alpha-mediated restricting of the Sertoli cell barrier in vitro involves matrix metalloprotease 9 (MMP9), membrane-bound intercellular adhesion molecules-1 (ICAM-1) and the actin cytoskeleton. Spermatogenesis. 2012;2:294–303.

Malenchenko AF, Barkun NA, Guseva GF. Effect of uranium on the induction and course of experimental autoimmune orchitis and thyroiditis. J Hygiene Epidemiol Microbiol Immunol. 1978;22:268–77.
Malolina EA, Kulibin AY, Kushch AA. Neonatal testicular cell transplantation restores murine spermatogenesis damaged in the course of herpes simplex virus-induced orchitis. Reprod Fertil Dev. 2014;17 doi:10.1071/RD14255.
Matthys P, Vermeire K, Mitera T, Heremans H, Huang S, Schols D, De Wolf-Peeter C, Billiau A. Enhanced autoimmune arthritis in IFN-gamma receptor-deficient mice is conditioned by mycobacteria in Freund's adjuvant and by increased expansion of Mac-1^+ myeloid cells. J Immunol. 1999;163:3503–10.
McDermott MF, Aksentijevich I, Galon J, McDermott EM, Ogunkolade BW, Centola M, Mansfield E, Gadina M, Karenko L, Pettersson T, McCarthy J, Frucht DM, Ariger M, Torosyan Y, Teppo AM, Wilson M, Karaarslan HM, Wan Y, Todd I, Wood G, Schlimgen R, Kumarajeewa TR, Cooper SM, Vella JP, Amos CI, Mulley J, Quane KA, Molloy MG, Ranki A, Powelll RJ, Hitman GA, O'Shea JJ, Kastner DL. Germline mutations in the extracellular domains of the 55kDa TNF receptor, TNFR1, define a family of dominantly inherited autoinflammatory syndromes. Cell. 1999;97:133–44.
Mealy K, Robinson B, Millette CF, Majzoub J, Wilmore DW. The testicular effects of tumor necrosis factor. Ann Surg. 1990;211:470–5.
Mielcarek N, Hornquist EH, Johansson BR, Locht C, Abraham SN, Holmgren J. Interaction of Bordetella pertussis with mast cells, modulation of cytokine secretion by pertussis toxin. Cell Microbiol. 2001;3:181–8.
Miller FW. Non-infectious environmental agents and autoimmunity. The autoimmune diseases. 5th ed. Amsterdam: Elsevier Academic Press; 2014. p. 283–95.
Miyaso H, Komiyama M, Matsuno Y, Naito M, Hirai S, Itoh M, Mori C. The changes of cortactin p80/85 isoform profiles and tyrosine phosphorylation status during spermatogenesis in the mouse testis. J Androl. 2010;31:507–18.
Miyaso H, Naito M, Hirai S, Matsuno Y, Komiyama M, Itoh M, Mori C. Neonatal exposure to diethylstilbestrol causes granulomatous orchitis via epididymal inflammation. Anat Sci Int. 2014a;89:215–23.
Miyaso H, Nakamura N, Naito M, Hirai S, Matsuno Y, Itoh M, Mori C. Early postnatal exposure to a low dose of decabromodiphenyl ether affects expression of androgen and thyroid hormone receptor-alpha and its splicing variants in mouse Sertoli cells. PLoS One. 2014b;9:e114487.
Mochida K, Adachi S, Yamauchi K. Initial phase of an inflammatory reaction in testis caused by experimental testicular autoimmunity in the Nile tilapia, Oreochromis niloticus. Zool Sci. 1995;12:543–50.
Moraes AJ, Bonfa E, Cocuzza M, Borges CT, Saito O, Silva CA. Gonad evaluation in male dermatomyositis. A pilot study. Clin Exp Rheumatol. 2010;28:441–2.
Morrow CM, Hostetler CE, Griswold MD, Hofmann MC, Murphy KM, Cooke PS, Hess RA. ETV5 is required for continuous spermatogenesis in adult mice and may mediate blood testes barrier function and testicular immune privilege. Ann N Y Acad Sci. 2007;1120:144–51.
Morrow CM, Tyagi G, Simon L, Carnes K, Murphy KM, Cooke PS, Hofmann MC, Hess RA. Claudin 5 expression in mouse seminiferous epithelium is dependent upon the transcription factor ets variant 5 and contributes to blood-testis barrier function. Biol Reprod. 2009;81:871–9.
Mueller DL. Mechanisms maintaining peripheral tolerance. Nat Immunol. 2010;11:21–7.
Mukasa A, Itoh M, Tokunaga Y, Hiramine C, Hojo K. Inhibition of a novel model of murine autoimmune experimental autoimmune orchitis by intravenous administration with a soluble testicular antigen: participation of $CD8^+$ regulatory T cells. Clin Immunol Immunopathol. 1992;62:210–9.
Murphy CJ, Stermer AR, Richburg JH. Age- and species-dependent infiltration of macrophages into the testis of rats and mice exposed to mono-(2-ethylhexyl) phthalate (MEHP). Biol Reprod. 2014;91:18. doi:10.1095/biolreprod 113.115527.

Musha M, Hirai S, Naito M, Terayama H, Qu N, Hatayama N, Itoh M. The effects of adjuvants on autoimmune responses against testicular antigens in mice. J Reprod Develop. 2013;59:139–44.

Naito M, Hirai S, Mihara M, Terayama H, Hatayama N, Hayashi S, Matsushita M, Itoh M. Effect of a magnetic field on Drosophila under supercooled conditions. PLoS One. 2012;7:e51902.

Naito M, Hirai S, Terayama H, Qu N, Hayashi S, Hatayama N, Kawamura H, Nakano T, Itoh M. Neonatal estrogen treatment with beta-estradiol 17-cypionate induces in post-pubertal mice inflammation in the ductuli efferentes, epididymis and vas deferens, but not in the testis, provoking obstructive azoospermia. Med Mol Morphol. 2014;47:21–30.

Nandipati KC, Pasqualotto FF, Thomas AJ Jr, Agarwal A. Relationship of interleukin-6 with semen characteristics and oxidative stress in vasectomy reversal patients. Andrologia. 2005;37:131–4.

Natwar RK, Mann A, Sharma RK, Aulitzky W, Frick J. Effect of human gamma interferon on mice testis: a quantitative analysis of the spermatogenic cells. Acta Eur Fertil. 1995;26:45–9.

Ogawa Y, Itoh M, Hirai S, Suna S, Naito M, Qu N, Terayama H, Ikeda A, Miyaso H, Matsuno Y, Komiyama M, Mori C. Cadmium exposure increases susceptibility to testicular autoimmunity in mice. J Appl Toxicol. 2013;33:652–60.

Ohtomo T, Miyazawa K, Naito M, Moriya S, Kuroda M, Itoh M, Tomoda A. Cytoprotective effect of imatinib mesylate in non-BCR-ABL-expressing cells along with autophagosome formation. Biochem Biophys Res Commun. 2010;391:310–5.

Okabayashi A. Induction of a disease resembling systemic lupus erythematosus in later stage of prolonged sensitization. Acta Path Jap. 1964;14:345–71.

Okabayashi A. Degenerative conversion of glomerulitis in the later stage of prolonged sensitization; experimental studies. Jap J Nephrol. 1967a;9:29–32.

Okabayashi A. Dysimmunization and the concept of sensitization disease. In: Oshima Y, editor. Clinical allergology. Tokyo: Asakura Shoten; 1967b. p. 67–77.

Okabayashi A. Hematologic- and immunologic-central organs in a systemic lupus erythematosus-like disease of the rabbit experimentally induced in the later stage of prolonged sensitization. Acta Haem Jap. 1972;35:83–100.

Okabayashi A. Pathogenesis of autoimmunity; experimental induction of a systemic lupus-like disease in the later stage of prolonged antigenic stimulation and its pathogenetic suggestion (in Japanese). RInsho Men-eki. 1973;5:683–92.

Okabayashi A. Concept of immunologic disorder (in Japanese). In: Immunopathology and disease. Tokyo: Bunkodo; 1979. p. 165–223.

Okabayashi A, Kondo Y, Tada T. Nephrotoxic serum nephritis and some other immunologically induced experimental models: a coherent view. In: Okabayashi A, Kondo Y, editors. Masugi nephritis and its immunopathologic implications. Tokyo: Igaku-Shoin; 1980. p. 162–79.

Pelletier RM, Nemirovsky RC, Hugon JS. Effects of immunization with Freund's complete adjuvant and isologous spermatozoa on the seminiferous epithelium and blood-testis barrier in guinea pigs. Anat Rec. 1981;199:197–211.

Pelletier RM, Yoon SR, Akpovi CD, Silvas E, Vitale ML. Defects in the regulatory clearance mechanisms favor the breakdown of self-tolerance during spontaneous autoimmune orchitis. Am J Physiol Regul Integr Comp Physiol. 2009;296:R743–62.

Perez C, Sobarzo C, Jacobo P, Jarazo Dietrich S, Theas M, Denduchis B, Lustig L. Impaired expression and distribution of adherens and gap junction proteins in the seminiferous tubules of rats undergoing autoimmune orchitis. Int J Androl. 2011;34:e566–77.

Perez CV, Sobarzo CM, Jacobo PV, Pellizzari EH, Cigorraga SB, Denduchis B, Lustig L. Loss of occludin expression and impairment of blood-testis barrier permeability in rats with autoimmune orchitis: effect of interleukin-6 on Sertoli cell tight junctions. Biol Reprod. 2012;87:122. doi:10.1095/biolreprod.112.101709.

Perez CV, Pellizzari EH, Cigorrage SB, Galardo MN, Naito M, Lustig L, Jacob PV. IL17A impairs blood-testis barrier integrity and induces testicular inflammation. Cell Tissue Res. 2014;358:885–98.

Person PL, Snoek M, Demant P, Woodward SR, Teuscher C. The immunogenetics of susceptibility and resistance to murine experimental allergic orchitis. Reg Immunol. 1992;4:284–97.

Plotkin SR, Banks WA, Maness LM, Kastin AJ. Differential transport of rat and human interleukin-1 alpha across the blood-brain barrier and blood-testis barrier in rats. Brain Res. 2000;88:57–61.

Poletaev A, Churilov L, Stroev Y, Agapov M. Immunophysiology versus immunopathology: Natural autoimmunity in human health and disease. Pathophysiology. 2012;19:221 31.

Poletaev A. The natural autoimmunity: self-recognition, self-interaction, and self maintenance. J Autoimmun Res. 2014;1:1001–3.

Qu N, Naito M, Li J, Terayama H, Hirai S, Itoh M. Xenogeneic and endogenous spermatogenesis following transplantation of rat germ cells into testes of immunocompetent mice. Reprod Fertil Dev. 2012;24:337–43.

Qu N, Naito M, Terayama H, Hirai S, Musha M, Itoh M. Chronological changes of delayed-type hypersensitivity in mice immunized with testicular germ cells alone. Andrologia. 2014;46:556–63.

Qu N, Terayama H, Hirayanagi Y, Kuramasu M, Ogawa Y, Hirai S, Naito M, Itoh M. Induction of experimental autoimmune orchitis induced by immunization with xenogeneic testicular germ cells in mice. J Reprod Immunol. 2017;21:11–16.

Raghavendra V, Tanga FY, DeLeo JA. Complete Freund's adjuvant-induced peripheral inflammation evokes glial activation and proinflammatory cytokine expression in the CNS. Eur J Neurosci. 2004;20:467–73.

Randolph SSB, Gooley TA, Warren EH, Appelbaum FR, Riddel SR. Female donors contribute to a selective graft-versus-leukemia effect in male recipients of HLA matched, related hematopoietic stem cell transplants. Blood. 2004;103:347–52.

Riccioli A, Starace D, D'Alessio A, Starace G, Padula F, De Cesaris P, FIlippini A, Ziparo E. TNF-alpha and IFN-gamma regulate expression and function of the Fas system in the seminiferous epithelium. J Immunol. 2000;165:743–9.

Rival C, Theas MS, Guazzone VA, Lustig L. Interleukin-6 and IL-6 receptor cell expression in testis of rats with autoimmune orchitis. J Reprod Immunol. 2006;70:43–58.

Sakaguchi S, Ermak TH, Toda M, Berg LJ, Ho W, de St Groth BF, Peterson PA, Sakaguchi N, Davis MM. Induction of autoimmune disease in mice by germline alteration of the T cell receptor gene expression. J Immunol. 1994;152:1471–84.

Sakamoto Y, Himeno K, Sanui H, Yoshida S, Nomoto K. Experimental allergic orchitis in mice. I. A new model induced by immunization without adjuvants. Clin Immunol Immunopathol. 1985;37:360–8.

Sakamoto Y, Nomoto K. Suppression of delayed-type hypersensitivity to syngeneic testicular cells in mice: involvement of suppressor T cells which act at the induction stage. Cell Immunol. 1986;102:168–76.

Sarkar O, Mathur PP, Cheng CY, Mruk DD. Interleukin 1 alpha is a novel regulator of the blood-testis barrier in the rat. Biol Reprod. 2008;78:445–54.

Sato K, Hirokawa K, Hatakeyama S. Experimental allergic orchitis in mice. Histopathological and immunological studies. Virchows Arch A Pathol Anat Histol. 1981;392:147–58.

Schlesser HN, Simon L, Hofmann MC, Murphy KM, Murphy T, Hess RA, Cooke PS. Effects of ETV5 (ets variant gene 5) on testis and body growth, time course of spermatogonial stem cell loss, and fertility in mice. Biol Reprod. 2008;78:483–9.

Schuppe HC, Meinhardt A. Immune privilege and inflammation of the testis. Chem Immunol Allergy. 2005;88:1–14.

Schuppe HC, Meinhardt A, Allam JP, Bergmann M, Weidner W, Haidl G. Chronic orchitis: a neglected cause of male infertility? Andrologia. 2008;40:84–91.

Secombes CJ, Needham EA, Laird LM, Lewis AE, Priede IG. The long-term effects of autoimmunologically induced granulomas on the testis of rainbow trout, Salmo gairdneri Richardson. J Fish Biol. 1985a;26:483–9.

Secombes CJ, Lewis AE, Needham EA, Laird LM, Priede IG. Appearance of autoantigens during gonad maturation in the rainbow trout (Salmo gairdneri). J Exp Zool. 1985b;233:425–31.

Sewell WA, Moerloose PA, McKimm-Breschkin JL, Vadas MA. Pertussigen enhances antigen-driven interferon-r production by sensitized lymphoid cells. Cell Immunol. 1986;97:238.

Shibahara H, Shiraishi Y, Suzuki M. Diagnosis and treatment of immunologically infertile males with antisperm antibodies. Reprod Med Biol. 2005;4:133–41.

Shinohara T, Orwig KE, Avarbock MR, Brinster RL. Restoration of spermatogenesis in infertile mice by Sertoli cell transplantation. Biol Reprod. 2003;68:1064–71.

Shiraishi Y, Shibahara H, Koriyama J, Hirano Y, Okazaki H, Minota S, Suzuki M. Incidence of antisperm antibodies in males with systemic autoimmune diseases. Am J Reprod Immunol. 2009;61:183–9. doi:10.1111/j 1600-0897.

Shoenfeld Y, Agmon-Levin N. 'ASIA'-Autoimmune/inflammatory syndrome induced by adjuvants. J Autoimmun. 2011;36:4–8.

Sun B, Qi N, Shang T, Wu H, Deng T, Han D. Seroli cell-initiated testicular innate immune response through toll-like receptor-3 activation is negatively regulated by Tyro3, Axl, and Mer receptors. Endocrinology. 2010;151:2886–97.

Tanaka A, Nagayoshi M, Awara M, Mawartari Y, Tanaka I, Sofkins N. Conclusions from the transplantation of human or hamster spermatogonia/primary spermatocytes to rat or mouse testis. Fertil Steril. 1997;68(Suppl):S61.

Taurog JD, Rival C, van Duivenvoorde LM, Satumira N, Dorris ML, Sun M, Shelton JM, Richardson JA, Hamra FK, Hammer RE, Tung KSK. Autoimmune epididymoorchitis is essential to the pathogenesis of male-specific spondylarthritis in HLA-B27-transgenic rats. Arthritis Rheum. 2012;64:2518–28.

Terayama H, Yoshimoto T, Hirai S, Naito M, Qu N, Hatayama N, Hayashi S, Mitobe K, Furusawa J, Mizoguchi I, Kezuka T, Goto H, Suyama K, Sakabe K, Itoh M. Contribution of IL-12/IL-35 common subunit p35 to maintaining testicular immune privilege. PLoS One. 2014;9(e):96120.

Teuscher C, Smith SM, Goldberg EH, Shearer GM, Tung KSK. Experimental allergic orchitis in mice, I: Genetic control of susceptibility and resistance to induction of autoimmune orchitis. Immunogenetics. 1985a;22:323–33.

Teuscher C, Potter M, Tung KS. Differential susceptibility to experimental autoimmune orchitis in BALB/c substrains. Curr Top Microbiol Immunol. 1985b;122:181–8.

Tokunaga Y, Hiramine C, Itoh M, Muaksa A, Hojo K. Genetic susceptibility to the induction of murine experimental autoimmune orchitis (EAO) without adjuvant. I. Comparison of pathology, delayed type hypersensitivity, and antibody. Clin Immunol Immunopathol. 1993a;66:239–47.

Tokunaga Y, Hiramine C, Hojo K. Genetic susceptibility to the induction of murine experimental autoimmune orchitis (EAO) without adjuvant. II. Analysis on susceptibility to EAO induction using F1 hybrid mice and adoptive transfer system. Clin Immunol Immunopathol. 1993b;66:248–53.

Tonon S, Goriely S, Aksoy E, Pradier O, Del Giudice G, Trannoy E, Willems F, Goldman M, De Wit D. Bordetella pertussis toxin induces the release of inflammatory cytokines and dendritic cell activation in whole blood: impaired responses in human newborns. Eur J Immunol. 2002;32:3118–31125.

Tung KS, Yule TD, Mahi-Brown CA, Listrom MB. Distribution of histopathology and Ia positive cells in actively induced and passively transferred experimental autoimmune orchitis. J Immunol. 1987;138:752–9.

Tyagi G, Carnes K, Morrow C, Kostereva NV, Ekman GC, Mekling DD, Hostetler C, Griswold M, Murphy KM, Hess RA, Hofmann MC, Cooke PS. Loss of Etv5 decreases proliferation and RET levels in neonatal mouse testicular germ cells and causes an abnormal first wave of spermatogenesis. Biol Reprod. 2009;81:258–66.

Wagner AM, Beier K, Christen E, Hollander GA, Krenger W. Leydig cell injury as a consequence of an acute graft-versus-host reaction. Blood. 2005;105:2988–00.

Wang Y, Lui WY. Opposite effects of interleukin-1 alpha and transforming growth factor-beta2 induce stage-specific regulation of junctional adhesion molecule-B gene in Sertoli cells. Endocrinology. 2009;150:2404–1412.

Wentworth BC, Mellen WJ. Active immunity induced and spermatogenesis suppressed by testicular antigen in the male Japanese quail. J Reprod Fertil. 1964;8:215–23.

Yokoyama T, Miyazawa K, Naito M, Toyotake J, Tauchi T, Itoh M, You A, Hayashi Y, Georgescu MM, Kondo Y, Kondo S, Ohyashiki K. Vitamin K2 induces autophagy and apoptosis simultaneously in leukemia cells. Autophagy. 2008;4:629–40.

Yi K, Hatayama N, Hirai S, Qu N, Hayashi S, Kawata S, Nagahori K, Naito M, Itoh M. Developmental of heterotopic transplantation of the testis with the epididymis to evaluate an aspect of testicular immunology in rats. PLoS One. 2017;12(5):e0177067.

Yoshida S, Nomoto K, Himeno K, Takeya K. Immune response to syngeneic or autologous testicular cells in mice. I. Augmented delayed footpad reaction in cyclophosphamide-treated mice. Clin Exp Immunol. 1979;38:211–7.

Yoshida S, Nomoto K, Himeno K, Sanui H. Delayed hypersensitivity to syngeneic or xenogeneic cells in guinea-pigs. Immunology. 1981;42:445–9.

Yule TD, Montoya GD, Russell LD, Williams TM, Tung KSK. Autoimmunogenic germ cells exist outside the blood testis barrier. J Immunol. 1988;141:1161–7.

Zhao S, Zhu W, Xue S, Han D. Testicular defense systems: immune privilege and innate immunity. Cell Mol Immunol. 2014;11:428–37.

Zhang D, Liu X, Peng J, He D, Lin T, Zhu J, Li X, Zhang Y, Wei G. Potential spermatogenesis recovery with bone marrow mesenchymal stem cells in an azoospermic rat model. Int J Mol Sci. 2014a;15:13151–65.

Zhang H, Yin Y, Wang G, Liu Z, Liu L, Sun F. Interleukin-6 disrupts blood-testis barrier through inhibiting protein degradation or activating phosphorylated ERK in Sertoli cells. Sci Rep. 2014b;4:4260. doi:10.1038/srep04260.

Zhang M, Nii T, Isobe N, Yoshimura Y. Expression of Toll-like receptors and effects of lipopolysaccharide on the expression of proinflammatory cytokines and chemokine in the testis and epididymis of roosters. Poult Sci. 2012;91:1997–2003.

Zhang X, Wang T, Deng T, Xiong W, Lui P, Li N, Chen Y, Han D. Damaged spermatogenic cells induce inflammatory gene expression in mouse Sertoli cells through the activation of toll-like receptors 2 and 4. Mol Cell Endocrinol. 2013a;365:162–73.

Zhang X, Li N, Chen Q, Yan K, Liu Z, Zhang X, Liu P, Chen Y, Han D. Breakdown of immune homeostasis in the testis of mice lacking Tyro3, Axl and Mer receptor tyrosine kinases. Immunol Cell Biol. 2013b;91:416–26.

Zhang Z, Shao S, Shetty G, Meistrich ML. Donor Sertoli cells transplanted into irradiated rat testes stimulate partial recovery of endogenous spermatogenesis. Reproduction. 2009;137:497–508. doi:10.1530/REP-08-0120.

Erratum to: Testicular Autoimmunity – A Cause of Male Infertility

Masahiro Itoh

Erratum to:
M. Itoh, *Testicular Autoimmunity – A Cause of Male Infertility,*
https://doi.org./10.1007/978-4-431-54460-9

This book was initially published with error in the following Figures, which has now been corrected.

Chapter 1
https://doi.org/10.1007/978-4-431-54460-9_1
Fig. 1.13 - The image of "Blood capillary Endothelium" has been changed.

Chapter 3
https://doi.org/10.1007/978-4-431-54460-9_3
Fig. 3.7 - "Obstroction of blood flow" changed to "Obstruction of blood flow".

Chapter 4
https://doi.org/10.1007/978-4-431-54460-9_4
Fig. 4.6 - "Postnatal days of donor mice from which TGC was obtained for sensitization" has been changed to "Postnatal days of donor mice from which TGC were obtained for sensitization".

The updated online version of these chapters can be found at
https://doi.org/10.1007/978-4-431-54460-9_1
https://doi.org/10.1007/978-4-431-54460-9_3
https://doi.org/10.1007/978-4-431-54460-9_4

M. Itoh, *Testicular Autoimmunity*, DOI 10.1007/978-4-431-54460-9_9

MIX
Papier aus verantwortungsvollen Quellen
Paper from responsible sources
FSC® C105338
FSC
www.fsc.org

If you have any concerns about our products,
you can contact us on
ProductSafety@springernature.com

In case Publisher is established outside the EU,
the EU authorized representative is:
Springer Nature Customer Service Center GmbH
Europaplatz 3, 69115 Heidelberg, Germany

Printed by Libri Plureos GmbH
in Hamburg, Germany